AF621285

# HANDBUCH DER UROLOGIE
# ENCYCLOPEDIA OF UROLOGY
# ENCYCLOPÉDIE D'UROLOGIE

HERAUSGEGEBEN VON · EDITED BY
PUBLIÉE SOUS LA DIRECTION DE

C. E. ALKEN
HOMBURG (SAAR)

V. W. DIX
LONDON

W. E. GOODWIN
LOS ANGELES

E. WILDBOLZ
BERN

XIII/2

SPRINGER-VERLAG BERLIN · HEIDELBERG · NEW YORK 1970

# Handbuch der Urologie
# Encyclopedia of Urology · Encyclopédie d'Urologie

*Gesamtdisposition · Outline · Disposition générale*

| | Allgemeine Urologie | General Urology | Urologie générale |
|---|---|---|---|
| I | Anatomie und Embryologie | Anatomy and embryology | Anatomie et embryologie |
| II | Physiologie und Pathologische Physiologie | Physiology and pathological physiology | Physiologie normale et pathologique |
| III | Symptomatologie und Untersuchung von Blut, Harn und Genitalsekreten | Symptomatology and examination of the blood, urine and genital secretions | Symptomatologie et examens du sang, de l'urine et des sécrétions annexielles |
| IV | Niereninsuffizienz | Renal insufficiency | L'insuffisance rénale |
| V/1 | Radiologische Diagnostik | Diagnostic radiology | Radiologie diagnostique |
| V/2 | Radiotherapie | Radiotherapy | Radiothérapie |
| VI | Endoskopie | Endoscopy | Endoscopie |
| | **Spezielle Urologie** | **Special Urology** | **Urologie spéciale** |
| VII/1 | Mißbildungen | Malformations | Malformations |
| VII/2 | Die urologische Begutachtung und Dokumentation | The urologist's expert opinion and documentation | L'expertise et documentation en urologie |
| VIII | Entleerungsstörungen | Urinary stasis | La stase |
| IX/1 | Unspezifische Entzündungen | Non-specific inflammations | Inflammations non-spécifiques |
| IX/2 | Spezifische Entzündungen | Specific inflammations | Inflammations spécifiques |
| X | Die Steinerkrankungen | Calculous disease | La lithiase urinaire |
| XI/1 | Tumoren I | Tumours I | Les tumeurs I |
| XI/2 | Tumoren II | Tumours II | Les tumeurs II |
| XII | Funktionelle Störungen | Functional disturbances | Troubles fonctionnels |
| XIII/1 | Operative Urologie I | Operative urology I | Urologie opératoire I |
| XIII/2 | Operative Urologie II | Operative urology II | Urologie opératoire II |
| XIII/3 | Operative Urologie III | Operative urology III | Urologie opératoire III |
| XIII/4 | Operative Urologie IV | Operative urology IV | Urologie opératoire IV |
| XIV | Traumatologie | Traumatology | Traumatologie |
| XV | Die Urologie des Kindes | Urology in childhood | Urologie de l'enfant |
| XVI | Gynäkologische Urologie | Gynaecological urology | Urologie de la femme |
| XVII | Geschichte der Urologie<br>Schlußbetrachtungen<br>General-Register | History of urology<br>Retrospect and outlook<br>General index | Histoire d'urologie<br>Conclusions<br>Table des matières |

# OPERATIVE UROLOGY II

TH. BURGHELE · R. F. GITTES
V. ICHIM · J. KAUFMAN · A. LUPU
D. C. MARTIN

MIT 132 ABBILDUNGEN

SPRINGER-VERLAG BERLIN · HEIDELBERG · NEW YORK 1970

ISBN-13: 978-3-642-65062-8 e-ISBN-13: 978-3-642-65060-4
DOI: 10.1007/978-3-642-65060-4

This work is subject to copyright. All rights are reserved, whether the whole or part of the material is concerned, specifically those of translation, reprinting, re-use of illustrations, broadcasting, reproduction by photocopying machine or similar means, and storage in data banks.
Under § 54 of the German Copyright Law where copies are made for other than private use, a fee is payable to the publisher, the amount of the fee to be determined by agreement with the publisher.
© by Springer-Verlag Berlin · Heidelberg 1970. Library of Congress Catalog Card Number 75-135956.
Softcover reprint of the hardcover 1st edition 1970 . Stürtz AG, Würzburg.
The use of general descriptive names, trade names, trade marks, etc. in this publication, even if the former are not especially identified, is not to be taken as a sign that such names, as understood by the Trade Marks and Merchandise Marks Act, may accordingly be used freely by anyone.

## Contents

## Contributors to Vol. XIII/2

THEODOR BURGHELE, Prof. Dr., The Clinic of Urology, Panduri Hospital, Bucharest/Rumania

R. F. GITTES, M. D., Professor, University of California, University Hospital of San Diego County, School of Medicine, Dept. of Surgery — Division of Urology, 225 West Dickinson Street, San Diego, CA 92103/U.S.A.

VASILE ICHIM, D.M.S., Senior Lecturer, The Clinic of Urology, Panduri Hospital, Bucharest/Rumania

JOSEPH J. KAUFMAN, M. D., Professor and Chairman, Division of Urology, Dept. of Surgery, University of California, School of Medicine, Center for Health Science, Los Angeles, CA 90024/U.S.A.

ANDREI N. LUPU, M. D. Senior Investigator of the Los Angeles County Heart Association, University of California, Dept. of Surgery, School of Medicine, Center for Health Science, Los Angeles, CA 90024/U.S.A.

DONALD C. MARTIN, M. D., Associate Professor of Surgery, Chief of the Division of Urology, University of California, Irvine, CA 92664/U.S.A.

# Renovascular Surgery

Joseph J. Kaufman and Andrei N. Lupu[1]

With 22 Figures

## Introduction

Surgical operations on the renal vessels for renovascular hypertension, renal artery aneurysms, renal artery embolism and renal vein thrombosis, have been made feasible during the last decade as a result of improved diagnostic techniques as well as improved surgical skills. These technical advances have developed at an equal pace with the increasing awareness of the existence of vascular problems affecting the kidney.

# A. Renovascular Hypertension

Renovascular hypertension is estimated to exist in 5% to 15% of persons with high blood pressure. Hence, it affects some 2,000,000 persons in the United States alone and constitutes the most prevalent form of curable high blood pressure. The duration of hypertension tends to be shorter in patients with renovascular hypertension than in those with essential hypertension, and the majority of patients with renovascular hypertension do not have a family history of high blood pressure whereas most essential hypertensives *do*. There are no pathognomonic clinical features of renovascular hypertension, but an upper abdominal bruit can be detected in 55% or more of patients with stenosing lesions of the renal artery. The incidence of such murmurs is higher in patients with fibromuscular renal artery disease than in those with atherosclerotic stenosis. Secondary features of hypertension such as retinopathy, cardiac hypertrophy, cerebrovascular accidents, and secondary hyperaldosteronism are found no more characteristically with hypertension from renal artery stenosis than with other forms of hypertension. Since there is a generous overlap in the clinical features of essential and renovascular hypertension, special diagnostic tests must be relied upon, including the radioactive renogram, Anger scintillation renal photoscan, intravenous urogram, renal arteriogram, individual kidney function tests, assay of renal vein plasma for pressor substances, determinations of pressure gradients and flow at operation, and renal biopsies. These specialized but invaluable diagnostic aids make possible the recognition of stenosing lesions of the renal vessels, their functional impact, and the predictability of cure by appropriate surgical methods.

---

1 From the Department of Surgery/Urology, UCLA School of Medicine, Los Angeles, California 90024 and Wadsworth Hospital, Veterans Administration Center, Los Angeles.

# I. Diagnostic Tests

## 1. Radioactive Renogram

Although the isotope renogram has gained wide popularity as a simple means of recognizing the disparate kidney diseases and was initially heralded as a particularly useful screening test in the recognition of renovascular hypertension, it has been found in recent years that the renogram lacks sufficient specificity to make it indispensable. The most important abnormal parameter of the renogram in patients with renovascular hypertension is the time elapsed from the injection of the radioactive iodohippurate-$I^{131}$ to the peak of maximum radioactivity over the respective kidneys (Fig. 1). In a recent collation of 348 cases

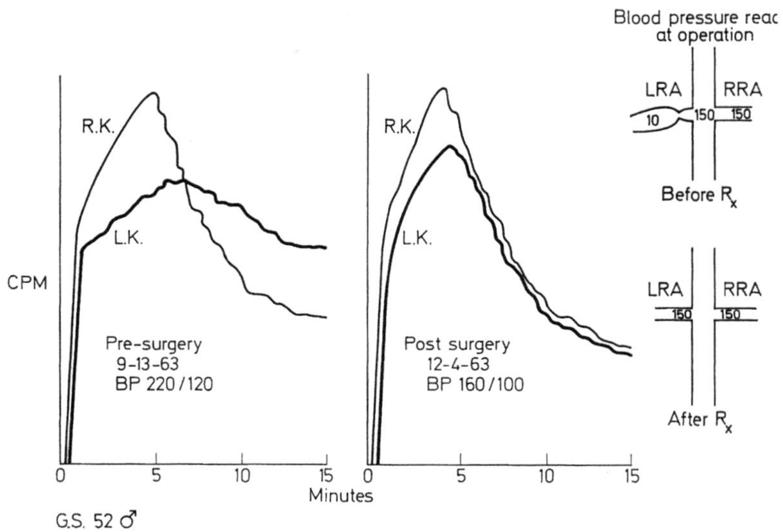


Fig. 1. Radioisotope renogram before and after surgery for left renal artery stenosis. There is a delay in the time elapsed from injection of the radioactive iodohippurate-$I^{131}$ to the peak of maximum radio-activity over the left kidney in the preoperative film which is largely corrected in the postoperative study

from the literature in which renal artery stenosis was proved by surgery or arteriography or both, 86% of subjects had positive renograms. In 357 control subjects with essential hypertension (negative arteriograms), 19% had false positive renograms (MAXWELL, LUPU and TAPLIN, 1968). Alterations in the renogram curve are not specific for renovascular lesions and hence reliance must be placed on other, more specific tests.

## 2. Renal Scanning

Renal scanning with chlormerodrin $Hg^{203}$ or chlormerodrin $Hg^{197}$ is useful in defining kidney mass and contour, but no practicable means has been found of applying the test to assess renal function. Recent refinements of scanning technique using technetium-iron complex $Tc^{99m}$ and iodohippurate-$I^{131}$, have found greater usefulness in demonstrating functional features of disparate kidney disease, but despite the ease of performance and certain characteristic findings in renovascular hypertension, the test still lacks sufficient specificity in its present form. A delay in the uptake and a prolongation of transit time of the tracer substance from the parenchymal cells to the renal pelvis occurs in such unilateral lesions as renal artery stenosis and obstructive uropathy (Fig. 2). The test is useful, however, in the immediate postoperative evaluation of renal function to assess the success of surgical repair.

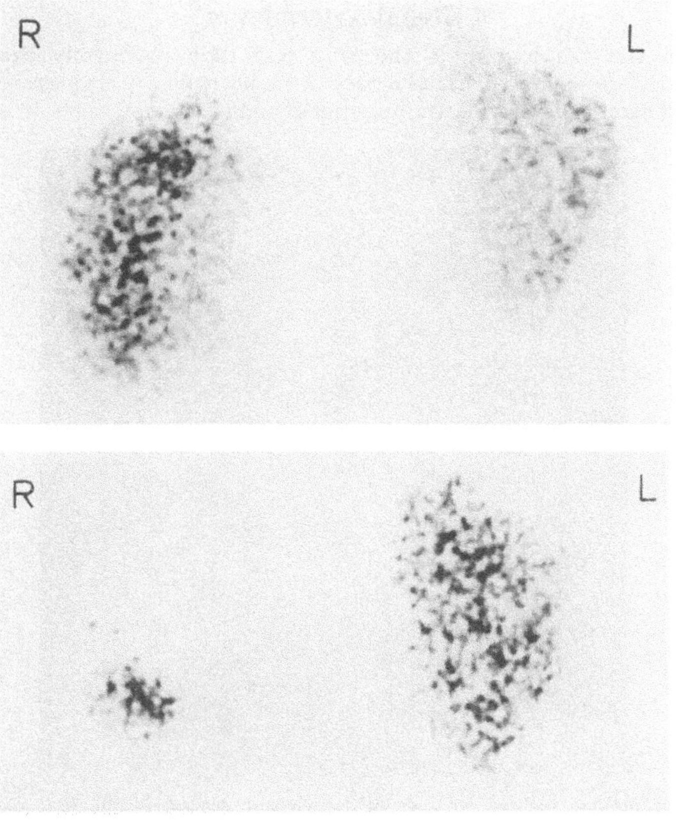


Fig. 2. Anger camera scan of a patient with left renal artery stenosis showing a delay in the uptake and a prolongation of transit time of the iodohippurate-$I^{131}$

## 3. Intravenous Urography

In most studies in which the intravenous urogram has been evaluated, the following criteria have been analyzed: kidney size, early nephrogram, pyelocalyceal appearance time, and differential pyelocalyceal concentration with dehydration, hydration or drug induced diuresis. In a recent analysis of 748 cases of renal artery stenosis it has been found that the diagnostic yield of the individual urographic parameters did not correlate with angiographic and surgical findings in more than 69% of cases. When all these parameters were considered together, however, a positive correlation was found in 93% (MAXWELL and LUPU, 1968). Hence, the intravenous urogram seems to be the most practical and useful diagnostic test for hypertensive patients with suspected renal artery stenosis, providing that rapid sequence studies are done and that all parameters of the pyelogram are analyzed: a disparity in kidney size of 1 cm or more, a delay in the appearance time of the contrast medium in the minor calyces, a relative hyperconcentration of the contrast medium on the involved side, and a delay in washout of the contrast medium from the ischemic kidney in response to a diuretic agent.

## 4. Renal Arteriogram

Although the arteriogram is the only test that specifically demonstrates the presence of a lesion of the renal artery or its branches, it is generally accepted that alone it cannot determine the functional significance of such an anatomical

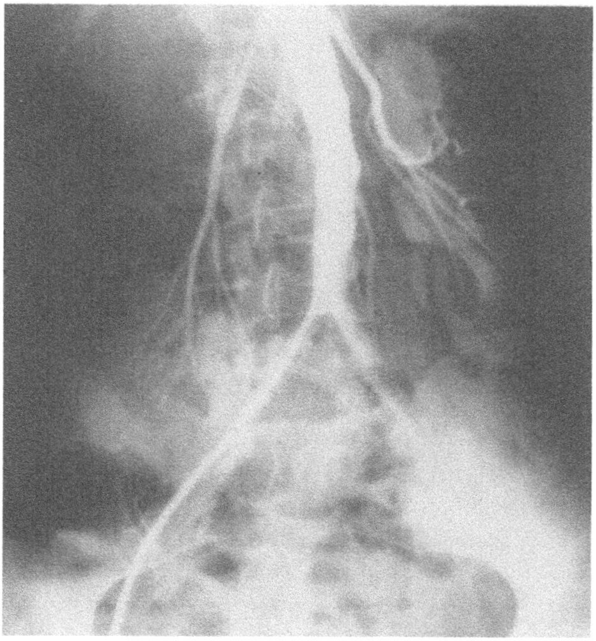

Fig. 3. Aortogram in a patient with an atherosclerotic plaque in the first portion of the right renal artery

finding. Constrictions of less than 50% of the luminal diameter are not likely to be of functional importance, except in the presence of multiple stenoses which act as a summation of resistances in series.

Improvements in the technique of aortography and renal arteriography have reduced the morbidity of the test to a relatively insignificant amount. In experienced hands, arteriography need not be an uncomfortable nor a hazardous procedure for the patient. Upright aortography has been particularly useful to demonstrate excessive renal mobility and stretching of the renal arteries and to produce better delineation of stenosing lesions that may be obscured unless the artery is placed on stretch. Aortography with the patient performing the Valsalva maneuver shows some of the same features seen in the upright aortogram but in selected cases the orthostatic study is more critical (Kaufman and Maxwell, 1963; Kaufman, Hanafee and Maxwell, 1964). Selective catheterization of the renal arteries has become routine in the study of patients with suspected renovascular lesions, since it provides the best definition of the finer details of the renal vasculature. Newer techniques employing radiological magnification permit demonstration of very fine architecture of intrarenal vascular aborization. With these techniques it is possible to visualize small aneurysms (periarteritis nodosa), small areas of infarction and scarring, as well as minute arteriovenous shunts.

It is usually easy to distinguish mural dysplasias from atheromatous lesions by considering their location and type of constriction. Atherosclerotic plaques usually, but not always, occur in the proximal third of the renal artery or at its orifice, and they tend to be asymmetrical in appearance (Fig. 3). There is often atherosclerosis evident in the aorta and iliac vessels. Fibrous and fibromuscular dysplasias seldom occur solely in the first third of the renal artery,

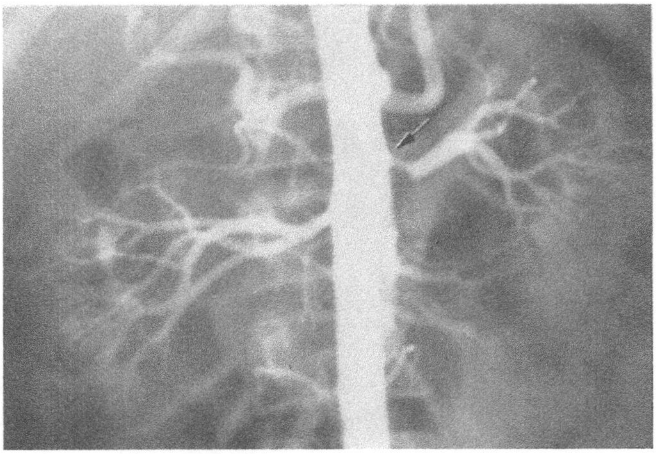

Fig. 4. Congenital coarctation of the first portion of the left renal artery

but subadventitial fibrosis (periarterial fibrosis), congenital coarctations, and extrinsic compression of the renal artery by the crus of the diaphragm or adhesive bands constrict the proximal third of the renal artery (Figs. 4 and 5). Middle and distal renal artery stenoses are likewise confusing at times, but the corrugation or "string of beads" effect of fibromuscular dysplasias (subintimal fibrous dysplasias and medial fibrous or fibromuscular dysplasias) are easily recognized (Fig. 6). Fibromuscular dysplasia of the renal arteries often coexists with atherosclerosis. McCormack, Poutasse, Meany, Noto, and Dustan (1966) and Crocker (1968) have described the various mural dysplasias of the renal arteries and have classified them according to the site of involvement (subintimal, medial, subadventitial), and according to whether the thickening is essentially fibrous or fibromuscular. It appears that muscular dysplasia of the media or subadventitia may precede fibroplasia which predominates in many of the advanced stenotic lesions. Various degrees of disruption of the internal elastica are seen. No specific cause of fibrous or fibromuscular dysplasia has been found. Several of the proposed explanations are: trophic disturbances of the vessel wall caused by abnormalities of the vasa vasorum, dissections of the arterial wall with subsequent fibrosis, traction or torsion of the renal artery in cases of excessive renal mobility, autoimmune vasculitis, and hormonal disturbances. It has been found in experiments on animals that the characteristic radiological and histological appearance of fibromuscular dysplasias can be produced by mobilizing the kidney and placing the renal artery on excessive stretch. The cause of fibrous and fibromuscular dysplasias of the renal vessels may well be multifactorial.

It is important to distinguish fibromuscular dysplasia, atherosclerosis, and periarterial fibrosis because of the variable rate of progression of these diseases.

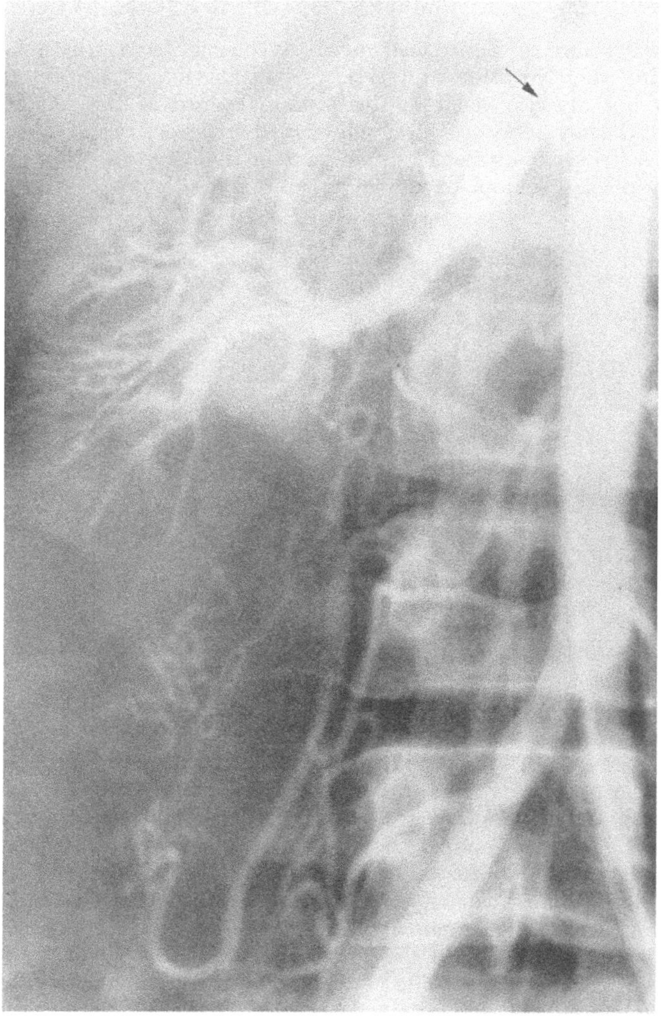

Fig. 5. Proximal right renal artery stenosis caused by extrinsic compression secondary to crossing of the artery by the crus of the diaphragm. In addition there is occlusion disease of the branch to the lower pole

Periarterial fibrosis seems to progress most rapidly and new or recurring lesions have been witnessed in some patients over a period of one to two years. Fibromuscular dysplasias affecting the media and subintima appear to progress more slowly; marginal lesions have been observed to become critical over periods of four to eight years. Atherosclerosis seems to progress at a rate intermediate between that of periarterial fibrosis and fibromuscular dysplasias.

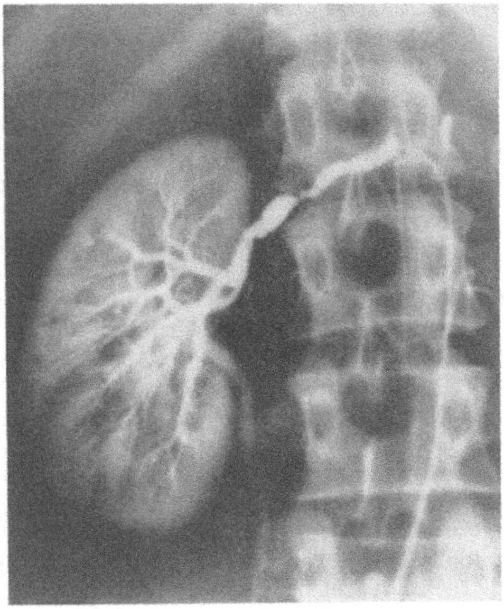

Fig. 6. Selective right renal arteriogram showing stenosis of the middle and distal thirds of the renal artery caused by fibrous dysplasia

## 5. Individual Kidney Function Tests

The historical background and physiology of divided kidney function tests have been covered in the literature (Maxwell, Lupu and Kaufman, 1968). Partial occlusion of the renal artery leads to decreased excretion of sodium and water by the ischemic kidney. This may be explained by the fact that a reduction in glomerular filtration rate produces a lower filtered load of sodium and hence, a reduced volume of isotonic tubular fluid delivered to the loop of Henle. The loop of Henle functioning normally as a counter-current multiplier, abstracts a larger than normal proportion of sodium in achieving hypertonicity of the medullary interstitium. The fluid in the first portion of the distal tubule is thereby reduced both in volume and in tonicity and if the distal tubules and collecting ducts function normally with regard to sodium reabsorption and back-diffusion of water, the final volume of urine will be reduced and the sodium concentration decreased. This increased fractional reabsorption of sodium and water will lead to a higher osmolality of the final urine and to a hyperconcentration of those solutes that are poorly reabsorbed (para-aminohippurate, inulin, and creatinine). Another explanation for the reduced water and sodium excretion of the ischemic kidney is that there is a reduction in renal blood flow with correlative reduction in medullary blood flow. In the presence of reduced medullary blood flow (therefore decreased medullary washout) the counter-current exchange mechanism becomes more efficient, increases the hypertonicity of the medullary interstitium, and abstracts by osmosis a larger amount of water from the collecting ducts.

Three tests commonly employed in divided kidney function studies are those proposed by Howard and Connor (1964), Stamey (1961), and Rapoport (1960). In the Howard test the criteria for ischemia and unilateral main renal artery stenosis are 60% or greater reduction in urine volume, 15% or greater reduction in urine sodium concentration and/or 50% or greater increase in urine creatinine concentration on the suspected side. Rapoport devised a test which does not depend upon measurements of urine volume for its interpretation, but instead, upon urine creatinine concentration and sodium concentration. Since for practical purposes creatinine is neither reabsorbed nor secreted by the renal tubules, its concentration in the urine will vary directly with the percentage of reabsorbed water. In renal ischemia, therefore, the urine-to-plasma sodium concentration ratio ($U_{Na}/P_{Na}$) will move in the opposite direction to the urine-to-plasma creatinine ratio ($Ue_r/P_{Cr}$). The formula derived by Rapoport is as follows: $LU_{Na}/LU_{Cr} \times RU_{Cr}/RU_{Na} = TRFR$, where LU and RU refer to urines collected from the left and right kidneys respectively. The resultant figure is called the tubular rejection fraction ratio (TRFR), which in normal subjects should theoretically be equal to 1.0. It has been found that normal subjects, patients with essential hypertension, and patients with chronic pyelonephritis have a TRFR between 0.6 and 1.6. Values higher than 1.6 imply relative arterial obstruction of the right kidney, whereas values below 0.6 implicate the left kidney.

The Stamey test is based largely upon observations indicating the importance of urea by the urinary concentrating mechanism. The urinary urea is presumed to be osmotically balanced by the urea in the medullary interstitium rather than by sodium chloride which is concentrated within the medulla by an active transport process. The technique utilizes a rapid infusion of hypertonic urea (4%), antidiuretic hormone (ADH) and sodium para-aminohippurate (PAH), or insulin in isotonic saline during collection of ureteral specimens. The comparative urine volumes and PAH or inulin concentrations are measured. Stamey's current modified criteria are (for unilateral main renal artery stenosis), at least a 2:1 difference (increase) in the concentration of PAH on the affected side and (for segmental renal artery stenosis), at least 2:1 difference in urine flow rates (decrease) and a 16% or greater difference (increase) in the concentration of PAH.

With regard to individual kidney function tests the terms "diagnostic" and "predictive" must be defined. It is true that the terms are synonymous in most stenosing lesions of the renal artery that are curable by surgery. Discrepancies occur perhaps by virtue of the fact that the early mechanism of hypertension resulting from renal artery stenosis is humoral and that at later stages extrarenal factors may become dominant and sufficient to sustain the elevated blood pressure. In the past it has been held that positive individual kidney function tests are predictive of surgical cure and that in the presence of negative divided renal function tests, surgery should not be performed. Recent evidence has accumulated, however, to indicate that positive divided renal vein renin values and pressure gradients may exist with negative individual kidney function tests and cures have resulted in some of the cases, casting doubt on the validity of the divided renal function test as an absolute criterion of operative results (Kropp and O'Conor, 1968).

It is generally agreed that even with unilateral main renal artery stenosis the divided kidney function test has a positive correlation with operative findings in only 80% of cases. Even when the tests are positive, a consistently valid predictive value of the divided kidney function test has been challenged by the following figures: among patients who have been cured by appropriate surgical means, positive divided kidney function tests have been obtained in only 70% to 75% of cases, and in 15—20% of cases in which a positive divided kidney function test has been obtained, surgery has failed to correct the hypertension. Fifty per cent of subjects with negative divided kidney function tests have been cured or improved. These figures indicate that older doctrines attributing predictive and absolute values to the divided kidney function tests have been erroneous and misleading.

These discrepancies notwithstanding, the divided kidney function test continues to be employed in clinical research centers, since it is, to date, the most practical means of obtaining quantitative data of the respective kidneys and in assessing the relative contribution of each kidney to global renal function.

## 6. Assay of Renal Vein Plasma for Pressor Substances

No laboratory test for plasma renin activity or circulating angiotensin has yet been perfected to the degree that makes it readily available, practical, and inexpensive. Pending the development of a critical radioimmunoassay for angiotensin, most tests rely on the determination of plasma renin activity, i.e., liberation

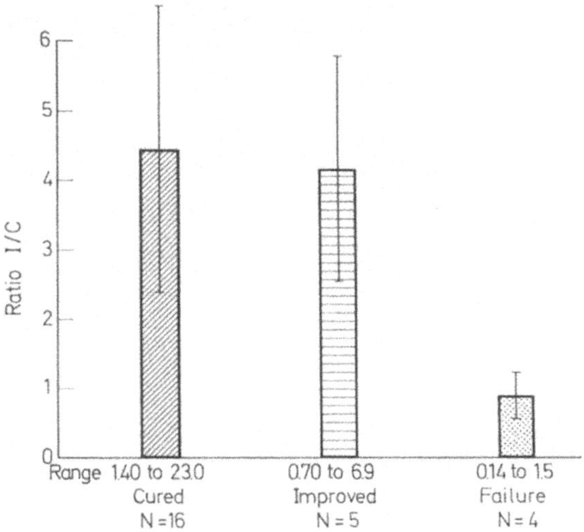


Fig. 7

of angiotensin by the action of renin in the presence of plasma substrate and with subsequent biological determination of the angiotensin yield against known standards of angiotensin amide. Some of the tests which have simply involved the determination of crude pressor activity of plasma have not shown reproducibility or recovery obtained by other methods.

At present there are eleven proposed methods of which we will mention those of Helmer and Judson (1963), Boucher, Veyrat, Champlain and Genest (1964), Lever, Robertson and Tree (1964) and Pickens et al. (1965).

In our laboratory we have utilized the method of Boucher et al. In this method, plasma is incubated at 37° C for three hours at pH 5.5 in the presence of moist Dowex. The angiotensin formed is then absorbed on Dowex columns and eluted. The lyophilized dry residue is repeatedly washed with 80% and 50% ethanol, concentrated to dryness under high vacuum, recovered in 1 ml of saline and assayed in the bilaterally nephrectomized, ganglion-blocked rat. Results are expressed at nanograms of angiotensin per 100 ml plasma per 3 hours incubation. Values of peripheral plasma renin activity obtained from normotensive subjects on restricted sodium diet ranged from 70 ng% to 470 ng% with a mean of 162ng%.

Table 1

| | Patient | Age | Sex | Duration of HBP (years) | Diagnosis | Average pre-op BP | IVP | Divided kidney function tests Stamey | Howard | Rapoport | $U_V$ C/I | $U_{PAH}$ I/C | $U_{Na}V$ C/I |
|---|---|---|---|---|---|---|---|---|---|---|---|---|---|
| 1. | J.K. | 33 | F | 2 | FMD (R) | 230/145 | + | Pos (R) | Pos (R) | Pos (R) | 5.4 | 3.2 | 24.3 |
| 2. | S.K. | 44 | F | 3 | FMD (R) | 200/115 | + | Pos (R) | Pos (R) | Pos (R) | 4.5 | 3.6 | 39.0 |
| 3. | J.P. | 23 | F | 1 | FMD (R) | 250/130 | + | Pos (R) | Pos (R) | Pos (R) | 8.7 | 4.2 | 48.0 |
| 4. | R.L. | 50 | F | 1 | FMD (R) | 200/100 | + | Pos (R) | Pos (R) | Pos (R) | 4.4 | 3.0 | 7.5 |
| 5. | N. Q. | 34 | F | 1 | FMD (R) | 190/120 | + | Pos (R) | Pos (R) | Pos (R) | 3.0 | 2.3 | 3.7 |
| 6. | K.H. | 37 | F | 1 | FMD (R) s stenosis | 180/120 | — | Neg | Neg | Neg | 1.4 | 1.1 | 1.4 |
| 7. | K.C. | 42 | F | 1 | FMD (R) | 200/120 | NI | Neg | Neg | Neg | 1.1 | 1.1 | 1.1 |
| 8. | L.N. | 16 | F | 1 | Coarct (R) | 210/150 | + | Pos (R) | Pos (R) | Pos (R) | 3.5 | 2.0 | 3.7 |
| 9. | G.C. | 56 | F | 5 | FMD (L) | 210/120 | + | Pos (L) | Pos (L) | Pos (L) | 5.0 | 6.1 | 51.0 |
| 10. | B.C. | 41 | M | 1 | PAF (L) | 210/130 | + | Pos (L) | Pos (L) | Pos (L) | 6.9 | 4.8 | 100.0 |
| 11. | G.B. | 50 | M | 5 | AS R > L | 190/100[a] | — | Pos (R) | Pos (R) | Pos (R) | 2.8 | 2.7 | 3.7 |
| 12. | R.F. | 28 | M | 2 | SMD L > R | 180/110 | + | Neg | Neg | Pos (L) | 1.4 | 1.4 | 1.9 |
| 13. | B.B. | 50 | F | 4 | AS (R) | 230/120 | + | Non functioning right kidney | | | | | |
| 14. | M.R. | 43 | F | 1 | FMD (R) | 190/115 | + | | | Not done | | | |
| 15. | T.L. | 33 | F | 1 | FMD (R) | 190/125 | + | | | Not done | | | |
| 16. | L.F. | 17 | M | 1 | SMF (R) | 170/120 | + | | | Not done | | | |
| 17. | D.B! | 41 | F | 3 | FMD (R) | 170/110 | + | Pos (R) | Pos (R) | Pos (R) | 5.7 | 2.3 | 5.6 |
| 18. | P.P. | 41 | F | 1 | FMD R > L | 165/115 | + | Pos (R) | Pos (R) | Pos (R) | 3.9 | 2.6 | 8.3 |
| 19. | T.C. | 34 | F | 2 | FMD (R) | 230/130[a] | + | Pos (R) | Pos (R) | Pos (R) | 2.8 | 2.4 | 65.0 |
| 20. | G.H. | 44 | F | 10 | FMD L > R | 220/130 | — | Neg | Neg | Neg | 1.3 (L) | 1.3 (L) | 1.5 (L) |
| 21. | L.R. | 22 | M | 7 | SMF Br (R) | 210/110 | + | | | Not done | | | |
| 22. | T.H. | 52 | M | 1 | AS (L) | 150/105 | — | Neg | Pos | Pos | 2.2 | 2.1 | 2.3 |
| 23. | B.E. | 57 | M | 2 | Hypopl. k (L) | 165/120 | + | Neg | Neg | Neg | 7.9 | 0.8 | 9.1 |
| 24. | P.G. | 31 | M | 7 | FMD Bil. | 235/130 | + | | | Not done | | | |
| 25. | R.C. | 43 | F | 2 | AS (L) | 185/125 | + | Pos (L) | Pos (L) | Pos (L) | 6.2 | 2.0 | 23.0 |

FMD: Fibromuscular dysplasia. SMF: Single mural fibrosis. SMD: Single mural dysplasia. PAF: Periarterial fibrosis. AS: Atherosclerosis. S: Supine. U: Upright (tilt). $\Delta$: Test not done. PRA: Plasma renin activity Ng-%/3° incubation. I: Ipsilateral. C: Contralateral. P: Peripheral. HAB: Free hypogastric artery autograft. DB: Dacron bypass. SVB: Free saphenous vein autograft. SRB: Splenorenal bypass. END Endarterectomy. Nx: Nephrectomy. E/E: End-to-end anastomosis graft to renal artery. E/S: End-to-side anastomosis graft to renal artery. Aneur: Aneurysmectomy. Art-Art: Arterio-arteriostomy. Dil: Dilation of renal artery.

It is now clear that absolute values of peripheral plasma renin activity are relatively high in such conditions as malignant hypertension and some cases of renal parenchymal disease, but that they have little or no value in the diagnosis of renovascular hypertension. When renal vein plasma samples are obtained by selective catheterization of the renal veins, however (percutaneous transfemoral Seldinger technique), the ratio of the suspected ischemic side to the normal side provides a more meaningful criterion. In our laboratory chronic hypertension has been produced in the dog by constricting one renal artery while the reduction in blood flow was monitored with the electromagnetic flowmeter. When flow was reduced by greater than 75% of the baseline and less than 90% of the baseline, chronic hypertension almost invariably ensued. In these animals, renal vein plasma renin activity was always found to be higher on the constricted side

(continued)

| Pressure gradient (mm/Hg) | | Blood flow (ml/min) | | Operative procedure | PRA | | | PRA ratio I/C | Result | Average post-op BP |
|---|---|---|---|---|---|---|---|---|---|---|
| Pre | Post | Pre | Post | | I | C | P | | | |
| 125 | 40 | 12 | 238 | HAB E/E | 1,000 | 180 | 200 | 5.6 | Cure | 120/80 |
| 100 | 0 | Δ | Δ | HAB E/S | 5,000 | 2,000 | 2,500 | 2.5 | Cure | 120/70 |
| 90 | 0 | 13 | 124 | D.B. E/S | 2,500 | 1,100 | 1,000 | 2.3 | Cure | 130/80 |
| 170 | 0 | 15 | 187 | D.B. E/S | 600 | 400 | 340 | 1.5 | Cure | 120/80 [c] |
| 95 | 0 | Δ | Δ | SVB E/S | 500 | 100 | 100 | 5.0 | Cure | 130/85 |
| 30 | 5 | 113 | 313 | HAB E/E | 6,000 | 260 | 200 | 23.0 | Cure | 125/85 [c] |
| 20 | 0 | 300 | Δ | HAB E/S | 2,000 | 330 | 500 | 6.1 | Cure | 120/80 [c] |
| Δ | Δ | Δ | Δ | Nx | 750 | 165 | 150 | 4.8 | Cure | 140/90 |
| 70 | 40 | 100 | 200 | Nx (L) [b] | 2,000 | 1,080 | 400 | 1.9 | Cure | 140/80 |
| 30 | 25 | 170 | 440 | HAB E/E | 1,200 | 450 | 600 | 2.7 | Cure | 135/85 |
| 70 | 0 | 15 | 187 | DB E/S | S 2,500 | 1,500 | 880 | 1.7 | Cure | 140/90 |
| | | | | | U 5,000 | 1,650 | 937 | 3.0 | | |
| 55 | 0 | 240 | 390 | SRB E/S | S 325 | 180 | 238 | 1.8 | Cure | 140/90 [c] |
| | | | | | U 1,090 | 500 | 485 | 2.0 | | |
| Δ | Δ | Δ | Δ | Nx | 2,000 | 1,400 | 800 | 1.4 | Cure | 120/70 |
| 80 | 100 | Δ | Δ | HAB E/E | 1,000 | 500 | 600 | 2.0 | Cure | 135/90 |
| 100 | 0 | 50 | 138 | HAB E/E | 140 | 50 | 20 | 2.8 | Cure | 130/80 |
| 80 | Δ | Δ | Δ | Nx | 200 | 30 | 0 | 6.6 | Cure | 130/85 |
| Δ | Δ | Δ | Δ | Nx | 200 | 200 | 180 | 1.0 | Impr | 140/95 |
| 25 | 15 | 31 | 200 | HAB E/E | 1,200 | 200 | 50 | 6.0 | Impr | 170/100 |
| 55 | 0 | 60 | 210 | SVB | 220 | 320 | 200 | 0.7 | Impr | 160/110 [c] |
| (R) (L) | (R) (L) | (R) (L) | (R) (L) | (L) (R) | (L) | (R) | 1,500 | 6.2 | Impr | 180/105 [c] |
| 25 85 | 0 0 | 232 13 | 206 147 | DB E/S | 1,500 | 240 | | | | |
| | | | | Dil. | | | | | | |
| 70 | 15 | 10 | 20 | Art-Art | 1,280 | 175 | 185 | 6.9 | Impr | 160/100 |
| | | | | 2° Nx (R) | | | | | | |
| Δ | Δ | Δ | Δ | EHD (L) | 480 | 600 | 525 | 0.8 | Failure | 150/105 [c] |
| Δ | Δ | Δ | Δ | Nx (L) | 1,200 | 1,200 | 720 | 1.0 | Failure | 165/120 |
| Δ | Δ | Δ | Δ | Nx (L) | 1,200 (L) | 800 (R) | 750 | 1.5 | Failure | 240/140 |
| | | | | Aneur (R) | | | | | | |
| 90 | 40 | Δ | Δ | END (L) | 145 | 1,000 | 100 | 0.14 | Failure | 190/110 [c] |

$U_V$C/I: Ratio urine flow rate contralateral kidney Pos = 1.5.
$U_{PAH}$ I/C: Ratio urine PAH concentration ipsilateral kidney Pos = 1.25.
$U_{Na}V$ C/I: Urinary sodium × minute volume contralateral kidney mEq/l pos = 1.5.
[a] On drug therapy.
[b] Nephrectomy after unsatisfactory repair.
[c] Patients with negative DKF tests but positive PRA ratios or with negative PRA ratios but positive DKF tests.

and the elevation remained for long periods of time. Over a 12-month period of observation, the absolute amounts of renin from the constricted and the normal side showed a gradual decline, but the ratio remained above 1.5:1 between the constricted and the control kidney (Kaufman, Lupu and Maxwell, 1969). Clinical studies also suggest that a ratio above 1.5 between the ipsilateral and contralateral renal vein plasma renin activities is a helpful criterion for predicting the outcome of surgery. Our clinical results appear in Table 1. Of 25 treated patients there were 16 cures, five improved subjects and four failures. The four failures had ipsilateral/contralateral ratios of plasma renin activity had values of 0.14, 0.8, 1.0 and 1.5. The ratios for the five improved patients were 0.7, 1.0, 6.0, 6.2 and 6.9, respectively, whereas the lowest ratio obtained from the group of cures was 1.4. The mean values and the ranges for renal vein plasma renin activity appear in Fig. 7. It is possible to enhance the values of plasma renin assay by postural and physiological preparation of the patient. Salt deprivation or diuretics (natriuretics) appear to augment renin activity both in the peripheral plasma as well as in the renal vein plasma. Such augmentation appears to occur more on the ischemic side than in the contralateral renal vein effluent. Thus it may be possible to effect disparate renal vein renin augmentation.

In summary, it is now clear that despite lack of specificity and wide availability differential renal vein plasma renin determinations provide one of the most valuable means of determining the functional significance of stenosing lesions of the renal artery found on arteriography. The test also promises to be of more predictive value than any other test devised thus far. Because absolute values of renal vein plasma renin activity have less meaning than the relative values between the ischemic and control sides, the ratio remains the most important criterion of the presence of a functionally significant lesion and of the prospect for surgical cure. With future refinements of renin assay, it is to be expected that this test will become the touchstone of diagnosis and surgical prognosis.

## 7. Pressure Gradient and Renal Blood Flow Determinations

It is generally held that the determination of pressure gradients between the aorta and the poststenotic renal artery is necessary to confirm the functional significance of the renal artery stenosis. By and large, the tenet is valid that a pressure differential of 25 mm Hg or more correlates with a significant lesion and in many cases with a situation curable by nephrectomy or repair. In a recent correlation of pressure gradients with the results of surgical cure, it was found that four of thirteen patients (30%) were cured despite pressure gradients below 10 mm Hg. Of 25 patients with pressure gradients between 25 and 50 mm Hg, 8 (31%) were cured; of 65 patients with pressure gradients over 50 mm Hg, 38 (58%) were cured (Statistical Report, 1966). In some cases, however, the pressure gradient alone may be a misleading determinant. Experiments in animals have shown that intrarenal resistance can be increased pharmacologically (with norepinephrine or angiotensin) and that this may minimize or obliterate the gradient while renal blood flow is being significantly impeded (LUPU, KAUFMAN and MAXWELL, 1968). Conversely, with vasodilating agents it is possible to widen an equivocal pressure gradient (THOMAS, BROCKMAN and FOSTER, 1968). Placing acetylcholine in the renal artery will increase renal blood flow and at the same time widen the pressure gradient. The concomitant measurement of renal blood flow with an electromagnetic flowmeter is highly desirable, and recent improvements in probes and flowmeters have made this a practical procedure. It is our practice to determine both gradients and flows before and after arterial repair, whenever possible. When the flow has not been improved, repairs have sometimes been revised with better results. In other cases, a low flow indicates small vessel disease and increased intrarenal resistance thus vitiating the value of any major renal artery repair.

## 8. Renal Biopsy

Several types of renal histopathology are associated with renovascular hypertension: changes in the juxtaglomerular apparatus (hypercellularity and hypergranulation), ischemic tubular atrophy, interstitial fibrosis, round cell infiltration and arteriolar changes. It is generally accepted that these changes are inconstant and that they exist to different degrees at various stages in the development of renovascular hypertension. Our studies have shown a good correlation between the results of angioplastic surgery vis-a-vis the degree of tubular atrophy and interstitial fibrosis (Barajas, Lupu, Kaufman, Latta and Maxwell, 1967). Other pathological criteria, including juxtaglomerular size and granularity and arteriolar hyalinosis, had little or no prognostic significance. From this study we concluded that in the presence of significant unilateral renal artery stenosis, severe ipsilateral tubular atrophy and interstitial scarring oblige nephrectomy, whereas minimal ipsilateral tubular atrophy suggests that revascularization may be successful in curing the hypertension. Pathological changes in the contralateral kidney appeared to have less correlation with prognosis, and contrary to prevalent opinion, many of the changes, including those of small vessel disease in the contralateral ("unprotected") kidney, are apparently reversible after the hypertension is relieved by removal or repair of the offending kidney.

## II. Surgical Treatment

It has been over three decades since Butler (1937) demonstrated that nephrectomy may cure hypertension caused by unilateral renal disease and 16 years since Freeman, Leeds, Elliott and Roland (1954) successfully introduced

Table 2. *Renovascular hypertension surgical results (to 10/1/68)*

| | | |
|---|---|---|
| Unilateral procedures<br>Bilateral procedures | 149<br>20 | 169 patients (179 procedures) |
| Nephrectomy (primary)<br>Partial nephrectomy | 48<br>8 | 31% |
| Reconstructive procedures | 123 (113 pts) | 69% |
| Secondary nephrectomy<br>(after unsuccessful repair) | 15/123 | 12% |

Table 3. *Renovascular hypertension, surgical results (to 10/1/68), 179 procedures in 169 patients*

| | Cured improved | Failed |
|---|---|---|
| Ablative surgery (31%) | 86% | 14% |
| Reconstructive surgery (69%) | 77% | 23% |

Table 4. *Renovascular hypertension, surgical results (to 10/1/68), unilateral procedures*

| | | Cured | Improved | Failed |
|---|---|---|---|---|
| Primary nephrectomy | 42 | 22 | 17 | 3 |
| Partial nephrectomy | 7 | 2 | 2 | 3 |
| Nephropexy (alone) | 6 | 2 | 2 | 2 |

vascular repair for renal artery stenosis. Considerable progress has been made n vascular surgery but surgeons are still frequently confronted with the task of selecting the treatment most likely to succeed for an individual patient. Not all patients are cured or improved by nephrectomy, the sacrifice of a "good" kidney distal to the renal artery stenosis is anathema to surgeons, and many angioplasties are inadequate or otherwise unsuccessful. Between 1958 and 1962, among 383 patients collected from the literature, the proportion of nephrectomy to arterioplasty was 2:1 (Kaufman, Lupu and Maxwell, 1969). In a National Cooperative Study between 1962 and 1966, 427 cases were subjected to operation for renal artery stenosis in the United States (Statistical Report, 1967). Of these patients 211 were treated by nephrectomy, 16 by partial nephrectomy, and 200 by arterioplasty, a ratio of ablative to reconstructive procedures of approximately 1:1. The greatest need at present is for clarification of factors that have predictive value in regard to blood pressure response following ablative or reconstructive renal surgery. The results of surgical treatment of renovascular

Table 5. *Renovascular hypertension surgical results (to 10/1/68) unilateral procedures*

| | | Cured | Improved | Failed | Deaths |
|---|---|---|---|---|---|
| Endarterectomy | 17 | 5 | 5 | 7 | |
| Resection and anastomosis | 9 | 5 | 3 | 1 | |
| Bypass | 45 | | | | |
| Vein | 12 | 4 | 3 | 5 | |
| Artery | 6 | 6 | 0 | 0 | |
| Dacron | 27 | 15 | 4 | 5 | 3 |
| Splenorenal | 9 | 5 | 3 | 1 | 0 |
| Arteriolysis | 2 | 0 | 1 | 1 | 0 |
| Reno-aortic reimplantation | 2 | 0 | 0 | 0 | 2 |
| Aneurysmorrhaphy | 3 | 0 | 2 | 1 | |
| Patch plasty | 3 | 1 | 0 | 2 | |

Table 6. *Renovascular hypertension bilateral surgical procedures. One stage: 14*

| | | Cured | Improved | Failed |
|---|---|---|---|---|
| Bilateral endarterectomy | (6) | 2 | 4 | 0 |
| Bilateral resection and anastomosis | (1) | | 1 | |
| Nephrectomy and repair | (3) | 1 | 1 | 1 |
| Splenorenal and bypass (Dacron) | (1) | 1 | | |
| Nephrectomy and autotransplantation | (1) | 1 | | |
| Bypass (Dacron) and dilation | (1) | | 1 | |

Table 7. *Renovascular hypertension bilateral surgical procedures. Two stages: 6*

| | | Cured | Improved | Failed |
|---|---|---|---|---|
| Endarterectomy | (1) | | 1 | |
| Splenorenal and Dacron bypass | (1) | | 1 | |
| Endarterectomy and resection and anastomosis | (1) | 1 | | |
| Resection and anastomosis (bilat) | (1) | | | 1 |
| Nephrectomy and autotransplantation | (1) | | | 1 |
| Partial nephrectomy and nephrectomy | (1) | 1 | | |

hypertension do not clearly indicate the relative superiority of nephrectomy as opposed to angioplasty. Undoubtedly, some of the failures with angioplasty are attributable to inadequate repair. The results of our personal series of 169 cases are listed in Tables 2 to 3. In this group there were 48 primary nephrectomies and 15 secondary nephrectomies after unsuccessful arterioplasties among the 179 procedures for renal artery stenosis (169 patients). There were eight partial nephrectomies. One hundred and twenty-three reconstructive procedures were done on 113 patients. Although there were 48 cases of bilateral renal artery stenosis, only 12 patients have had bilateral reconstructive operations (shown in Tables 6 and 7). In the other 36 cases of bilateral disease, the grade of stenosis on the unoperated side was not considered to be of sufficient magnitude to justify intervention.

Criteria of cure, improvement and failure were as follows: patients were considered cured if the blood pressure was 140/90 mm Hg or less without drugs six months or longer after operation. Improved patients were those showing a reduction in diastolic blood pressure of 15 mm Hg or more, evidence of cardiovascular improvement or who were normotensive on medications to which they had been unresponsive previously. Failures were those patients who do not quality in the other two categories.

## 1. Nephrectomy

The indications for nephrectomy are: 1. unilateral renal infarction or nonfunction; 2. multiple branch lesions, i.e., stenosis, aneurysms, infarcts; 3. severe unilateral parenchymal disease with or without associated renal artery stenosis; 4. unsuccessful previous arterioplasty or partial nephrectomy; 5. poor flow through a repaired vessel after vascular repair; and possibly 6. open biopsies showing severe or moderately severe ischemic tubular atrophy ipsilaterally with absent or minimal tubular atrophy contralaterally.

In the presence of bilateral disease the need for renal conservation is more compelling and the surgeon must be willing to gamble on a favorable result from reconstruction. In our series of 63 patients undergoing primary or secondary nephrectomy (Table 3), there were 86% cures or improvements and 14% failures.

## 2. Partial Nephrectomy

It appears that the indications for partial nephrectomy for branch disease are relatively uncommon. Although theoretically sound, the results even in well-defined cases have not been dramatic. There were three cures and four failures in our series of seven patients. Persistence of hypertension may be related at times to the incomplete removal of ischemic tissue.

## 3. Nephropexy

Nephropexy should be done in all cases in which there is excessive renal mobility or in which the kidney has been freed during the procedure. Fig. 6 is an (p. 7) arteriographic study of a patient with subadventitial fibroplasia of the right renal artery associated with renal ptosis (excessive mobility). This patient was treated with a Dacron bypass graft and nephropexy. As the sole treatment for rare cases of hypertension secondary to ptosis which caused renal artery traction and torsion, nephropexy has been somewhat disappointing, even though preoperative studies showed that orthostatic hypertension was clearly related to renal ptosis.

## 4. Surgical Approaches to the Renal Vessels

The customary approach to the renal vessels is through an anterior abdominal incision. With the patient in the supine position, the abdomen is opened by a midline incision extending from the xyphoid to the mid-lower abdomen; *or* by a transverse incision in the upper abdomen, cutting both rectus muscles and incising the external and internal oblique muscle on the side of the intended repair. Occasionally extending the incision through the costal cartilage between the eighth and ninth or the ninth and tenth ribs may be indicated. For obese or muscular patients the thoraco-abdominal approach provides the best exposure. There are two good approaches to the renal vessels: by colonic reflection (Figs. 8

and 9) or by duodenal mobilization (Fig. 10). In the first method the peritoneum is incised along the paracolic reflection. On the left side the splenic flexure must be mobilized by incising the lienocolic ligament. This will allow retraction of the descending colon medially. On the right side the incision is continued through the hepatocolic ligament and the duodenum is mobilized by Kocher's maneuver after incising the peritoneum along the lateral border of the duodenum. If it is not sufficiently free to be retracted, the cecum is also mobilized. The right colon is reflected medially together with the duodenum, exposing the vena cava.

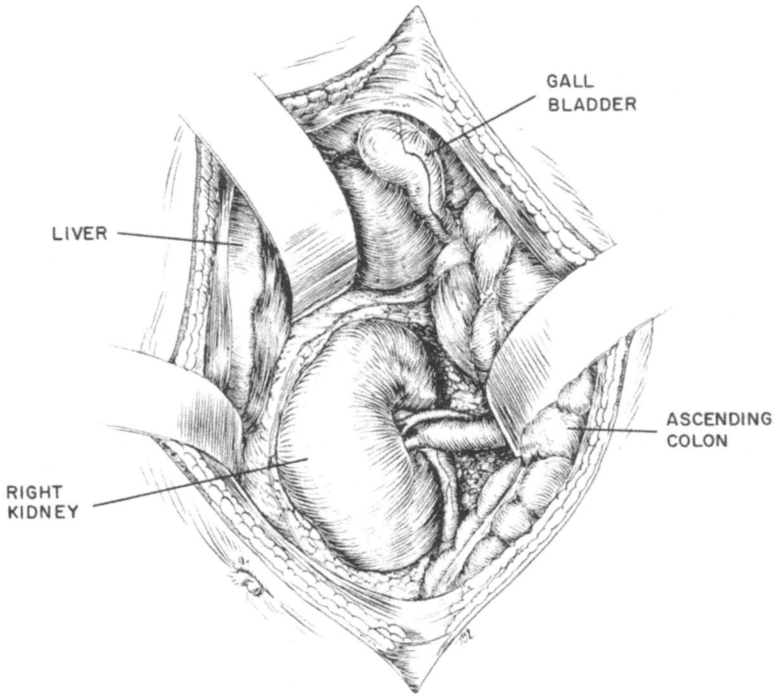


Fig. 8. Exposure of the right kidney and distal portion of the right renal vessels by transperitoneal approach. Hepatic flexure and ascending colon are retracted medially

The most direct approach to the aorta, vena cava, and proximal portions of the renal vessels is afforded by mobilizing the duodenum upward as shown in Fig. 10. The small bowel is eviscerated and packed in a plastic bag and the transverse colon is lifted upward and cephalad. The peritoneal reflection along the inferior border of the ascending portion of the duodenum is incised and the duodenum is rotated upward. This will open the retroperitoneal area and give direct exposure to the great vessels. The ovarian or spermatic veins should be severed, particularly on the side of the repair, since this will allow freer retraction of the vena cava on the right side and of the renal vein on the left side.

A variety of reconstructive surgical techniques has been described and used for repair of stenosing lesions of the renal arteries. These include: 1. thromb-endarterectomy, with or without a patch graft; 2. resection of the diseased arterial segment with primary end-to-end anastomosis; 3. bypass grafts from the aorta to the distal portion of the renal artery with free autologous artery

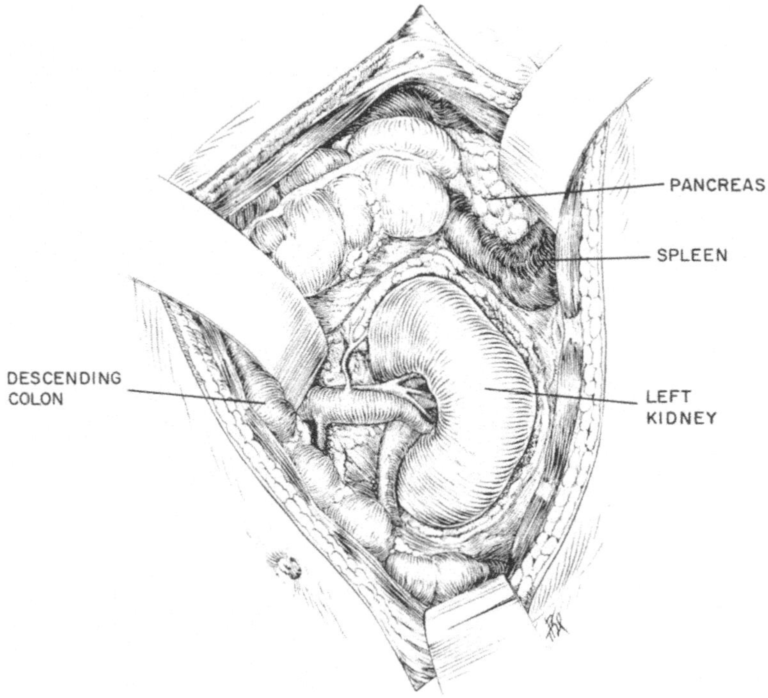


Fig. 9. Exposure of left kidney and renal vessels by transperitoneal approach. Splenic flexures mobilized and descending colon reflected medially

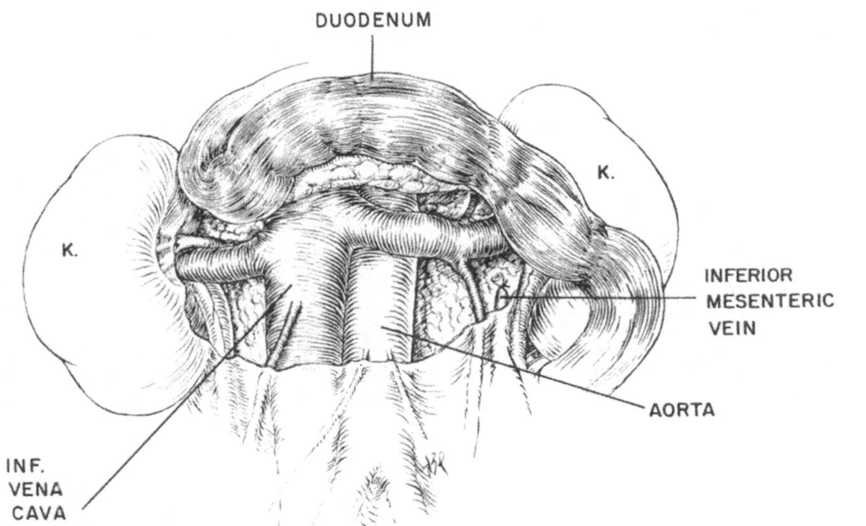


Fig. 10. Exposure of renal vessels by duodenal mobilization. Posterior parietal peritoneum is incised under ascending portion of duodenum, and duodenum is rotated upward. Inferior mesenteric vein and ovarian or spermatic veins are ligated to gain additional mobility

(hypogastric), autologous vein, synthetic prosthesis or *in situ* splenic artery; 4. transection of the renal artery with renoaortic reimplantation; 5. arteriotomy and patch graft; and 6. renal autotransplantation.

Some patients with extensive disease of the renal arteries (e.g., diffuse fibromuscular dysplasia) often have involvement of the primary and secondary branches and require partial or total nephrectomy. Similarly, diffuse atheromatous disease with multiple areas of renal infarction also dictates nephrectomy. Associated disease of the aorta, or superior mesenteric, celiac or iliac vessels sometimes requires surgical management at the time of renovascular operation in patients with atheromatous disease.

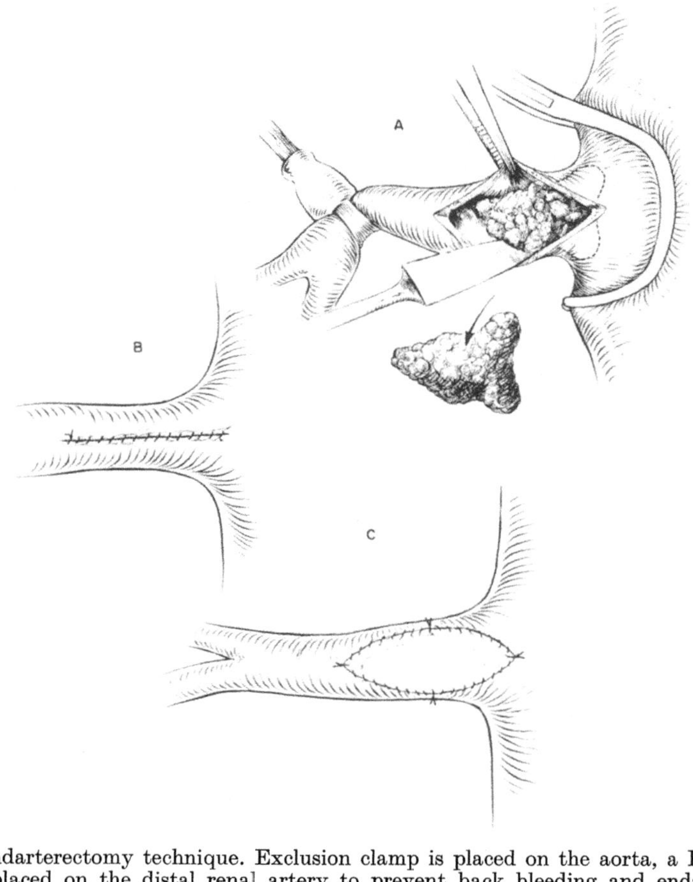


Fig. 11. Endarterectomy technique. Exclusion clamp is placed on the aorta, a Rumel tourniquet is placed on the distal renal artery to prevent back bleeding and endarterectomy is done with a spatula as shown

## a) Endarterectomy

Thrombendarterectomy is applicable in patients with localized atheromatous stenosis of the renal artery occurring unilaterally or bilaterally. Between 55% and 65% of hypertensive patients with renal artery disease have atheromatous occlusions. There are several methods of performing endarterectomy on the renal artery. Exposure of the aorta and the first portion of the renal artery is customarily required. An arteriosclerotic plaque in the proximal portion is easily felt

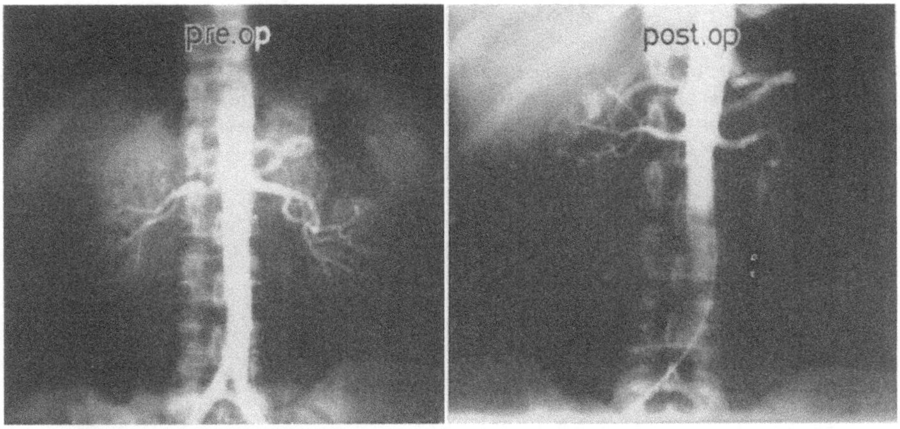


Fig. 12. Pre-and-postoperative appearance of arteriograms of a patient with right renal artery atherosclerotic plaque. Primary closure of the renal artery was done following endarterectomy

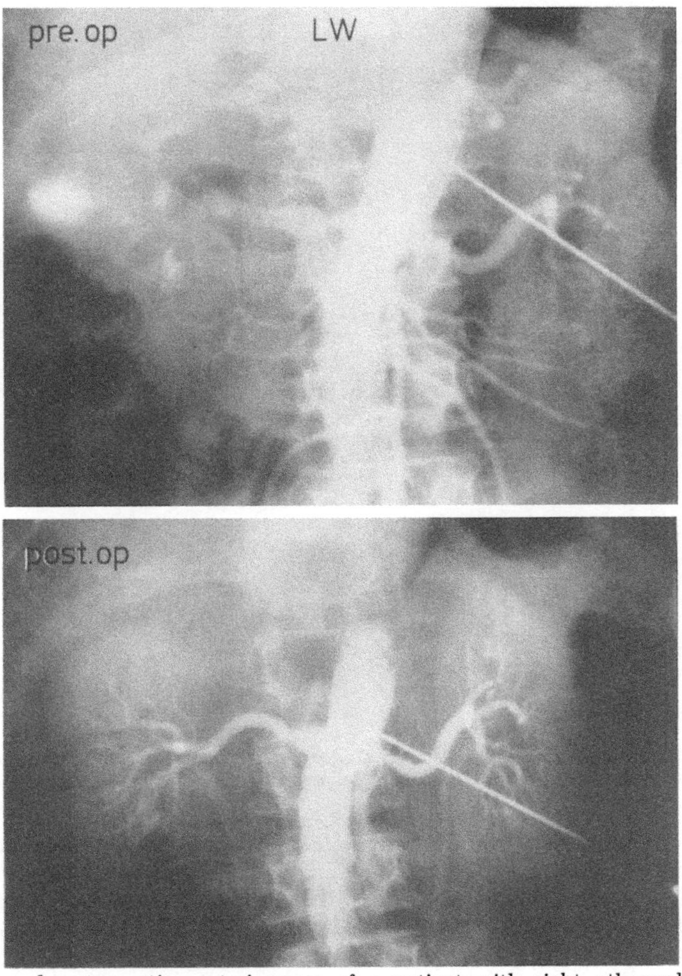


Fig. 13. Pre-and-postoperative arteriograms of a patient with right atherosclerotic renal artery plaque treated by endarterectomy and insertion of a Dacron patch

and a thrill is often palpated in the area of stenosis. The method most commonly employed consists of placing an exclusion clamp tangentially about the aorta, cutting off the renal artery flow without interrupting flow through the aorta (Fig. 11). A longitudinal arteriotomy is made on the anterior wall of the renal

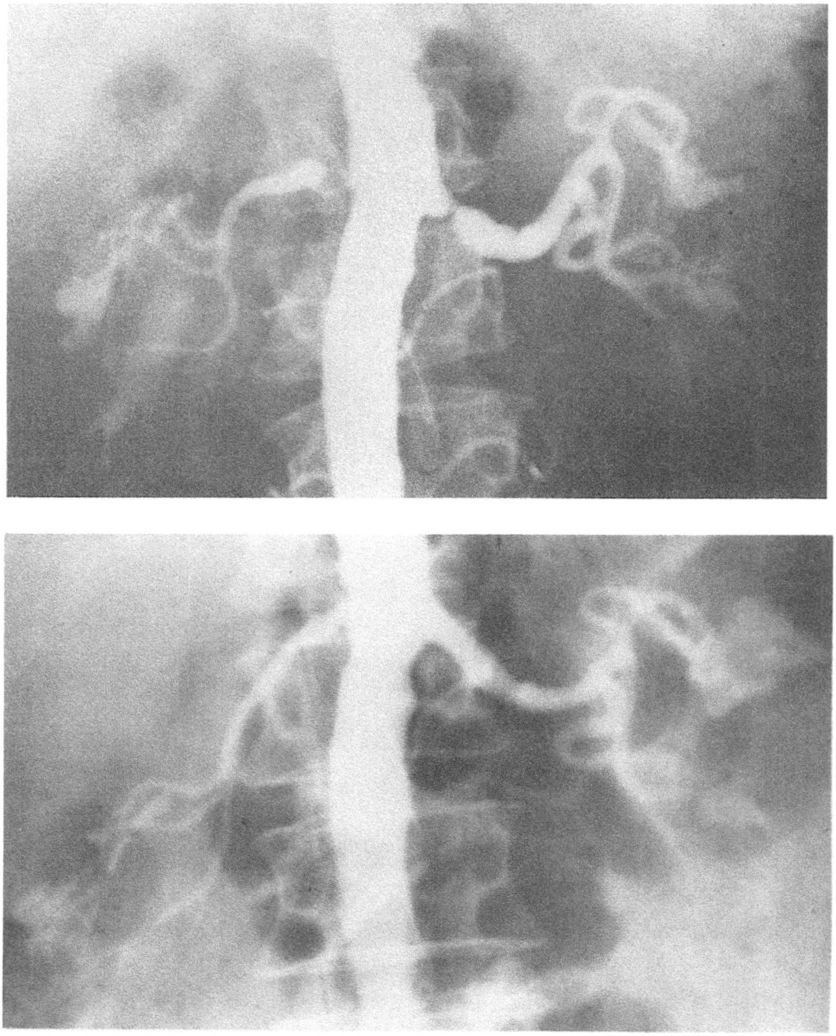

Fig. 14. Bilateral high grade renal artery stenosis secondary to atheromatous disease, preoperative arteriogram and postoperative arteriogram (one year after operation)

artery extending it into the aorta if necessary. Dissection of the plaque from the wall of the renal artery, using a Cannon arterial dissector or an ear curet, must be done meticulously. After the atheromatous plaque has been removed, the wall of the renal artery may be closed primarily with a continuous 5—0 or 6—0 suture of silk or Teflon-coated Dacron, but when the lumen appears inadequate or when there is a tendency for a thin-walled vessel to buckle, a gusset of vein, hypogastric artery or synthetic material should be used (Fig. 11). It is important to leave a smooth arterial wall to minimize the tendency for post-operative thrombosis and distal dissection of the intima. Occasionally it may be necessary to tack down a fold of intima at the distal end of the endarterectomy in order to prevent "lifting" and dissection.

Bilateral endarterectomy is indicated when there is significant stenosis in the proximal portions of both renal arteries. The technique is more difficult

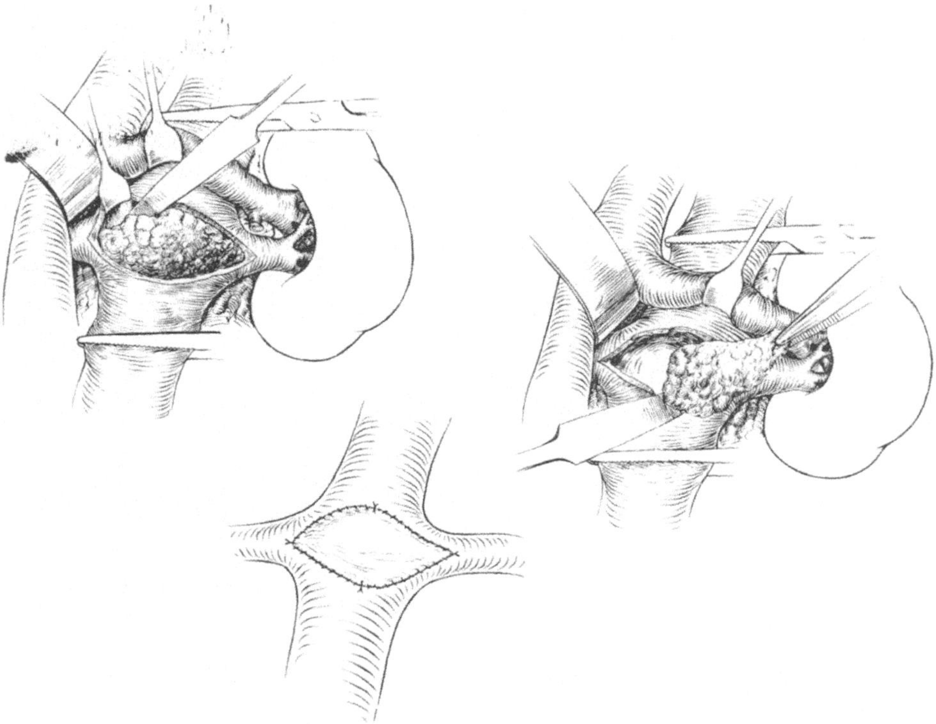

Fig. 15. Bilateral transaortic endarterectomy. Cross clamping of aorta, transverse aortotomy, endarterectomy and aortic closure with gusset of Dacron are shown

than that for unilateral renal artery endarterectomy, since it requires cross-clamping of the aorta above and below the renal arteries and a vertical or transverse aortotomy extending, when necessary, out into the proximal portions of the renal arteries on either side. The plaque within the aorta is gently lifted up and its extensions into the renal ostia are meticulously dissected from the vessels. Occasionally it may be possible to repair the incision in the aortic wall by direct closure with 4—0 silk or Tev-Dek. When the aortic wall is thin, however, and will not hold sutures well, it is preferable to insert a gusset of vein or Dacron.

Endarterectomy is easier in younger patients who have good residual vessel walls after the plaque has been removed. Some surgeons have advocated transection of the renal artery distal to the plaque with proximal endarterectomy and end-to-end anastomosis of the vessels after the obstructing plaque has been removed. We have not found this necessary and because the vessel wall is often thin in elderly patients after endarterectomy, such end-to-end anastomosis may be difficult and the results unsatisfactory. Fig. 12 shows pre-and-postarterectomy arteriograms in a patient who had a plaque removed from the first portion of the right renal artery and primary closure of the arteriotomy. Fig. 13 shows pre-and-postoperative aortograms in a patient who had a right renal endarterectomy and insertion of a Dacron gusset at the arteriotomy site. Eight years postoperatively the patient continues to be normotensive with a good anatomical result. Fig. 14 shows pre-and-postoperative aortograms in a patient with bilateral renal artery stenosis secondary to atherosclerosis affecting the aorta and both right and left renal arterial ostia. The patient was treated by a transaortic endarterectomy as shown in Fig. 15.

### b) Segmental Resection and End-to-End Anastomosis of the Renal Artery

Well localized stenosing lesions of the renal artery or aneurysm in the midportion of the renal artery, may be successfully treated by segmental resection

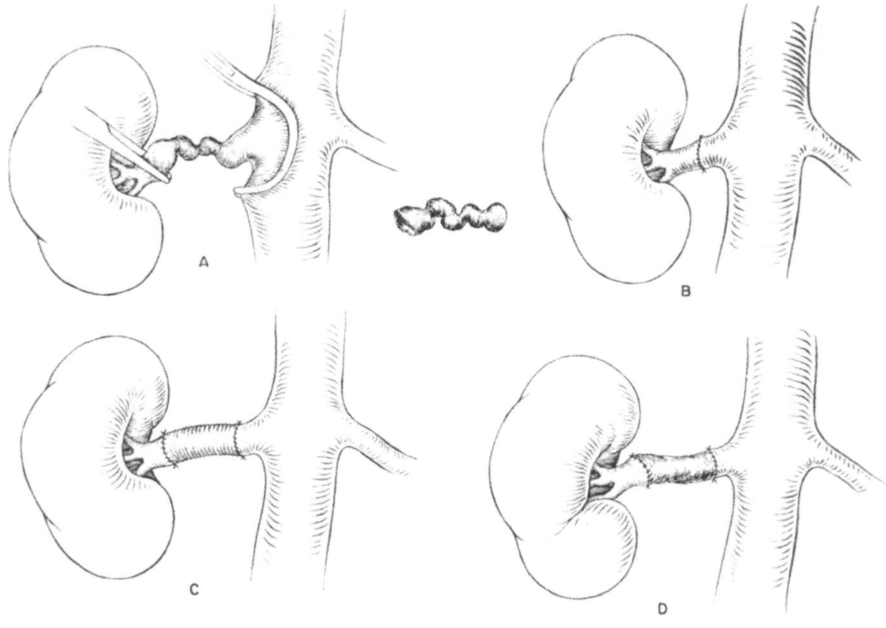


Fig. 16. Method of segmental renal artery resection and reanastomosis. C and D indicate interposition graft of Dacron and autologous artery respectively

and reanastomosis. When applicable, this operation is an ideal procedure, since the diseased segment of vessel wall is excised and a minimum of roughened surface is left to invite subsequent thrombotic occlusion. Cases must be selected prudently, however, because the disease of the renal artery wall is frequently more extensive than its appearance on the arteriogram would indicate. Sutures do not hold well in a diseased vessel, and unless delicate and accurate approximation of the two ends is made without compromising the luminal size, the results of repair will be unsatisfactory. If primary reanastomosis is impractical because of the short length of the renal artery, it is possible to insert a length of Dacron or autologous artery (Fig. 16). In rare instances it may be possible to join two branches of the renal artery and to anastomose the newly made single artery to the proximal stump. Such procedures are infrequently indicated, however, because the disease often extends into primary branches, and even when it is possible, the operation requires prolonged periods of renal ischemia.

It is important to fix the kidney position after repair to prevent nephroptosis and traction on the suture line since there is evidence to suggest that traction

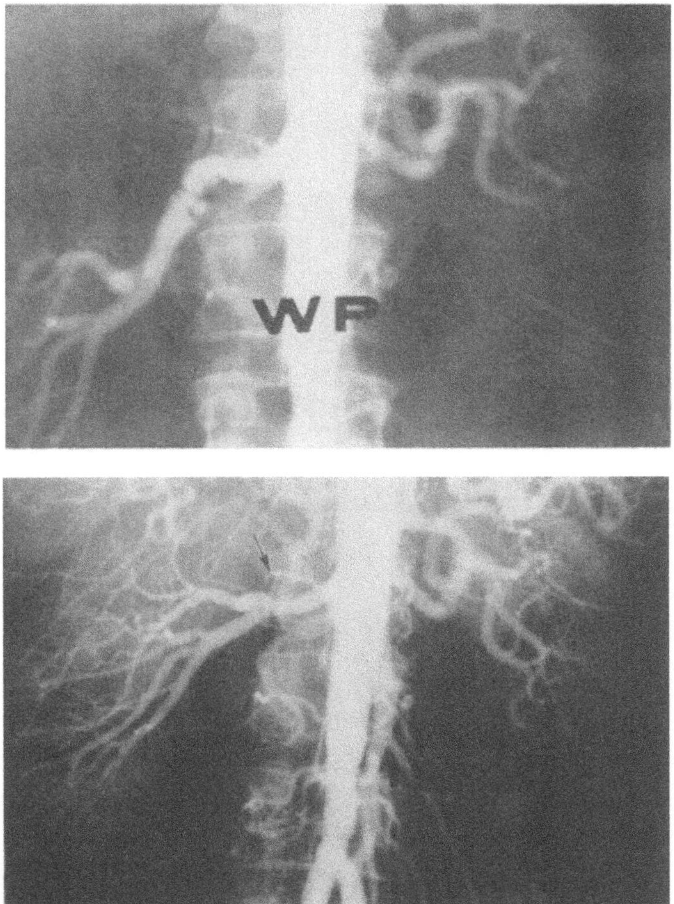


Fig. 17. Pre-and-postoperative arteriograms in a case of fibromuscular hyperplasia. Zone of anastomosis is shown. Approximately one-third of the length of the renal artery was resected

may result in restenosis in the area of the surgical union. Fig. 17 shows pre-and-postoperative arteriograms in a case of fibromuscular hyperplasia and severe ptosis. Approximately one-third of the length of the renal artery was resected in this case

### c) Aorterenal Bypass Grafts

The bypass graft has become the most popular reconstructive operation because it is the simplest technically, because extensive involvement of the renal arteries frequently precludes other types of repair, and because the grafts appear to function well. Although they offer theoretical advantages over synthetic materials, we have continued to have some disappointing early thromboses and late closures when autologous vein grafts were employed. Fig. 18a illustrates a saphenous vein bypass two months after operation (arteriogram) and Fig. 18b

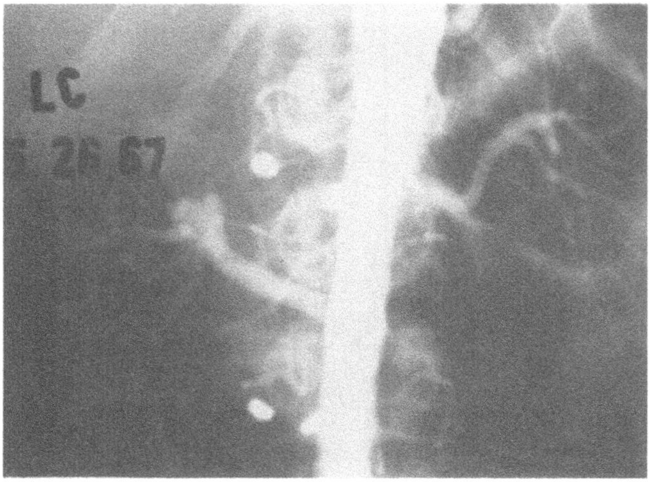


Fig. 18a. Arteriogram two months after operation showing patent venous (saphenous) aorto-renal bypass graft

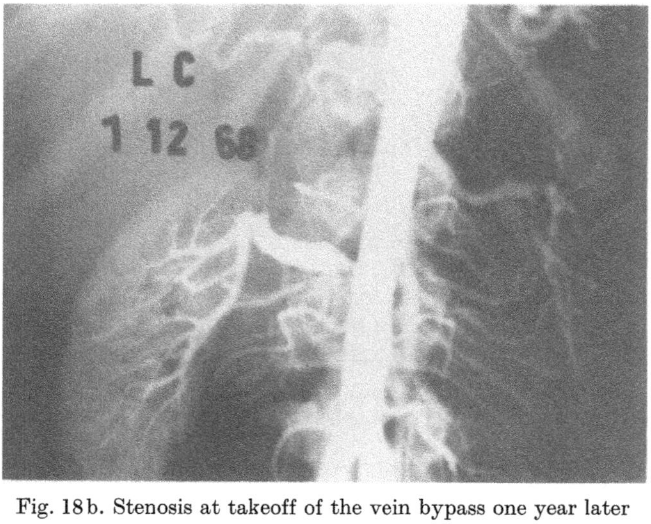


Fig. 18b. Stenosis at takeoff of the vein bypass one year later

shows stenosis of the take off of the vein bypass one year later. General rules of using vein grafts have been followed, i.e., reversal of the saphenous vein segment to prevent obstruction to flow by valves, use of local and systemic heparin, and avoidance of intimal trauma.

The following principles applying to the use of synthetic grafts are recommemded: 1. use only Dacron (preferably microweave); 2. avoid excessive lengths and kinking; 3. avoid septum formation at anastomotic areas by careful suturing; 4. use a graft whose diameter is between $1^1/_2$ and $2^1/_2$ times that of the vessel; and 5. use antibiotics prophylactically during the postoperative period.

Some vascular surgeons have deprecated synthetic renal bypass grafts because of alleged occlusion hazards. These opinions are based largely on experience with synthetic tubes used to replace other vessels over long distances or when there

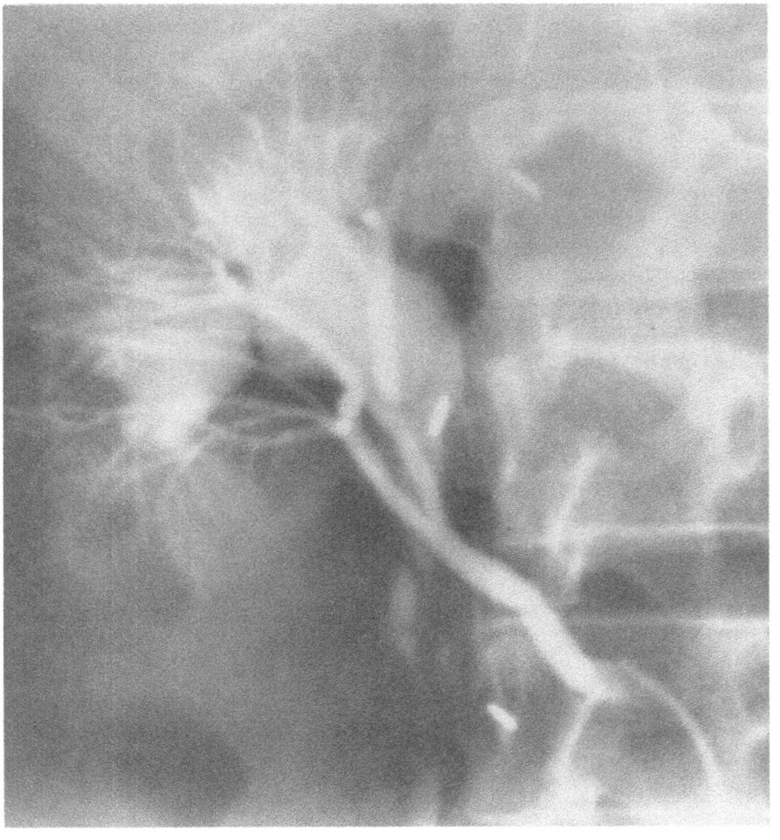

Fig. 19. Selective arteriogram showing hypogastric artery substitution graft. Autologous hypogastric artery has been attached to the aorta and an end-to-end anastomosis between the graft and the renal artery was done

has been mobility of the graft or runoff has been poor. These circumstances do not generally occur in aortorenal bypass grafts, wherein lengths are short, the graft is fixed, and flow is exceptionally high. We have witnessed three complete occlusions in synthetic grafts, each occurring because of technical and avoidable details. One occurred early (three months) after using a Teflon graft; one occurred immediately following a yearly follow-up selective catheterization of the bypass for X-ray visualization and probably resulted from lifting the pseudointima and producing a septum; and one occurred because of angulation of the graft behind the vena cava. The latter event was discovered on routine aortogram one year postoperatively and since the renal artery was still intact (end-to-side graft to vessel anastomosis) and only the aortic half of the tube was occluded, we were able to reoperate, attach another tube to the patent portion, and to transpose the graft anterior to the vena cava. The patient is well, more than one year later, with normal blood pressure and kidney function. One graft is showing gradual occlusion over a five-year period of observation, probably because of arterial branch disease, high resistance, and poor runoff.

Since 1967 we have employed the hypogastric artery as a free bypass autograft and have experience with eight cases. The hypogastric artery was too short to bridge the distance in an additional case in which a prosthetic graft was used alternatively. Of course, the hypogastric artery should be normal when it is being considered as an autologous bypass. For this reason, we now make arteriograms to include the iliac vessels when performing renal angiography. When it is normal, the hypogastric artery is ideally suited to serve as a bypass. It is one of the large arteries that can be sacrificed with impunity. The substitution of an artery for an artery is appealing. Most of the patients requiring bypass grafts are young individuals with fibroplasias, and the coexistence of disease of the hypogastric arteries in such patients appears to be infrequent. The viscoelastic properties of the hypogastric artery duplicate those of the normal renal artery and constrictions at the aortic anastomotic site might be expected to be infrequent. All of the cases in which we have employed the hypogastric artery as a bypass have had excellent technical and clinical results, and we are encouraged to continue using this technique (Fig. 19).

### d) Splenorenal Anastomosis

Splenorenal arterial bypass is an excellent procedure, providing certain requisites are met. The splenic artery must be healthy, and in this regard it is important to obtain preoperative lateral or oblique aortograms to insure that there

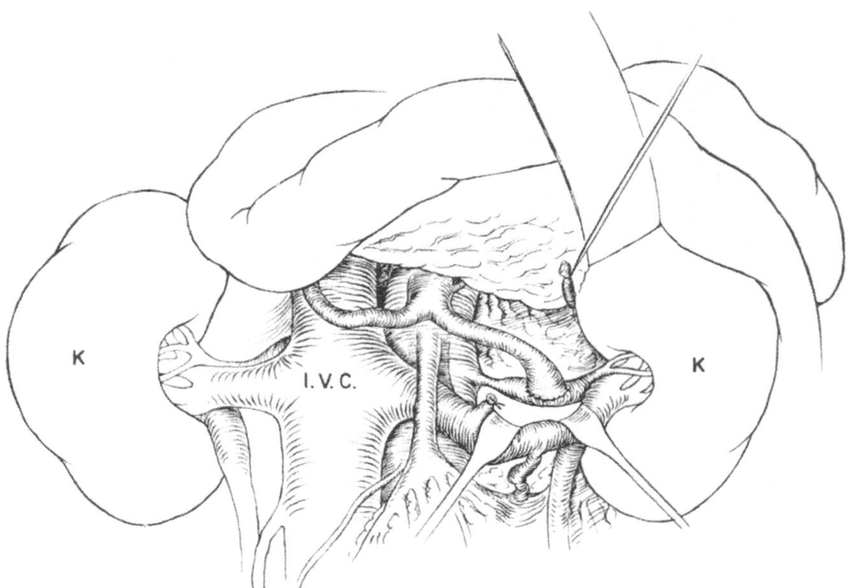


Fig. 20. Drawing to show technique of splenorenal bypass operation. End-to-side anastomosis of the splenic artery to the renal artery is shown

is no stenosis of the celiac axis or the splenic artery. The lesion must be on the left side and of the type suggesting that bypass is preferable to endarterectomy or resection and reanastomosis. Splenorenal bypass is somewhat more difficult to perform than a free bypass of Dacron, artery or vein, and for that reason it has not gained as much popularity as the latter type of angioplasty.

Sufficient length of the splenic artery should be mobilized to permit it to reach the renal artery without tension. It is not necessary to remove the spleen since it receives sufficient blood supply from short gastric vessels and collaterals

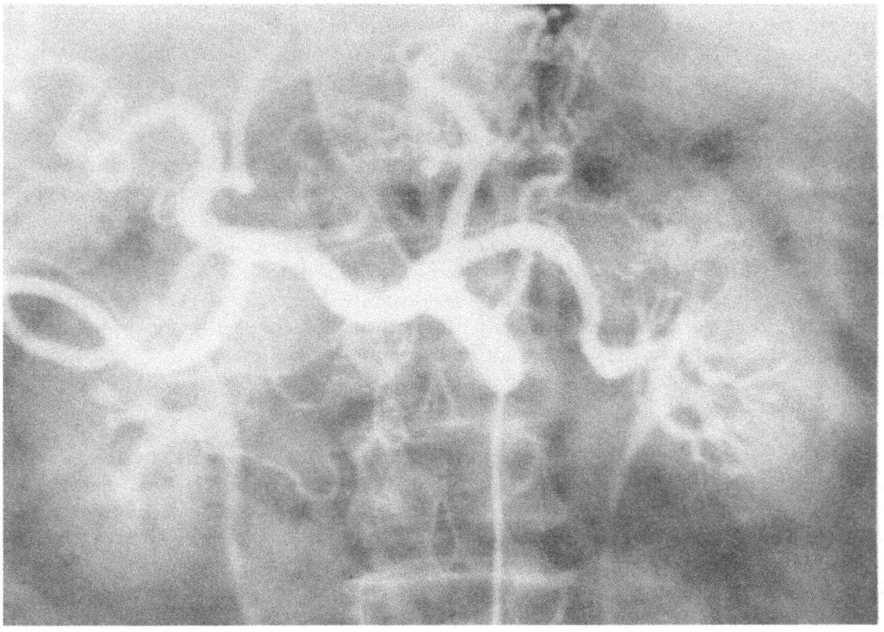

Fig. 21. Postoperative celiac arteriogram showing anastomosis of the splenic artery to the renal artery for left renal artery stenosis. An end-to-end anastomosis between the splenic artery and the renal artery was done in this case

originating from the gastroepiploic artery to insure its viability. The majority of surgeons prefer an end-to-side anastomosis, relying on an auxiliary flow rather than a substitution blood supply (Fig. 20). Moreover, it is generally recognized that there is less tendency to stenosis with end-to-side arterial anastomosis than with end-to-end anastomosis. Fig. 21 is a postoperative arteriogram in a case in which splenorenal anastomosis was curative of the hypertension.

### e) Reimplantation (Renal-Aortic)

The chief indication for this infrequently used procedure is stenosis limited to the orifice of the renal artery and an aorta reasonably free of atheromatous disease. The distal renal artery must also be free of significant disease. The chief disadvantage of renoaortic reimplantation is that in suturing the renal artery to a thick walled aorta, it is usually difficult to produce a satisfactorily wide bore anastomotic lumen. Furthermore, on the right side it usually requires freeing of the kidney in order to approximate the renal artery to the aorta, thus depriving the kidney of collateral blood supply.

### f) Arteriotomy and Patch-Plasty

Arteriotomy and insertion of a patch of vein, artery, or synthetic material is occasionally employed. It is particularly suited for isolated narrowings of the renal artery such as occur in congenital coarctation and single mural fibrosis. Following a longitudinal incision through the area of stenosis, a triangular patch of vein, artery or woven Dacron is fashioned to the appropriate size and is sutured in place. Caution must be exercised to avoid making the patch too large and predisposing to aneurysm formation. Unfortunately the indications for this procedure are not common and the results, in our hands, have not been as good as might be expected from the simplicity of the procedure.

Segmental resection of the kidney needs only brief mention since it is not strictly a vascular procedure. It is necessary to determine the renal segment involved by isolating and occluding the branch vessel leading to the area of ischemia. This can be facilitated by injecting the main renal artery with indigo carmine (2—3 $cm^3$) or by injecting the artery leading to the ischemic segment of kidney with the dye (Poutasse, 1962). In the former case all of the kidney except the ischemic area will be stained blue. In the latter only the ischemic area will be stained. When there is complete occlusion of the branch leading to the involved segment, injection of the main renal artery is obviously necessary. This type of mapping of the kidney is possible because of end-distribution of the renal blood supply to the kidney. It is thus possible to remove not only an ischemic pole of the kidney but middle segments as well.

### g) Autotransplantation

Occasionally a renal artery stenosis may be unusually difficult to repair *in situ*. In such cases the kidney may be transposed to the iliac fossa where the renal artery is anastomosed to the hypogastric or common iliac artery and the renal vein is joined to the common iliac vein or the vena cava (without interrupting ureteral continuity). If there is abundant collateral supply, we would caution against this type of operation. We have performed two autotransplantations on solitary functioning kidneys affected by renal artery stenosis. The first case was a seven-year-old boy with a high-grade stenosis but without extensive collateral circulation. Transplantation of the kidney to the ipsilateral iliac fossa provided an excellent result with normal kidney function and return of blood pressure to normal (Kaufman, Alferez, Vela-Navarette). The second case was technically satisfactory but the patient had malignant nephrosclerosis and eventually died of this disease.

## 5. Bilateral Renal Artery Stenosis

When bilateral lesions appear to be functionally significant, better results may be obtained by performing repairs at one stage. Less well defined is the indication for repairing a contralateral lesion of doubtful functional significance at the time that a unilateral significant lesion is being treated. If the functional impact of such a marginal stenosis appears imminent and if the repair can be done with relatively little risk of failure in the opinion of the surgeon, it is advisable that bilateral procedures be done at one stage. When a transaortic approach is being used for endarterectomy it is easy to perform bilateral endarterectomy if there is an atheroma in the contralateral renal artery. Since the results of revascularization are not always predictable, elective angioplasties should be done only by experienced surgeons.

### 6. Medical Versus Surgical Treatment

It is generally accepted that patients who show relatively isolated renal arterial lesions and who do not have widespread arterial disease, should be treated by arterioplasty or nephrectomy according to the indications, and that patients with extrarenal vascular insufficiencies or with extremely difficult renal artery involvement, should be treated medically. Subjects with only suggestive renal artery disease and no functional stigmata of renal ischemia should be treated medically because of the probability in such cases that the arterial stenosis is coincidental with rather than causative of the hypertension. When the natural history of occlusive renal artery disease is better understood by long-range studies and when surgical techniques have been standardized to a predictable level, the respective merits of medical and surgical therapies will be better established. Thirty-six patients with proven renal artery stenosis and hypertension were treated with drugs for reasons of poor risk, severe extrarenal vascular disease, refusal to undergo operation, or because repair appeared technically impossible. Ten of these subjects were satisfactorily controlled for periods of two to six years, and 26 could not be controlled. In this group eight patients died of cardiovascular complications from one to four years after treatment was instituted. Four patients showed a progressive loss of renal function while on drug therapy (Table 8).

Table 8. *Blood pressure response in conservatively treated patients. 36 subjects*

| | |
|---|---|
| Normal diastolic pressure with therapy | 10 |
| Diastolic hypertension with therapy | 26 |
| Progressive loss of renal function | 4 |

Sufficient experience has now been gained in the study of renovascular hypertension to glean insight into the natural history of stenosing lesions of the renal artery. A large number of our patients have had arteriograms performed yearly or every other year for eight years. It has been our impression from these studies that the rate of progression of stenosis of the renal arteries depends upon the nature of the pathology. Periarterial fibrosis (Takayasu's disease) often affects aortic branches at their takeoff but in other instances seems to involve longer segments of the main renal artery. It appears to have a rapidly progressive course and stenoses have been witnessed to progress from minimal to complete occlusion over a period of one or two years. Atherosclerosis progresses somewhat more slowly. We have followed several cases in which lesions with under 50% compromise of luminal diameter have progressed to complete occlusion in two to four years. Fibromuscular dysplasias of the renal artery have a slower course but it is clear that these lesions, too, are progressive and minor compromises of the arterial lumen have become functionally significant during four to eight years of observation. It is evident, therefore, that until the nature of these stenosing diseases is elucidated and medical treatment devised, efforts must be directed at improving surgical techniques in the hope of salvaging kidney function.

## B. Surgery of Renal Artery Aneurysms

In the main, renal artery aneurysms are of two types: arteriosclerotic, and associated with fibromuscular arterial dysplasias. Miscellaneous types of aneurysm include the congenital, mycotic, and traumatic. Aneurysms may be soft and

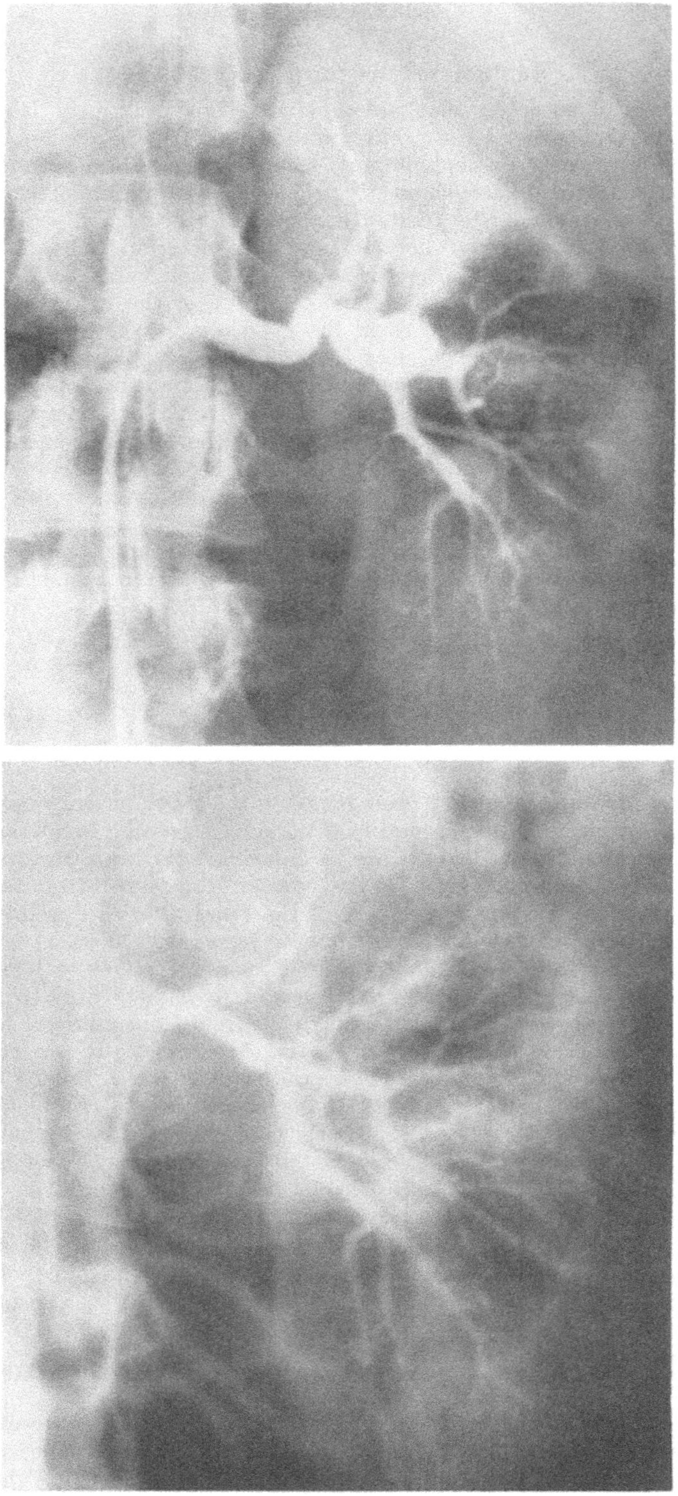

Fig. 22. Pre-and-postoperative arteriograms of patient who underwent aneurysmectomy for hypertension

thin-walled or calcified and they may be single or multiple. Calcification is more common with the arteriosclerotic variety than with other types. Commonly, arteriosclerotic aneurysms and aneurysms associated with fibromuscular arterial dysplasias occur at the branching of the renal artery where there is weakness of the vessel wall.

Formerly, renal artery aneurysms were treated expectantly or by nephrectomy. Only during recent years has vascular repair proven feasible and successful.

The simplest treatment is excision of the aneurysm and primary arteriorrhaphy. Occasionally it may be necessary to insert a patch of vein or synthetic material at the area of excision. The surgical treatment requires meticulous dissection of the main renal artery and its primary branches to gain good exposure and adequate control of the blood supply. Fig. 22a and b are reproductions of pre-and-postoperative arteriograms of a patient who underwent aneurysmectomy for hypertension.

# C. Renal Artery Embolism

Renal artery embolism is not as common as other forms of major arterial disease but Hoxie and Coggin (1940) found 205 cases among 14,411 autopsies. Most of the cases of renal infarction reported in the literature have been treated by nephrectomy but more aggressive attitudes toward this condition are evident in the number of case reports of renal artery embolectomy appearing in the literature.

Most patients with renal artery embolism have a past history of rheumatic heart disease. The majority are a result of thrombi dislodged from fibrillating atria or from a valvular site. Renal artery embolism should be suspected when a patient with heart disease complains of flank pain, hematuria and/or oliguria. The diagnosis is made presumptively by excretory urography showing non-function and a retrograde pyelogram showing normal pyelocalyceal architecture and definitively by renal arteriography.

Surgical removal of renal artery emboli depends on site and duration of the infarct. Emboli lodged in the main renal artery or in the primary branches can be satisfactorily removed while emboli in small branches cannot be satisfactorily removed. Although there are rare examples of successful late embolectomies, it is generally accepted that early intervention is mandatory and where unilateral anuria or oliguria have existed for longer than 48 hours, it is extremely rare to observe late good functional recovery. Systemic anticoagulant therapy is advisable with or without operation to prevent subsequent emboli from forming. Other conservative measures such as selective catheterization of the renal artery with infusion of fibrinolysin is of questionable value at this time.

## I. Technique of Embolectomy

The renal artery is best approached by the anterior incision previously described. The kidney is inspected and the artery palpated. After occluding the renal artery near its origin and without placing occluding clamps or tapes distally, a longitudinal arteriotomy is made. The Fogarty catheter is particularly useful to extract thrombi from the renal artery and the major branches. This device together with suction usually allows for complete extraction of the thrombus. Brisk back bleeding is a favorable sign. The absence of back bleeding often augurs a poor result but if the color of the kidney is good and its consistency firm, the outcome may eventually be excellent. Local heparin together with

Xylocaine or Cyclaine should be used to irrigate the renal vessels. The arteriotomy is closed primarily. If the condition of the vessel wall is poor, however, a gusset should be used as previously described for endarterectomy.

# D. Renal Vein Thrombosis

There are several clinical varieties of renal vein obstruction. *1. Thrombosis of the inferior vena cava with secondary involvement to the renal veins.* This type is commonly due to spread from pelvic and leg veins. *2. Obstruction of the inferior vena cava due to invasion by malignant neoplasm or external pressure.* In this type of case the middle caval segment is commonly involved. *3. Primary thrombosis of renal veins.* Except during infancy primary renal vein thrombosis is rare, probably because of the brisk blood flow which normally exists. The renal blood flow is relatively low in infancy and is liable to be further reduced by loss of water and salt from vomiting and diarrhea. Renal vein thrombosis, therefore, occurs especially as a complication of severe gastroenteritis. It may also be associated with acute pyelonephritis and thrombophlebitis of the renal vein. *4. Renal vein thrombosis secondary to primary renal disease.* In adults renal vein thrombosis may occur as a result of disease causing a reduction in renal blod flow. It is found rarely in association with acute glomerulonephritis and pyelonephritis but is more likely to occur in the nephrotic syndrome and renal amyloidosis.

The clinical picture of renal vein thrombosis consists of sudden pain in the flank radiating to the inguinal area of abdomen, enlargement and tenderness of the kidney. A nephrotic syndrome occurs in about 30% of cases. At operation the kidneys are often three to four times normal size and show diffuse hemorrhage and dilated lymphatics. The treatment depends on the location of the thrombus.

Nephrectomy is preferred in patients with proven unilateral thrombosis and a normal contralateral kidney, but restoration of renal venous return by removal of the thrombus may be quite effective if operation is carried out promptly (within 48 hours). Systemic heparin should not be used in patients in whom very low platelet counts are present subsequent to renal vein thrombosis (platelet consumption) since progression is unlikely in such patients.

## Conclusion

The current status of diagnosis and treatment of renovascular hypertension and related renal vascular problems has been described. A gratifying degree of diagnostic and therapeutic expertise has been achieved as a result of the combined efforts of internists, physiological chemists, urologists and vascular surgeons. The urologist of the future should be equipped to properly diagnose these problems and to deal effectively with the complicated surgery involved. He is in a unique position to grasp the full breadth of the disorders.

## References

Barajas, L., Lupu, A. N., Kaufman, J. J., Latta, H., Maxwell, M. H.: The value of the renal biopsy in unilateral renovascular hypertension. Nephron **4**, 231 (1967).

Boucher, R., Veyrat, R., Champlain, J. de, Genest, J.: New procedures for measurement of human plasma angiotensin and renin activity levels. Canad. med. Ass. J. **90**, 194 (1964).

Butler, A. M.: Chronic pyelonephritis and arterial hypertension. J. clin. Invest. **16**, 889 (1937).

CROCKER, D. W.: Fibromuscular dysplasias of renal artery. Arch. Path. **85**, 602 (1968).
FREEMAN, N. E., LEEDS, F. H., ELLIOTT, W. G., ROLAND, S. I.: Thrombendarterectomy for hypertension due to renal artery occlusion. J. Amer. med. Ass. **156**, 1077 (1954).
HELMER, O. M., JUDSON, W. E.: The quantitative determination of renin in the plasma of patients with arterial hypertension. Circulation **27**, 1050 (1963).
HOWARD, J. E., CONNOR, T. B.: Use of differential renal function studies in the diagnosis of renovascular hypertension. Amer. J. Surg. **107**, 58 (1964).
HOXIE, H. J., COGGIN, C. B.: Renal infarction: Statistical studies of 205 cases and detailed report of an unusual case. Arch. intern. Med. **65**, 587 (1940).
KAUFMAN, J. J., ALFEREZ, C., VELA-NAVARETTE, R.: Autotransplantation of a solitary functioning kidney for renovascular hypertension. J. Urol. (Baltimore) **102**, 146—150 (1969).
— HANAFEE, W., MAXWELL, M. H.: Upright renal arteriography in the study of renal hypertension. J. Amer. med. Ass. **187**, 977 (1964).
— LUPU, A. N., MAXWELL, M. H.: Renovascular hypertension: Clinical characteristics, diagnosis and treatment. Cardiovasc. Clin. **1**, 79—112 (1969).
— — — Further experiences in the diagnosis and treatment of renovascular hypertension: Surgical treatment of hypertension secondary to renal artery stenosis. Urol. int. (Basel) **24**, 12 (1969).
— MAXWELL, M. H.: Upright aortography in the study of nephroptosis. Stenotic lesions of the renal artery and hypertension. Surgery **53**, 736 (1963).
KROPP, K. A., O'CONOR, V. J., JR.: Results of surgery in renovascular hypertension with equivocal divided renal function studies. J. Urol. (Baltimore) **100**, 224 (1968).
LEVER, A. F., ROBERTSON, J. I. S., TREE, M.: The estimation of renin in plasma by an enzyme kinetic technique. Biochem. J. **91**, 346 (1964).
LUPU, A. N., KAUFMAN, J. J., MAXWELL, M. H.: Renal artery constriction: Physiological determinants of pressure gradients. Ann. Surg. **167**, 246 (1968).
MAXWELL, M. H., LUPU, A. N.: Excretory urography in renal arterial hypertension. J. Urol. (Baltimore) **100**, 395 (1968).
— — KAUFMAN, J. J.: Individual kidney function tests in renal arterial hypertension. J. Urol. (Baltimore) **100**, 384 (1968).
— — TAPLIN, G. V.: Radioisotope renogram in renal arterial hypertension. J. Urol. (Baltimore) **100**, 376 (1968).
MCCORMACK, L. J., POUTASSE, E. F., MEANY, T. F., NOTO, T. J., DUSTAN, H. P.: A pathologic arteriographic correlation of renal arterial disease. Amer. Heart J. **72**, 188 (1966).
PICKENS, P. J., et al.: Measurement of renin activity in human plasma. Circulat. Res. **17**, 438 (1965).
POUTASSE, E. F.: Partial nephrectomy: New techniques, approach, operative indications and review of 51 cases. J. Urol. (Baltimore) **88**, 153 (1962).
RAPOPORT, A.: Modification of the "Howard Test" for the detection of renal-artery obstruction. New Engl. J. Med. **263**, 1159 (1960).
STAMEY, T. A.: The diagnosis of curable unilateral renal hypertension by ureteral catheterization. Postgrad. Med. **29**, 496 (1961).
Statistical Report, Cooperative Study of Renal Arterial Hypertension, Annual Meeting, New York, May 1966.
— — Cooperative Study of Renal Arterial Hypertension, Annual Meeting, New York, May 1967.
THOMAS, C. S., BROCKMAN, S. K., FOSTER, J. H.: Variability of the pressure gradient in renal artery stenosis. Surg. Gynec. Obstet. **126**, 339 (1968).

# Renal Transplantation

DONALD C. MARTIN

With 60 Figures

## I. Renal Transplantation

### Historical Background

Successful transplantation of a vascular parenchymal organ depends upon the surgeon's ability to reconstruct the blood supply system. Thus the story of renal transplantation actually begins early in this century with the development of vascular anastomosis by ULLMANN, CARREL and GUTHRIE (ULLMANN [246]; CARREL, 1906 [42]). ALEXIS CARREL was a surgeon of great imagination and manual dexterity who did much of his work at the Rockefeller Institute in New York (SMITH [216]). These men performed autotransplantations and homotransplantations of kidneys in laboratory animals, principally dogs and cats, and proved the lifesupporting capacity of the autotransplant (CARREL, 1910 [41]). CARREL received a Nobel Prize for his achievements.

For a decade investigators were confused by the similarity between graft necrosis due to vascular occlusion and graft rejection in its late stages. Investigators who have performed canine renal transplantation are familiar with the similar late end result of these two processes. This problem was clarified by WILLIAMSON, a urologist working in the laboratories of the Mayo Clinic, who described and identified the inflammatory destruction of the homograft (WILLIAMSON [260]). Three decades later the immunological basis of this rejection was still not proven, although it was suspected. The presence of antibodies in the serum of graft recipients was not clearly established until recent years (MILGROM [151]); this finding, along with many other clinical observations, identifies the immunological basis of graft rejection.

Credit for the first human renal transplant is given to the Russian surgeon VORONOY for an operation performed in 1936 (VORONOY [250]); subsequent cases were reported from Chicago (LAWLER [123]), Paris (KÜSS [121]) and Boston (HUME [90]). The renal graft rarely functioned in these early cases; that function which did occur was transient. Although the ability of identical twins to exchange skin grafts had been reported by BAUER and BROWN as early as 1927 (BAUER [24]; BROWN [35]), this information lay dormant until 1954, when MURRAY, HARRISON and MERRILL in Boston performed the first kidney transplant between identical twins (MERRILL [149]). The dramatic recovery of these and subsequent patients was a great stimulus to the pursuit of successful organ grafting.

Total body irradiation of the recipient to suppress the immunological response was employed principally in Paris and Boston (DEALEY [53]; MURRAY, 1960 [163]). The European experience with this treatment was favorable in a few cases; however, the overall percentage of success was low and discouraging (HAMBURGER [79]). In 1959 SCHWARTZ and DAMASHEK reported that an antimetabolite drug

(6-mercaptopurine) would inhibit the rejection of rabbit skin grafts (SCHWARTZ [211]). ZUKOSKI in Richmond and PIERCE and VARCO in Minnesota confirmed this observation in canine renal transplants (ZUKOSKI [272]; PIERCE [189]). CALNE, working in the surgical laboratory of Harvard Medical School, studied azathioprine (similar to 6-MP) in canine renal grafts and laid the foundation for the clinical use of this drug (CALNE [39]).

PERSKY, Professor of Urology at Western Reserve University in Cleveland, attempted in 1951 to delay the rejection of canine renal grafts by administering the newly available hormone cortisone. The small doses he used failed to provide any salutary effect. It was not until 10 years later when another urologist — GOODWIN of U.C.L.A. — used massive doses of a potent synthetic corticosteroid (Prednisone) that the true value of this family of drugs in transplant therapy became apparent. The importance of these observations was quickly recognized throughout the United States.

The combination of an antimetabolite (azathioprine) and a corticosteroid (Prednisone) was found to inhibit graft rejection in 75% of cases involving close family members and in 40—50% of cases involving cadavers (ACKMAN [6]). The search for new drugs and techniques continues; local irradiation of the graft (MARTIN [139]; KAUFFMAN [102]), extra-corporeal irradiation of the blood (WOLF [263, 264, 265, 266]), thoracic duct fistula (SINGH [214]), intralymphatic injections (WHEELER [256]), alkylating agents (PARSONS [181]) or antibiotics (ALEXANDRE, 1963 [8, 9]), and other methods have been tried with mixed results.

That heterologous antilymphocyte sera demonstrate immunosuppressive activity was shown by WAKSMAN as early as 1961 (WAKSMAN [251]); however, this knowledge was not applied clinically until STARZL prepared canine and human antilymphocyte globulin in horses (IWASAKI [97]). After a beneficial effect in canine renal and hepatic grafts was established, clinical trials were undertaken. The material was found to be unsatisfactory when used alone and therefore was used with azathioprine and prednisone (STARZL [221, 224, 226]). The precise role and efficiency of this combination remain to be established.

In many of the early attempts to provide renal function with a graft the kidney was connected to the vessels of the thigh. KÜSS described anastomosis of the kidney to the iliac vessels combined with uretero-cutaneous anastomosis for placement of the graft in the iliac fossa. MURRAY and HARRISON used the iliac vessels but placed the donor ureter in the recipient bladder in the first transplantation between identical twins. This has become the standard technique of most surgeons.

The advances to this time have largely been the contributions of daring surgeons. The most significant observation to be made from experiences with whole organ transplants (modified by one or several of the methods described above) has been that the immunological reaction is not an "all-or-none" phenomenon but can be depressed or even stopped to allow continued function from the graft. Previous observations made of skin grafts in laboratory animals had indicated that this reaction was of an "all-or-none" nature, which suggested a discouraging outlook for the whole organ transplant.

The basic scientist, initially somewhat of a skeptic and critic, soon became a fascinated coworker. Identification of lymphocyte antigens by *in vitro* serologic methods appears to be a major advance. The results of many clinical organ grafts correlate well with the "match" of lymphocyte antigens between donor and recipient (TERASAKI [235, 237, 238]). Other laboratory and clinical methods of pairing donor and recipient have been suggested — for example, neutral leucocyte transfer (BRENT [33]), and mixed lymphocyte culture (HIRSCHHORN

[87]) but none is as practical as the lymphocyte cytotoxic test of Dr. PAUL TERASAKI (TERASAKI [234, 235]). Just as LANDSTEINER began with four red blood cell groups and we now have more than 100, so the number of recognized lymphocyte antigens increases annually.

The development of organ transplantation is one of the great advances in medical science of the 20th century. The story spans the present century and may not be complete at the end of 100 years. Present results fall far short of our desired goal and yet the valiant efforts of clinical surgeons have paid happy dividends for many patients.

# II. Evaluation of Patients

## A. Evaluation of the Recipient

Renal transplantation is not feasible nor advisable for all patients dying of chronic renal failure. Many factors must be considered in the selection of those patients who might benefit most from transplantation, and arbitrary limits will often be set in an attempt to produce optimum results.

### 1. Age

Although it is technically possible to make the required vascular anastomoses in infants, few centers have performed renal transplants in small children because of other considerations. We attempted to implant both kidneys with segments of aorta and vena cava from an anencephalic monster to a 12.0 kg child without success. Preadolescents have been transplanted with excellent results, and we have been gratified by the return of normal growth and development in previously growth-retarded children.

Patients in older age groups present more of a technical challenge to the surgeon, for a number of reasons. Older candidates are more likely to suffer from significant cardiac disease, diabetes or other systemic complications of long standing renal disease. Atherosclerosis may complicate the required arterial anastomosis. Recuperation is slower in older recipients than in young adults. The older patients must be evaluated carefully and judged individually; we have had little success with recipients over the age of 46 years. We have performed pre-transplantation arteriography in a few potential recipients. This provided a valuable warning of atherosclerosis in the internal iliac artery in a patient subsequently successfully transplanted with arterial anastomosis to the external iliac artery.

### 2. Diagnosis

It is likely that renal transplantation is not advisable in patients where renal failure is only one manifestation of a serious systemic illness such as diabetes mellitus, lupus erythematosis, amyloidosis, scleroderma, etc., since progression of the underlying illness will shorten the life expectancy of many of these patients. When renal failure is the major manifestation or is accompanied by few other complications, transplantation may be worthwhile. Selected patients with lupus and diabetes have been transplanted with some success.

1. Glomerulonephritis. It is desirable to have histologic or similar clear definition of the underlying nephropathy prior to planning transplantation. Glomerulonephritis is the cause of renal failure in the majority of cases requiring transplantation and is associated with the best prognosis. Patients with this

disease are usually young and rarely have anatomical defects of the urinary tract or urinary infection.

When the recipient has glomerulonephritis it is important to determine the activity of the pathological process. Patients with circulating antiglomerular basement membrane antibodies at the time of transplantation have been observed to develop glomerulonephritis in the graft. The detection of these antibodies is possible in a few sophisticated laboratories (LERNER [126]).

2. Pyelonephritis. In our experience, recipients with pyelonephritis have a slightly higher incidence of chronic infection than do those with glomerulonephritis. Those with active infection should be treated to sterilize the lower urinary tract prior to transplantation. Systemic antibiotics and mechanical bladder wash with the instillation of antibacterials may suffice in some cases (HINMAN [84]); preliminary bilateral nephro-ureterectomy may be necessary in others.

3. Polycystic renal disease. The adult form of polycystic renal disease presents a few candidates for transplantation. These are difficult to manage. Often the patient is older with many changes secondary to a slowly progressive chronic renal failure. Atherosclerosis seems to be accelerated by chronic uremia. This was dramatically brought to our attention in the case of a 37-year-old polycystic whose internal iliac artery contained a large atheromatous plaque requiring end-arterectomy while the renal artery of his 60-year-old donor (mother) was elastic and normal.

## 3. Urinary Tract Status

To minimize the risk of infection developing in the renal graft, the lower urinary tract of the recipient should function normally; thus, patients with noncorrectable uropathy are not good candidates. A moderate number of kidneys have been transplanted with urine drainage through an isolated iliac conduit (Bricker's operation) with a small percentage of success (KELLY [105]; KISER [111]). Our experience with this technique has resulted in infection, hemorrhage and death.

Evaluation of the recipient may be made by history alone. In the absence of symptoms, signs and urinary infection with clearly documented primary pathology, the urinary tract need not be instrumented prior to transplantation. Although vesicoureteral reflux might occasionally be missed by such a course, this risk must be weighed against the risk of introducing infection with catheter or cystoscope. Patients with a demonstrated uropathy must have this corrected, preferably prior to the transplantation. Refluxing ureters should be entirely removed. Bladder outlet obstruction can be corrected at the time of transplantation; however, this adds measurably to the length and complexity of the procedure, increasing the risk of hemorrhage, fistula or infection. Patients with severe bladder damage or uncorrectable lower urinary tract obstructions are probably best treated by chronic hemodialysis.

## 4. Circulating Antibodies

Antiglomerular basement membrane antibodies have been mentioned as a contraindication to transplantation. These are rare and must not be confused with cytotoxic antibodies, which are the result of prior pregnancy, abortion, repeated blood transfusions or organ grafts. Cytotoxic antibodies have been associated with immediate immunological destruction of the graft in a number of patients (STARZL [222]; WILLIAMS [257]). They may be detected by an in vitro serologic test in which recipient serum is incubated with lymphocytes from a number of different persons. This test should be performed as a routine prior to all transplants. Multiparous females and patients who have received many transfusions are most suspect. The presence of these antibodies is a serious contraindication to transplantation, unless a donor can be found who does not have those antigens to which the recipient reacts (PATEL, 1969 [184]; STEWART [229]).

Successful transplantation has been achieved in a few patients despite the presence of cytotoxic antibodies to the donor lymphocytes; however, more have failed. Recipients with circulating antibodies have not done well even when grafted with the kidney of a donor to whose lymphocytes they did not react. The development of such antibodies after grafting presents a major obstacle to repetitive transplantation.

### 5. Timing of the Transplant

Timing of the transplantation procedure must be considered in evaluation of the recipient. Therapy should be planned to avoid severe muscle wasting, neuropathy, pericarditis or peritonitis, since any of these late complications of uremia can jeopardize the outcome or prolong recovery. If a suitable donor is not immediately available, the patient must be supported by dialysis to avoid the complications of untreated uremia.

### 6. Psychological Factors

Organ transplantation makes many demands on the patient as well as the surgeon, and the full cooperation of the patient is necessary for success. The unstable or emotionally immature personality is a poor candidate for a renal transplant. Evaluation of a patient's personality is often complicated by the presence of chronic uremia.

The recipient must be mature and stable enough to follow the instructions of the physician regarding diet, fluid intake, medications and clinic visits. The restrictions on diet and fluid will usually be minimal compared with those of chronic dialysis. Because of the distressing side effects of corticosteroids, patients may attempt to reduce or regulate the dose in an undesirable fashion. We have observed deterioration in graft function in such cases.

## B. Evaluation of the Donor

### 1. Living Donors

The availability of a healthy organ from a willing family donor has advanced clinical renal transplantation immensely. The family donor provides not only a normally functioning organ but one which is genetically related to the recipient. The genetic transmission of antigens which determine the immunologic response to organ grafts, previously evident from the results of clinical experience, has now been documented in the laboratory; thus there are sound scientific as well as social and moral grounds for using close family members as living donors. Whatever the relationship of donor and recipient, it is essential that the donor be a willing volunteer. Unfortunately, most donors feel pressure from the recipient and from other family members. The physician should do nothing to increase such pressure; rather, he should attempt to minimize it.

1. Compatibility tests. Once convinced the donor is willing, the physician should begin to determine compatibility. The first compatibility test required

is the AB0 blood type. The pair should be of the same blood type or of types which will allow transfusion (e.g. 0→A, A→AB; not A→B nor A→0). The rhesus factor does not appear to be significant. If there is a difference in the Rh type and the recipient is negative, she could be tested for anti-Rh antibodies. We have no knowledge of this resulting in graft failure, but it might be considered as a possibility.

If several family members are willing and able to give kidneys, the physician can determine the lymphocyte antigen types (HL-A) of all concerned and choose the most favorable combination. The recognition of lymphocyte antigens gives promise of providing the means for significant improvement in the results of organ transplants (Terasaki) [238]. Six lymphocyte antigens are recognized by an international group of investigators. They are termed human leucocyte antigens (HL-A). The A designates the first locus on the chromosome found to be concerned with this system of histocompatibility antigens. All antigens recognized to date are at one locus of one chromosome; transmission follows mendelian principles.

Retrospective analysis of renal transplants from related and unrelated donors indicates these lymphocyte antigens are important in the results of organ grafts. Prospective matching of donor and recipient for cadaver renal transplantation is currently underway in a number of centers in the United States and Europe. Because of the great genetic variability, it is difficult to obtain a good "match" between random donors and even a large number of potential recipients.

2. Age. The renal donor should be over the age of 21 years, or over 18 years and married, to give legal consent in the United States. Identical twins under the age of 21 years have served as renal donors by obtaining a special court order. As not all identical twin renal transplants are successful, one might question the morality of this precedent.

The older donor has a greater surgical risk from nephrectomy. We have usually refused to accept a living donor over the age of 60 years; however, each case should be considered individually and the risks weighed. Renal function may be altered with aging (Orchardson [179]; Muether [161]; Adler [7]).

3. Informed consent. The physician should inform the prospective donor of the risks involved. We tell patients that they risk their lives by serving as renal donors. The risk takes two forms: the risk of a major operation with general anesthesia, and the continuing risk of having a solitary kidney. The mathematical expression of these risks is very difficult to obtain, but it is likely to be less than one in one thousand. The important responsibility of the physician is to inform the donor that these risks do exist, and then to do everything in his power to minimize them.

4. Medical evaluation. The medical evaluation of the donor is often best accomplished by a short hospitalization prior to the planned date of transplantation. Our evaluation consists of:

| | |
|---|---|
| History | $CO_2$ |
| Physical examination | Uric acid |
| Urinalysis | $Ca^+$ |
| Urine culture $^{\times 3}$ | Blood sugar |
| Serum creatinine | Chest X-ray |
| Serum $Na^+$ | Electrocardiogram |
| $K^+$ | Excretory urogram |
| Cl | Renal arteriogram |

The evaluation proceeds in this sequence. Further tests may be dictated by the history or by the results of the initial tests. Donors with major medical illness or any history of renal disease are excluded. Patients with a labile hypertension are difficult to evaluate; we have employed some as donors. The renal arteriogram must be obtained, as at least 25% of prospective donors have multiple renal arteries. To reduce the hazard of vascular complication and infarction, we have not taken a kidney from a living donor with two major arteries. A small accessory or polar vessel may be litigated without compromise in some cases. We have found vascular disease in a number of normotensive prospective renal donors and have excluded them on this basis.

## 2. Cadaveric Donors

1. Legal factors. The availability of kidneys for use in transplantation depends upon social, legal and medical factors. The legal aspects vary in the United States, but there is a trend toward establishing national standards and laws under the guidelines of the Anatomical Gift Act. This law, effective in a number of states, provides the legal basis for organ donation. In order to plan effectively, we find it necessary to obtain consent prior to the death of the donor. An entirely new approach to the legal problems may ultimately be necessary to provide the numbers of organs needed (DUKEMINIER [58]).

2. Medical factors. Medical evaluation of the prospective organ donor is made on the basis of history and condition of the patient. Those with infection or malignancy which could be transmitted must be excluded. We had the misfortune

*Cadaver kidney donors*

| | | |
|---|---|---|
| 1. CNS lesions (32 | | |
| Anencephalic monster | 2 | |
| Neoplasm | 17 | |
| Cerebral edema | 1 | |
| Vascular accidents | 5 | |
| Trauma | 6 | |
| Polio | 1 | |
| 2. Cardiovascular lesions (6) | | |
| Cardiac surgery | 3 | |
| Cardiac arrest | 2 | |
| Myocardial infarction | 1 | |
| 3. Cirrhosis (7) | 7 | |
| 4. Suicide (1) | 1 | |
| 5. Carcinoma of lung (1) | 1 | |
| 6. Unknown (1) | 1 | |
| | 48 | 73 Kidneys |

Fig. 1. Primary diagnosis in cadaveric renal donors of the U.C.L.A. series. 73 kidneys were transplanted from 48 donors

to observe transmission of malignancy in one of our early cases (MARTIN [138]). When the mode of death entails a prolonged interval of shock, there may be ante mortem renal damage. We have transplanted kidneys from cadaveric donors where hypotension and anuria occurred hours before death and have obtained satisfactory function in the graft (SMITH [217]). One must evaluate each case on its individual merits. The most favorable donors are those with intracranial pathology without sepsis. Fig. 1 shows the diagnoses on the first 48 cadaveric donors in our experience.

When consent has been obtained and the donor is found medically acceptable, the physician must determine whether there is a suitable recipient available. The AB0 blood type is the minimum matching which should be done. Donor and recipient should be of the same type or of a combination of types which will allow transfusion. We also determine the lymphocyte antigen type of the donor and select two recipients on the basis of red and white cell type.

Potential cadaveric donors with an indwelling urethral catheter and resultant bacteriuria are rejected by some surgeons. We have frequently employed kidneys from such donors and have not found urinary infections a problem.

A prompt autopsy may allow the use of organs considered of questionable value ante mortem (Ende [59]).

# III. Technique of Donor Nephrectomy

## A. Living Donor

### 1. Preparation

The removal of a kidney from a normal healthy patient is a procedure which many physicians and surgeons approach reluctantly, with the potential benefit to the recipient as the major motivating factor. Every effort is made to insure the safety of the donor and to provide an organ with minimal injury as a result of surgery. It is desirable to complete the evaluation of the donor at least three days prior to the planned nephrectomy as the arteriogram might cause some alteration in renal function. We prefer to make the donor evaluation several weeks prior to the planned nephrectomy.

To maintain a state of normal hydration and renal blood flow, we infuse $1^1/_2$ liters of 5% dextrose in $^1/_2$ normal saline overnight prior to nephrectomy. The efficacy of this regimen was established by Najarian (Najarian [168]).

Before positioning the donor on the operating table we pass a urethral catheter and connect it to gravity drainage. This is to prevent bladder distention as a result of fluids and mannitol given during nephrectomy.

### 2. Surgery

The nephrectomy is best accomplished through the standard renal flank approach. The left kidney is preferred because of the longer renal vein; the shorter right renal vein is more difficult to anastomose in the recipient. The patient should have endotracheal intubation to protect in the event of pneumothorax. The incision must provide access to the origin of the renal artery from the aorta and yet allow removal of a good length of ureter. We prefer an incision with resection of the 12th rib or intercostal above the 11th or 12th rib. The incision should be generous, as the dissection to the aorta requires good exposure and good vision "protects" the donor.

During dissection of the kidney, renal function is supported and maintained by an intravenous infusion of 50—100 g of mannitol. This osmotic diuretic will prepare the kidney for the 20—30 min of ischemia required for vascular anastomosis. If hypotension occurs due to position of the patient in lateral flexion or to anesthesia, we favor treatment by expanding the blood volume with fluids rather than by use of vasopressors, which may reduce renal tolerance to ischemia. When the transplanted kidney is diuresing in the donor at the time of removal, it will function immediately in the recipient, but when the kidney is not functioning in the donor it may not begin to function for many hours in the recipient.

The kidney must be handled with great care at all times. GOODWIN recommends nephrectomy in the donor similar to that for cancer, with removal of all envesting fat and fascia to minimize trauma. The renal hilus should not be dissected, as this might compromise the blood supply of the ureter. The renal artery must be skeletonized adjacent to its origin from the aorta. During this dissection the artery should not be compressed, pulled nor angulated. Surgeons have a tendency to retract the vessel they are dissecting or to place tapes about it. This must be avoided as it reduces renal blood flow and causes vascular spasm. Local anesthetic agents (e.g., lidocaine) may be applied topically to reduce vascular spasm.

The renal vein is similarly skeletonized to the vena cava. There will be several large tributaries (lumbar, spermatic and adrenal) of the left renal vein to be ligated. There are usually no such tributaries on the right.

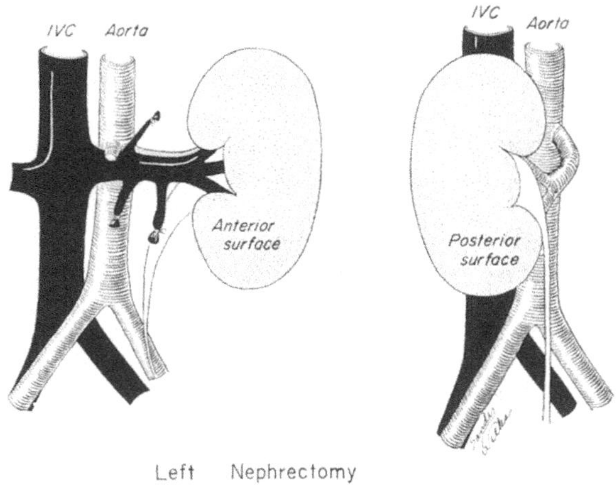


Fig. 2. Surgical anatomy seen in left nephrectomy for transplantation. The adrenal, spermatic (or ovarian) and lumbar tributaries of the left renal vein are ligated to obtain maximum length of the vein. The renal artery is dissected to its origin from the aorta

The ureter is dissected with its sheath to preserve blood supply. We transect the ureter as it passes into the anatomical pelvis to obtain a length of 15—20 cm. Urine should be spurting from the transected ureter if dissection has been gentle and fluid administration adequate. The kidney is not removed until the recipient has been completely prepared (see Chapter IV). We recommend systemic anticoagulation of the donor with 1.0 mg/kg body weight heparin intravenously just prior to nephrectomy. This will be reversed by an equal amount of protamine after the kidney is removed.

For maximum security we ligate the renal artery next to the aorta and then place a clamp on the vessel prior to transection. The artery may be ligated a second time or be oversewn with a vascular suture of 5—0 silk. We prefer to control the renal vein with a vascular clamp, transect and then close the vein with a running vascular suture. This latter suture may be placed after the kidney is removed and on its way to the recipient.

When the right kidney is employed in transplantation, the artery is handled in a similar manner after dissection behind the vena cava. To obtain maximum length of the right renal vein and to provide security for the donor, we control the lateral aspect of the vena cava with a vascular clamp and transect the renal vein at its junction with the vena cava. A scalpel allows a more controlled incision of the vein than does a scissor. The lateral vena cava is closed with one suture of 5—0 arterial silk placed in a simple over-and-over technique.

Hemostasis must be complete. The wound need not be drained. The flank is closed in layers with silk or catgut sutures. Because of the careful dissection required, it is not unusual for donor nephrectomy to entail $2^1/_2$ hours of operating time.

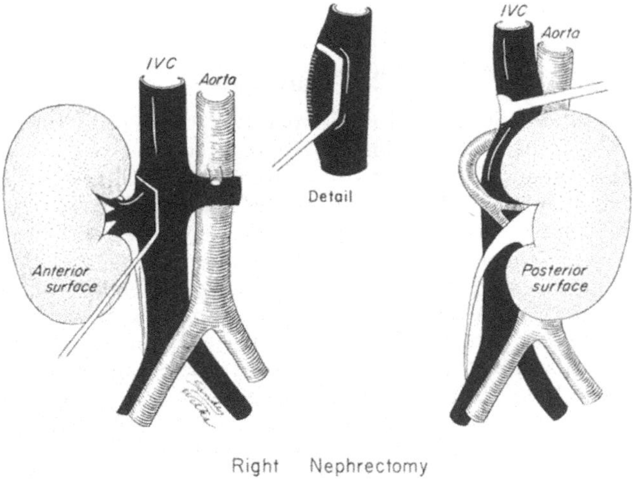


Fig. 3. Surgical anatomy seen in right nephrectomy for transplantation. There are no named tributaries of the right renal vein. The renal vein is transsected at its junction with the inferior vena cava to obtain maximum length. The right renal artery must be dissected from behind the vena cava to obtain optimum length

### 3. After Surgery

The patient should be checked clinically for signs of pneumothorax in the post anesthetic room. If there is any question of this condition existing, a chest X-ray must be obtained. Postoperative treatment of pneumothorax depends upon the extent of the collapsed lung.

The urethral catheter may be removed as soon as the patient is fully awake or on the morning following surgery. Closed drainage will protect against infection.

Following uncomplicated nephrectomy, it is not unusual for the donor to be ready for discharge from the hospital in 5—7 days.

## B. Cadaveric Donor

### 1. General Considerations

The transplantation of organs from cadaveric donors is complicated by the uncertainty of their availability and the time of donor death. The kidney must be preserved within an hour of donor death to ensure its subsequent functional potential. The interval between donor death and preparation of the recipient will vary; in our experience it is usually 1—3 hours. During this time the kidney must be preserved or its circulation maintained. It is possible to maintain circulation through the kidney with a mechanical device on the external surface of the heart (Attai [12]) or with an extracorporeal circuit and a pump oxygenator (Marchioro [132]). The latter carries the disadvantage of progressive renal damage inherent in all forms of extracorporeal circulation using whole blood. The former, only recently available, has the disadvantage of requiring that the chest be opened to apply the device, a major surgical maneuver.

The only proven modality of organ preservation apart from maintenance of circulation is cooling. This is very effective. We adopted the plan of providing cooling as rapidly as possible by removing the kidney in order to cool the organ alone rather than the entire donor.

## 2. Technique

The donor should be taken to the operating room or similar clean area immediately after death. The abdomen is prepared and draped as for surgery. With all sterile precautions, both kidneys are removed through a large transverse upper abdominal incision. Long segments of the renal vessels and ureters are obtained. The kidneys may be removed with segments of the aorta and vena cava, or the renal vessels may be divided adjacent to the great vessels. We divide the left renal vein adjacent to the vena cava between clamps to expose the aorta and origin of the renal arteries. The vein is clamped to minimize soiling of tissues with blood, which obscures the surgical anatomy. The surgeon must be alert to the possibility of multiple renal arteries as previous studies on such donors have not been made. Two renal arteries may be taken together with a segment of aorta or separately with a cuff of aorta to facilitate the subsequent vascular anastomosis. To provide maximum length, the right renal vein is always taken with a segment of vena cava; this segment can be trimmed later. A long segment of ureter should be taken with adjacent fascia and vessels.

Some surgeons prefer to remove both kidneys together with a segment of aorta and vena cava (Ackerman [4]). This has the advantage of preserving accessory arteries which might otherwise be transected near the kidney.

Once removed, the kidneys are preserved by cooling. This may be accomplished by immersion in a sterile ice bath or by intra-arterial infusion of a cold balanced salt solution. We have employed 500 ml lactated Ringer's solution at 4° C with added heparin (50 mg) and lidocaine (50 mg). This cold solution is infused into the renal artery by gravity with the solution 150 cm above the kidney. The plastic tubing used for routine intravenous fluid administration is sterilized with Ethylene oxide gas to be handled by the surgeon. The plastic tip of the tubing is suitable size for cannulation of the renal artery in most instances. Other tapered cannulae or even coronary artery perfusion cannulae have been employed. With this technique, the core temperature of the kidney is rapidly reduced. However, recent experiments in our laboratories suggest there is no advantage of perfusion cooling over surface cooling and, in fact, there is a greater likelihood of cortical infarcts from perfusion.

When the kidney has been cooled it may be cleaned of fat and extraneous tissue at leisure, and the accessory vessels may be ligated where appropriate. The kidney must be kept cold and sterile until the recipient is prepared. The optimum temperature for preservation has not been established. We have kept kidneys in a bath of Ringer's solution at 3.5—5° C with good results. Recent work in our laboratory indicates the canine kidney will tolerate eight hours of ischemia at 5° C and return to virtually normal function when re-implanted into the same animal. In clinical practice we implant the kidney as soon as possible; however, it would appear from laboratory results that there is ample time to complete laboratory tests such as lymphocyte antigen matching. Donor blood or a lymph node may be used to provide the cells for this test.

We have transplanted a kidney after 320 min of cold ischemia and observed good function after an interval of acute tubular necrosis. The principal injury to the kidney seems to occur prior to kidney cooling in most cases. To be useful in transplantation, the kidney should be cooled or otherwise preserved within an hour of death (where death is cessation of the circulation).

### 3. Evaluation of Cadaver Kidney

The precise moment of death or the effect of agonal death may be in doubt. To help clarify these uncertainties, we have employed a simple, subjective, metabolic test with a small piece of renal cortical tissue in a tetrazolium dye. The enzymatic activity of the renal tubular cells will cause adherence of the dye to renal cells and a color change in a time interval related to the metabolic activity. Preliminary work in the laboratory and with clinical cases suggests this procedure may be of value. The subjective nature of the end point obtained is the major drawback, since the physician must gain experience in the laboratory before he finds this test useful clinically (SMITH [218, 219]; TERASAKI [236]).

### 4. Utilization of both Kidneys

For maximum utilization of available organs, we have arranged to have two recipients ready for each cadaver kidney donor. All potential kidney recipients are typed by white and red cell antigens and their records kept in a central registry. The two recipients are selected on the basis of the best "match" by these tests. One or both kidneys are transported to the recipient(s) in sterile containers. We have found a 5-liter vacuum container convenient to handle and adequate to hold the kidney and cold solution sufficient to maintain the organ at 5—10° C.

The selection of organ and recipient by matching histocompatibility antigens promises improved results from cadaveric organ transplantation (PATEL [183]).

# IV. Technique of Recipient Implantation

## A. Adults

The surgical techniques employed in renal transplantation have become standardized in most centers. Placement of the graft in the iliac fossa using the iliac vessels is ideal for adults and adolescents. To minimize the time the kidney will be without circulation, the procedure should be systematized and carefully planned, with the surgical team working together as a unit. This requires practice and experience which is best achieved in the animal laboratory. We performed 100 canine renal transplants before our first clinical case and were rewarded by completing the arterial and venous anastomoses in 17 min.

### 1. Approach

The left kidney of the donor is placed in the contralateral iliac fossa to reverse the relation of artery and vein. The renal vein is anterior in the lumbar region while the iliac vein is posterior in the pelvis.

The iliac fossa is readily approached with an oblique lower abdominal incision just lateral to the rectus muscle. Extraperitoneal exposure is advantageous;

should urinary leak or wound infection occur it will be confined by the peritoneum. The incision is not placed too far lateral, as the origin of the internal iliac artery must be exposed near the midline. We routinely divide the inferior epigastric artery and vein for better exposure. The spermatic vessels can be mobilized and retracted medial by incising their lateral fascial bands. We divided the internal spermatic artery and vein in many of our early cases; three hydroceles resulted, but no other complication was observed. Ureteral obstruction from the spermatic

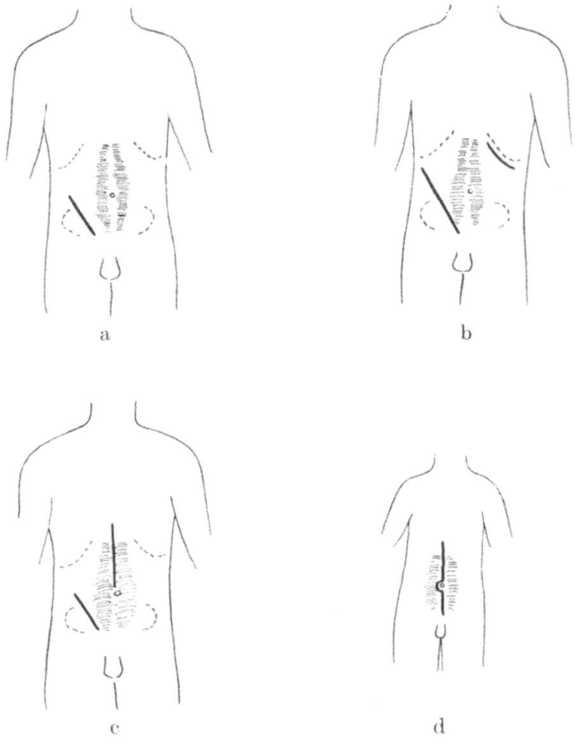

Fig. 4a—d. Surgical incisions employed for renal implantation and recipient nephrectomy. a Lower quadrant, extraperitoneal approach for renal implantation in adults. b Two incisions to allow extraperitoneal implantation and bilateral nephrectomy. c Two incisions to allow extraperitoneal implantation and transperitoneal bilateral nephrectomy. d Transperitoneal incision used for implantation and bilateral nephrectomy in small children

vessels has been reported, and this must be avoided. It is not difficult to pass the graft ureter posterior to the spermatic vessels. In the female the round ligament is divided to improve exposure.

The retroperitoneum is opened from the psoas muscle in the lumbar fossa superior to the lateral aspect of the bladder inferior. The peritoneum is reflected medial to expose the origin of the internal iliac artery.

## 2. Dissection

Dissection of the external iliac vein involves division and ligation of numerous lymphatic channels to reduce the accumulation of lymph postoperative. The external iliac vein is skeletonized from the inguinal ligament to its junction with the internal iliac vein. Occasionally a lateral or posterior tributary vein requires ligation and division in this procedure. The adequacy of venous exposure is tested by a trial application of the vascular clamp. We currently employ a rubber shod Satinsky for occlusion of the vein. Previously we used two rubber shod bull-dog clamps. The venous clamp should be nontraumatic to minimize the risk of venous thrombosis. We have seen four cases of marked venous thrombosis in 170 renal transplants. It should not be a frequent problem.

The internal iliac artery is skeletonized from its origin to major divisions. This vessel is quite variable. One or more large posterior divisions are ligated with silk, and the vessel is controlled proximal with a rubber shod bull-dog clamp or a Rummel tourniquet (umbilical tape with rubber sleeve). The internal

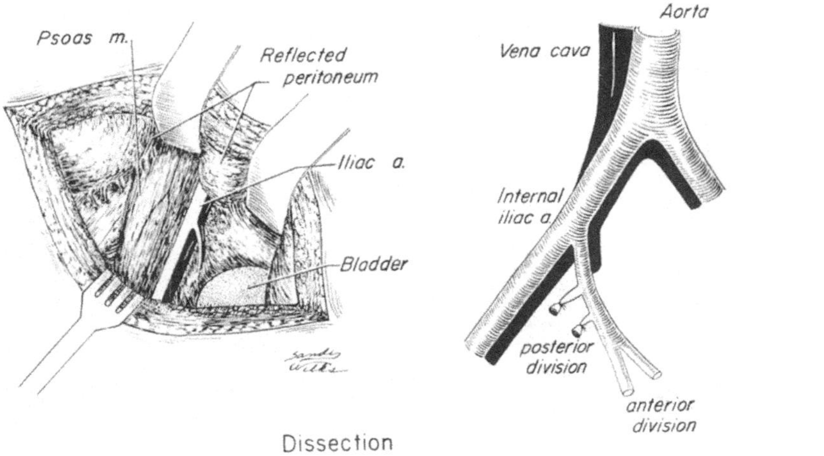


Fig. 5. Surgical anatomy in preparation of the recipient for transplantation to the iliac fossa

iliac artery is transected in a manner that will provide maximum length. We ligate the divisions of the artery and transect at the last major bifurcation. This may provide a slightly larger lumen for anastomosis if needed.

The internal iliac artery is subject to atheromatous plaques. This condition may be suspect and evaluated by palpation prior to dissection. In most patients an endarterectomy can be performed via the end of the transected vessel. If this is not feasible, the arterial anastomosis can be made to the common or the external iliac artery with an end-to-side technique. End-to-end anastomosis of the renal to the internal iliac artery is preferred ,however, as it is easier and therefore quicker and surer. In order to minimize any thrombus formation in relation to the vascular clamp, we do not occlude the artery until the graft is completely prepared in the donor. After the vessel is transected the lumen is washed with a dilute solution of heparin in saline. Endarterectomy is performed as required. After endarterectomy the vessel is flushed by release of the vascular clamp to clear fragments and demonstrate flow. This completes preparation of the artery.

## 3. Venous Anastomosis

The vein is occluded with a rubber shod clamp, and a longitudinal venotomy is made to correspond with the breadth of the renal vein. We frequently remove a narrow ellipse of tissue. The presence of venous valves is readily detected on inspection of the exterior of the vein, and the venotomy is made in an area free of valves whenever possible. Should there be valves present within the venotomy, their leaflets are carefully excised to obviate venous obstruction during suture anastomosis. The vein is washed with the dilute heparin solution and three sutures of 5—0 arterial silk are placed in the superior and inferior extremities of the venotomy and in the middle of the venotomy on the wall of the vein opposite the surgeon. These sutures are passed from outside in the iliac vein and will be passed through the renal vein to complete the anastomosis. We do not clamp the ends of the sutures but spread them on the side of the wound.

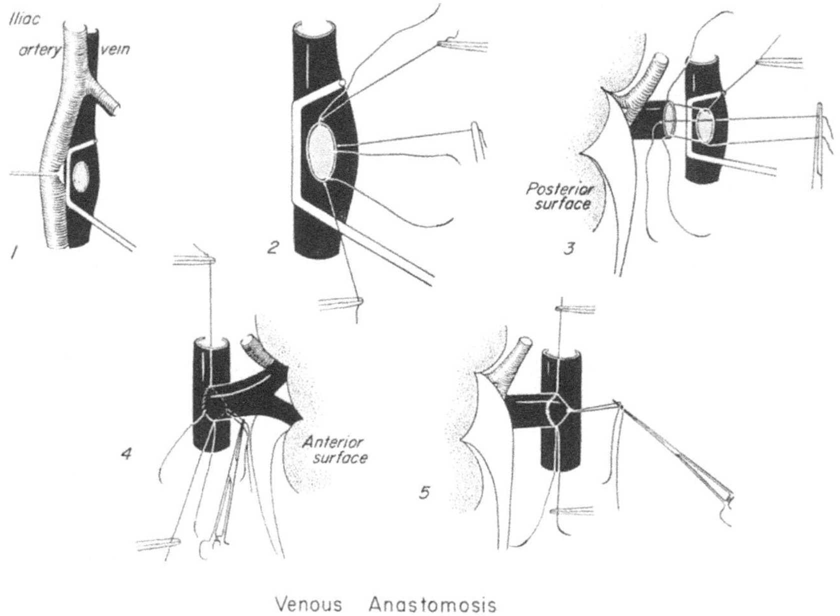


Fig. 6. Technique for venous anastomosis to the external iliac vein

The kidney from the donor is brought to the side of the wound and oriented with the renal pelvis anterior and renal vein posterior. The ureter is directed toward the bladder. It is important that the kidney be postured on the side of the patient adjacent to the surgeon in the technique to be described.

The renal vein is identified and held with two forceps by the assistant. The superior and inferior sutures are passed through the renal vein inside-out to place the knot external. As these sutures are 180° apart, it is simple to orient one from the other. The third suture — which is through the medial aspect of the iliac vein — is now passed through the anterior surface (nearest the surgeon) of the renal vein. The kidney is placed in the iliac fossa as the three sutures are held taut. These sutures are tied, and the non-needle ends are secured on holding clamps. The medial suture is pulled sufficiently to triangulate the venotomy. If this does not open the vein well, a fourth suture may be placed lateral to quadrangulate the vein; however, we rarely find this necessary. The kidney is supported to hold the renal vein on a sufficient tension to expose the interior surfaces of the veins to be anastomosed. The surgeon approximates the venous walls adjacent to him passing from renal to iliac vein with a simple over-and-over suture. To guard against inadvertent closure of the vein, the venous walls must be well triangulated. We find it helpful to grasp the medial traction suture with a clamp near the vein wall, since this traction deep in the wound is more effective than an external pull. The suture may be tied at the 180° point of anastomosis or continued about the entire 360°, with the latter being slightly faster. No ties are made to traction sutures, which are simply oversewn. We prefer to suture 180° and then pass the needle to an assistant on the other side as he has a better view (another advantage of having a trained team!). The venous anastomosis is completed and the suture tied. All ends are removed.

The venous anastomosis is logically performed first as it is deeper in the wound and in that sense posterior, while the arterial anastomosis is more superficial.

## 4. Arterial Anastomosis

The internal iliac and renal arteries are approximated with two sutures of 5—0 arterial silk 180° apart. These are placed first, then tied. The anastomosis

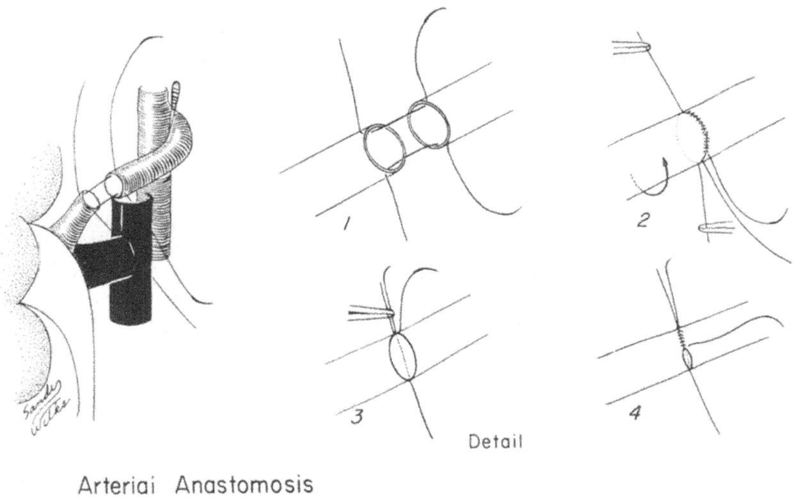


Fig. 7. Technique for arterial anastomosis to the internal iliac artery

is again a simple continuous suture. The first suture is positioned as close to the knot as possible. When 180° has been sutured, a tie is made to the non-needle end and the vessel rotated through 180° so the surgeon can continue toward himself. If one margin of the vessel tends to overlap the other and so obscure the lumen, an assistant can pull the vessel wall posterior with a vascular forceps and improve exposure. In the rotation of the vessel there will be three ends of suture at one end of the anastomosis and one at the other. Taking the three anterior will allow the single strand to be passed more readily posterior. When the arterial anastomosis is completed and tied, the suture ends are removed. The arterial and venous clamps should be removed simultaneously. This is best done by one person.

## 5. Hemostasis

Sponges packed next to the anastomosis will promote closure of any bleeding points. Persistent arterial suture line bleeding can be controlled by careful sutures, taking only the adventitia of the vessel. The vascular clamp should never be reapplied as this is conducive to thrombosis in the graft. Hemostatic sutures in the artery should be placed with the blood flowing, as this identifies the point of bleeding, and the full lumen protects against suture of the opposite wall.

The kidney should immediately assume normal color and turgor upon release of the vascular clamps. If this does not occur, one must suspect a faulty anastomosis, poor cardiac output, hypotension or even compression of the iliac artery with a retractor. When the kidney is well perfused and hemostasis is achieved, the graft is allowed to rest in the iliac fossa.

## 6. Ureteral Anastomosis

The ureteral anastomosis to the recipient bladder is commenced by cleaning the lateral surface of the bladder of any fascial bands which might interfere with the course of the ureter. The anterior bladder surface is exposed and a

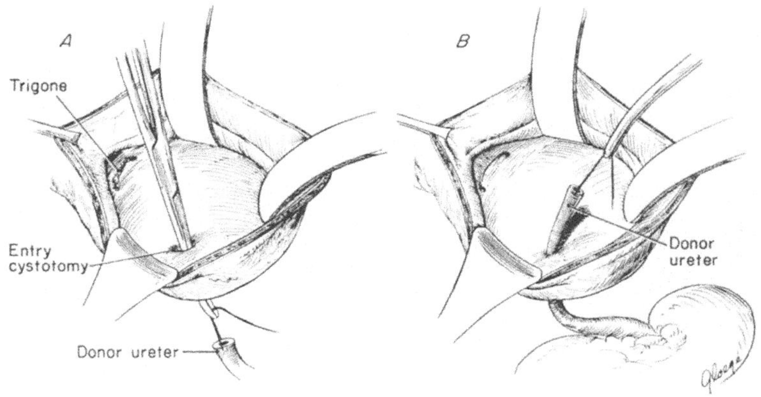


Fig. 8. Author's technique for ureterovesical anastomosis in renal transplantation

small cystotomy made. We always obtain a specimen of urine for bacteriological studies. The ureter is to be implanted on the floor of the bladder near the trigone and anatomical ureteral orifices, in order to obtain good support for an antireflux valve and to place the opening in a position which will allow endoscopic catheterization should it be indicated in the future. A separate entry cystotomy is made for the ureter at the junction of the lateral wall and bladder floor by incising the mucosa and pushing a clamp through the muscularis. This opening in the muscularis must be made large enough to accommodate the ureter with ease. The ureter is drawn into the bladder, and its extravesical course is then inspected for obstructing or angulating bands and for torsion of the ureter. These must be corrected. Obstruction of the ureter by the spermatic cord has been reported (MURRAY [162]), and this should be avoided by maintaining the ureter in a posterior position. A submucosal tunnel is developed in a medial and inferior direction for 2—2$^1/_2$ cm, which should place the end of the ureter near the trigone. We discard excess ureter, spatulate the terminal 1—1$^1/_2$ cm, and make a mucosa-to-mucosa anastomosis with 4—0 plain catgut. The sutures through the distal portion of the ureter must be secured to muscle of the bladder wall to prevent the ureter from withdrawing from the bladder. This is extremely important, as withdrawal of the ureter causes a ureterocutaneous fistula and such fistulas are associated with great morbidity and mortality (see Chapter VI). The ureteral entry cystotomy is closed at the mucosal level only with 4—0 plain catgut. We do not employ a ureteral catheter as we feel this may embarrass circulation in the transplanted ureter and add to the risks of infection. The anterior cysto-

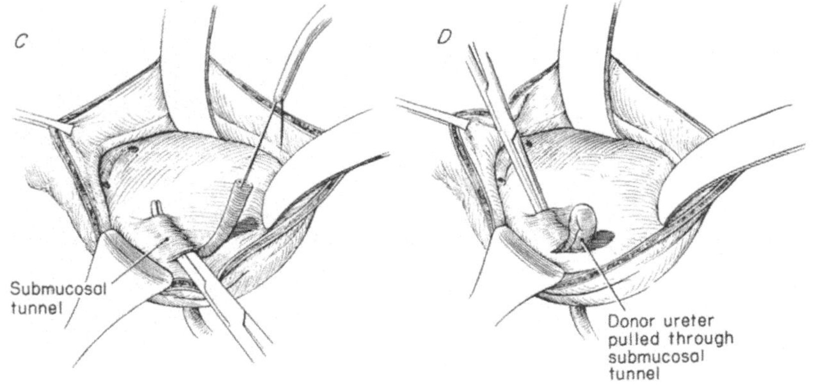


Fig. 9. Author's technique for ureterovesical anastomosis in renal transplantation

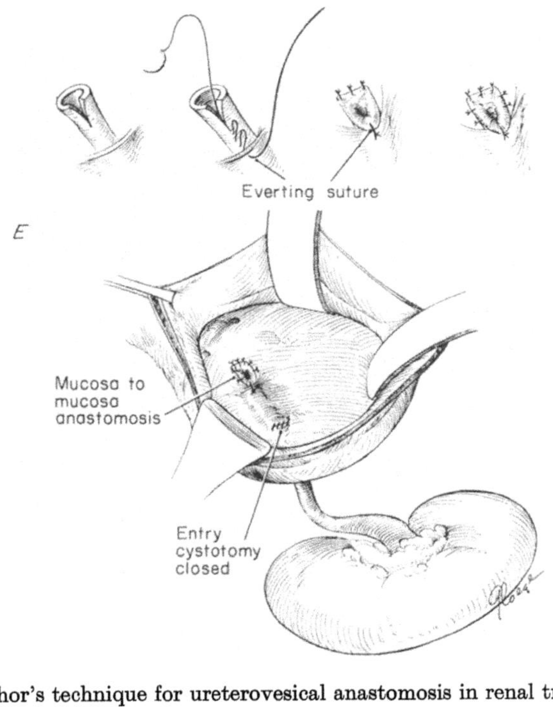


Fig. 10. Author's technique for ureterovesical anastomosis in renal transplantation

tomy is closed in three layers with great care. We use all running suture lines, 4—0 plain catgut in the mucosa and 3—0 chromic catgut in the muscularis and adventitia. A urethral catheter is placed in anticipation of profuse diuresis, for measurement of urine volumes and for patient comfort. Once the uretero-vesical anastomosis is complete, it is wise not to exert any traction on the ureter which might dislodge it from the bladder. The wound is carefully inspected for bleeding points, and these are controlled by ligation. We drain the ureterovesical area with a plastic tube to a closed vacuum container (Hemovac). This system

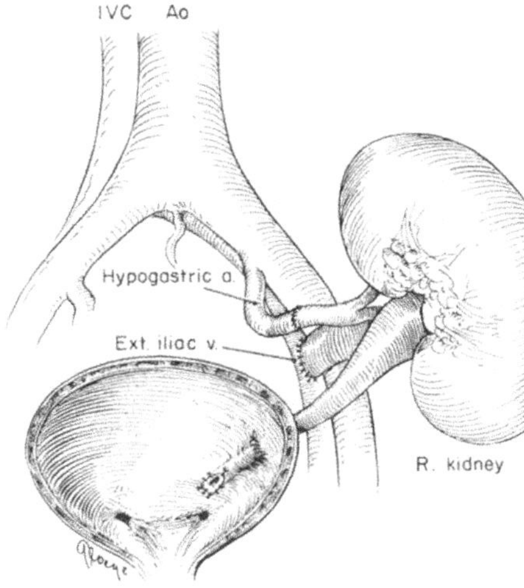


Fig. 11. Author's technique for transplantation of donor right kidney to the left iliac fossa with ureterovesical anastomosis

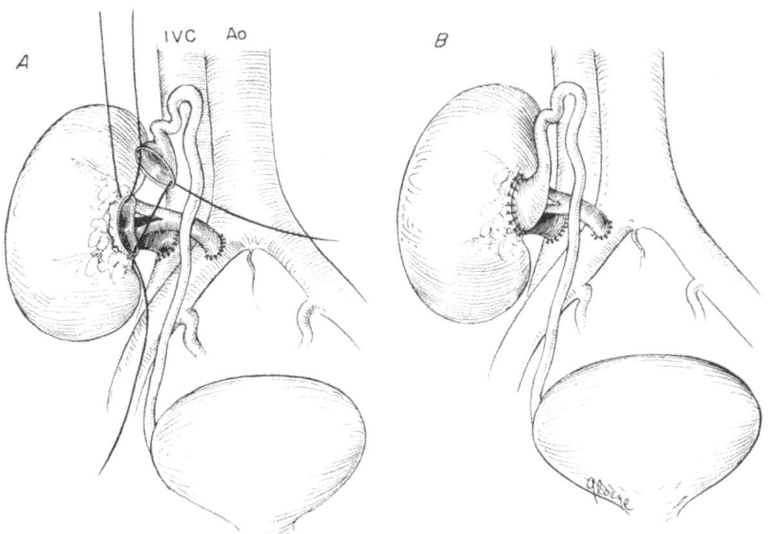


Fig. 12. Technique for renal transplantation described by Dr. GIL VERNET, Barcelona, with pyelopelvic anastomosis. The vascular anastomoses are similar to those used for transplantation in infants and small children

will often remove several hundred ml over the first 48 hours. Much of this drainage is lymph. The incision may be closed in layers with 2—0 silk or 0-Chromic catgut.

Implantation of the donor ureter into the recipient bladder has been the most predictable procedure for urine drainage in our experience. Several other techniques are available and are the procedures of choice for certain surgeons. These include ureteroureterostomy (STARZL [220]) and pyeloureterostomy (LEADBETTER [125]), employing the recipient ureter. Dr. GIL VERNET of Barcelona has described pyelopyelostomy with placement of the graft in the low lumbar fossa (GIL VERNET [67]). We prefer to reserve these techniques for organs in which the donor ureter is short or for reconstruction in repair of a fistula.

Ureteroureterostomy is usually made by spatulation of both ends of the ureters to be joined and a careful approximation. Fine catgut sutures of 5—0 chromic are placed through the full thickness and are spaced very close to one another. STARZL has made direct end to end ureteral anastomosis with vascular silk sutures passed through all layers except the mucosa. This technique calls for careful placement of each suture to avoid stenosis.

Pyeloureterostomy is made by careful suture of the spatulated recipient ureter to an appropriate opening in the graft renal pelvis. This technique is familiar to many urological surgeons as it is similar to the operation for the correction of ureteropelvic obstruction. Fine catgut sutures are placed through the full thickness of ureter and pelvis. Nephrostomy tubes and stenting catheters are not advised in transplant recipients.

Anastomosis of the graft ureter to an isolated ileac conduit has been performed in a number of patients with limited success (KELLY [105]; KISER [111]). We would strongly recommend preliminary preparation of the ileac conduit to minimize the risk of infection at the time of transplantation. This procedure can give a favorable long term result but several patients have developed hemorrhage at the graft site likely due to infected vascular anastomoses (KELLY [105]). This sequence of events occurred in our one experience with transplantation to an isolated ileac conduit (MARTIN [136]).

The renal vein may be anastomosed end-to-end with the common or external iliac vein if necessary. We have used this technique several times to improve exposure in a deep anatomical pelvis. Most patients suffer no untoward effects, but one or two have been troubled by persistent edema in the corresponding lower extremity.

## B. Infants

For transplantation of the kidney in infants or small children, an alternative approach and technique is required to obtain adequate vessel size for anastomosis and to accommodate the graft. These patients are approached transperitoneal via a longitudinal incision. The distal aorta and vena cava are skeletonized with reflection of the right colon medial. The renal vein is anastomosed end-to-side with the vena cava, using the suture techniques previously described. The renal artery is anastomosed to the side of the aorta or common iliac artery. The ureter of the graft may be implanted in the bladder or managed in one of the alternate ways previously described. If the donor ureter does not reach the bladder readily, we favor the pyelopyelostomy of GIL VERNET. The kidney lies in the low lumbar fossa.

## C. Nephrectomy in the Recipient

### 1. Indications

Infected kidneys should be removed prior to transplantation, but old pyelonephritic organs can be removed at the time of transplantation. If the recipient has not had his diseased kidney(s) removed prior to transplantation, there are several advantages to removing them at this time. With the old kidneys removed, the clinician is never in doubt about the origin of urine volume, urine protein, enzymes or cellular elements. The origin of hypertension is likewise not in question.

### 2. Techniques

We have found it convenient to remove the diseased kidneys at the time of transplantation. This is most frequently done through a separate midline incision in the epigastrium by a transperitoneal approach, although many alternatives are available. It is possible to remove the ipsilateral kidney through a superior extension of the transplant incision and the contralateral by a short subcostal incision. In this way all the dissection is retroperitoneal.

We have been able to prepare the graft site before the donor kidney is ready in many cases. In these, we remove one or both kidneys while the donor organ is being prepared. There is thus no loss of time, and the recipient has but one operation to complete two jobs.

# V. Postoperative Care

## A. Following Immediate Function of the Graft

### 1. Nursing

In the early experience, transplant patients were placed in separate rooms, and sterile technique was employed to guard against cross infection, a procedure which had been used after total body irradiation to suppress the immunological response. The procedure does not protect the patient from his own bacterial flora, however, and it soon became evident that special isolation procedures were neither effective nor necessary. Recipients may be nursed in an intensive care unit with other clean surgical patients or with special duty nurses for 2—3 days and then placed on ward care.

### 2. Fluid Balance

The graft from a living donor should function immediately at surgery. The urea, creatinine and other solutes result in an osmotic diuresis ranging from 100 to 2,000 ml/hour. Accurate measurement of hourly urine volume is the principal guide to fluid replacement, and the urine may also be analyzed for sodium and potassium concentration as a guide to replacement. In osmotic diuresis the sodium concentration is high, 80—100 milliequivalents/liter, while the potassium concentration is more variable, ranging from 5—35 milliequivalents/liter. When the patient is in a normal state of hydration, intravenous fluids are given each hour to replace urinary volume. If the patient shows evidence of overhydration with edema and hypertension, this condition may be reduced by regulating intravenous fluids to replace 75% of the urine output.

The hypertension of chronic renal failure is often the result of an expanded blood volume. This responds to fluid loss through the transplanted kidney. Intravenous fluid therapy is reduced to maintenance when the blood urea and serum creatinine are normal. The administration of excess fluid may perpetuate the diuresis, a condition which is recognized when blood urea is normal but urine volumes remain high. Persistent diuresis may also be caused by osmotic agents other than urea, such as glucose. For most patients, we have found it convenient to replace urinary volumes with 5% dextrose in $^1/_2$ normal saline to which 22 milliequivalents of sodium bicarbonate has been added. This solution closely approximates the sodium loss in the urine. Potassium is not added for several hours in most cases; it will usually be added to the intravenous fluid when there is evidence of a falling serum potassium. The urinary concentration of potassium will be a guide to intravenous replacement. We tend to replace less then the measured urinary loss, to guard against hyperkalemia.

The serum and urinary electrolytes may be determined at 4—8 hour intervals in the first 24 hours after surgery to ensure that replacement is adequate and accurate.

## 3. Immunosuppressive Agents

The standard method of suppressing host immunological responses and graft rejection is to employ the antimetabolite azathioprine (Imuran, Burroughs-Wellcome) in combination with a potent corticosteroid, prednisone (CALNE [39]; MURRAY [162]). A loading dose of azathioprine (4 mg/kg body weight) may be given for 1—2 days starting on the day of surgery. This is usually reduced to 2 mg/kg body weight for maintenance therapy. The white blood count is determined daily to detect evidence of drug toxicity. Leucopenia is a toxic effect rather than a desired sequel of azathioprine action. Prednisone has a marked lympholytic and immunosuppressive action. It is given in a large dose (100 mg/24 hours) initially. This can be gradually reduced to 40 mg/day two weeks postoperative for an adult patient.

A number of adjuvant agents and techniques are employed to increase immunosuppression:

1. Local irradiation. Location irradiation of the graft with 150 rads on alternate days commencing on the day of surgery has long been advocated by HUME (HUME [89]; KAUFFMAN [102]; WOLF [265]). We found evidence of an immunosuppressive effect on canine renal grafts by this technique (MARTIN [139]). Local radiation is used in many centers at the time of clinical graft rejection crisis in the dose schedule recommended by HUME (150 rads alternate days for 3—4 doses).

2. Thoracic duct fistula. Drainage of thoracic duct lymph has been demonstrated to have an immunosuppressive effect in laboratory animals (SINGH [214]; SAMUELSON [208]; MCGREGOR [142]; MAYER [141]) and man (TUNNER [245]). This method has been used clinically by FRANKSSON, MURRAY and others with somewhat inconclusive results (FRANKSSON [66]; TILNEY [242], 1967; FISH [64]).

3. Irradiation of the blood. Irradiation of peripheral blood by means of an extracorporeal circuit has been suggested as an immunosuppressive adjuvant. There is little laboratory and clinical evidence to support this procedure, which has been used in Richmond and other centers (WOLF, 1965 [263]; WOLFE, 1966 [264]). We had no favorable experience in three patients treated (WINKLESTEIN [262]).

4. Antilymphocyte globulin. Heterologous antilymphoid globulin has demonstrated immunosuppressive action in rodent skin grafts (LEVEY [127]; RUSSELL, 1967 [207]) and canine renal grafts (LAWSON [124]; ABBOTT [1]; SHANFIELD [212]; HUNTLEY [96]; STARZL, 1967 [224, 226]). It is the most promising new agent for use in clinical transplantation. The methods of production, refinement and dosage remain to be elaborated (MONACO [156]): at the present time numerous investigators are using a variety of materials, which may cloud the data and render conclusions difficult to reach.

The only established test of immunosuppressive activity is a biological one with primate skin grafts (BALNER [22]). Cytotoxicity titers rise very high in the immunized animal, but this cannot be equated with immunosuppressive activity. Until these factors are standardized, this agent cannot be evaluated well (BACH [18]; GREAVES [75]). STARZL used it clinically in 20 patients and reported good results (STARZL, 1967 [226]). However, subsequent attempts to produce a refined gamma globulin resulted in loss of immunosuppressive activity. Work continues in a number of laboratories (STARZL, 1969 [221]; TRAEGER [243]; NAJARIAN [169]; KASHIWAGI [101]). The material is not yet commercially available.

### 4. Antibiotics

Patients with chronic renal failure placed on immunosuppressive drugs are susceptible to infection by yeast and other opportunistic organisms. The addition of a broad spectrum antibiotic to these patients increases the likelihood of such an infection. We do not, therefore, employ antibacterial agents routinely after renal transplantation, but only for specific, defined, clinically significant infections.

In the presence of a severe or significant infection with good renal function, the physician need not hesitate to use potent agents. Colistin, Kanamycin and other potentially nephrotoxic agents can be given in doses appropriate for patient size and the status of renal function.

## B. Following Delayed Function from the Graft

When transplantation involves a prolonged interval of renal ischemia, as may occur with cadaveric donors, the physician must anticipate delayed function from the graft. Typical histologic changes of acute tubular necrosis are seen in these organs; the recovery interval is governed to some extent by the duration of ischemia. In 50 cases of the U.C.L.A. series the mean interval of anuria or

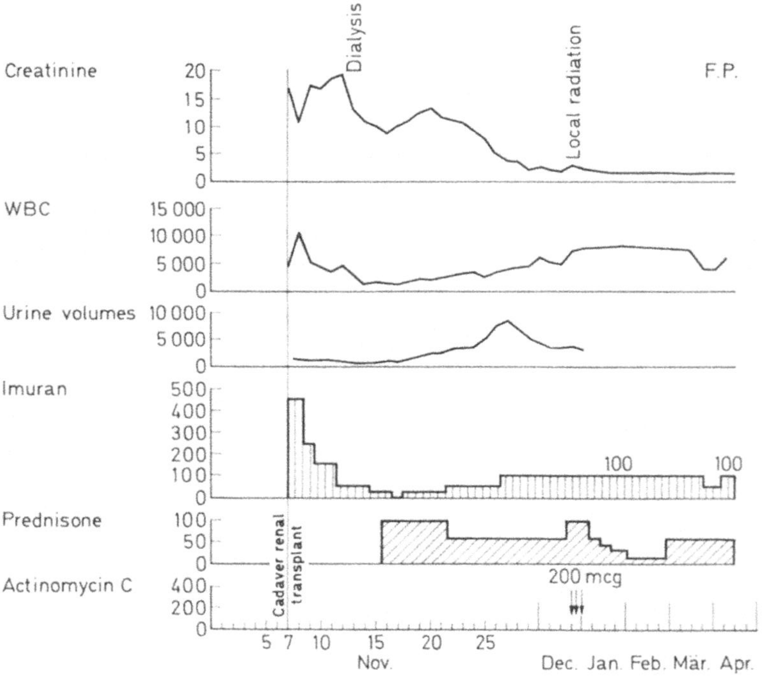


Fig. 13. Clinical course of a patient who received a cadaveric kidney Nov. 7, 1964. This patient continues to take azathioprine 100 mg and prednisone 20 mg per day. Renal function remains stable with a serum creatinine of 1.3 mg-% and endogenous creatinine clearance of 56 ml/min

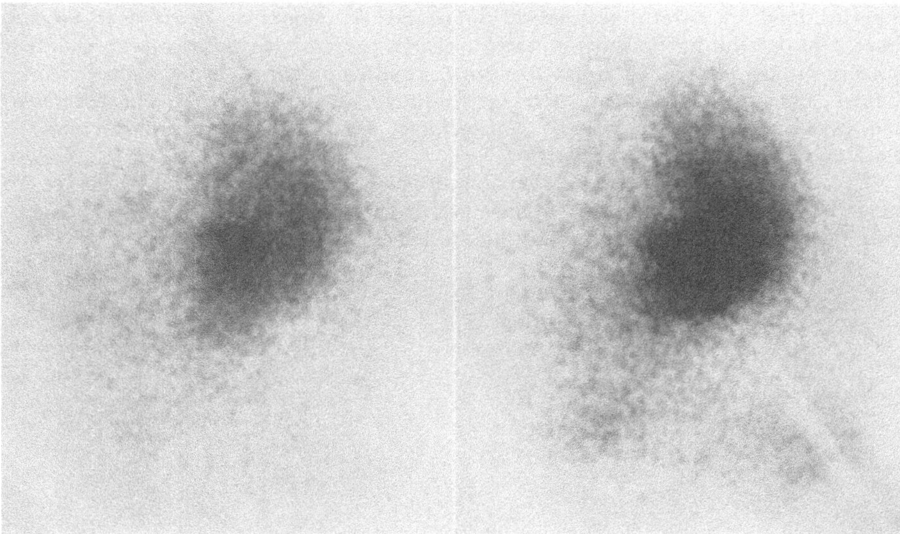

a b

Fig. 14 a and b. Radiohippuran renal scan with the gamma (anger) camera 2 days following renal transplantation from a cadaveric donor (a, b). The scan shows vascularization and tubular function in the absence of urine volumes

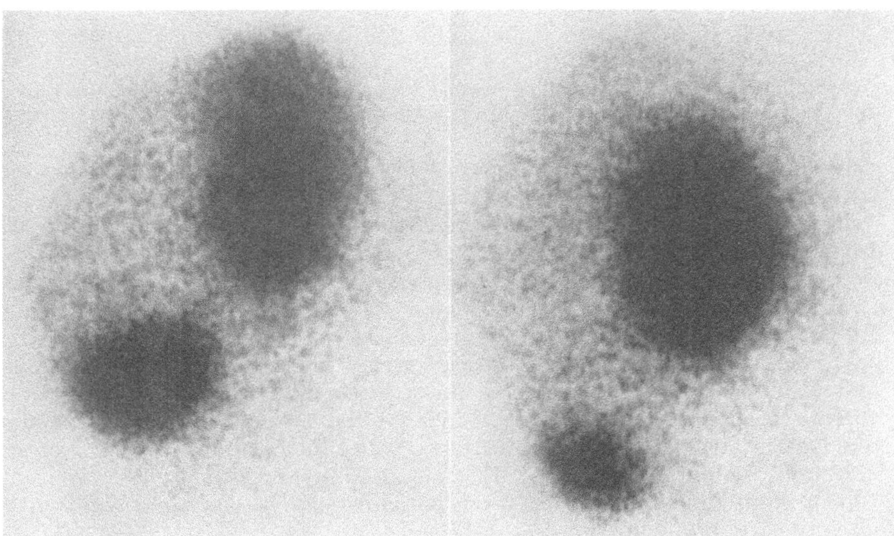

a b

Fig. 15 a and b. Repeat scan 10 days following transplantation reveals excretion into the bladder

oliguria was 11 days. The interval of oliguria is critical for the patient. Hyperkalemia may be marked as a result of blood transfusion and surgery and is controlled with ion exchange resins given as enemata in sorbitol. Fluid balance is maintained by careful restriction of intake. Azathioprine is given in reduced dose (1.0—1.5 mg/kg body weight) to oliguric patients, as tolerance to this drug appears to be related to renal function; prednisone may be used in standard dosage. The patient is supported by frequent hemodialysis. In the first week postoperative there is a risk of hemorrhage, so regional heparinization of the machine is used.

The anuric cadaveric renal transplant is always of uncertain viability. The status of the graft in the anuric phase can be determined by biopsy but we have found isotopic studies to give valuable information.

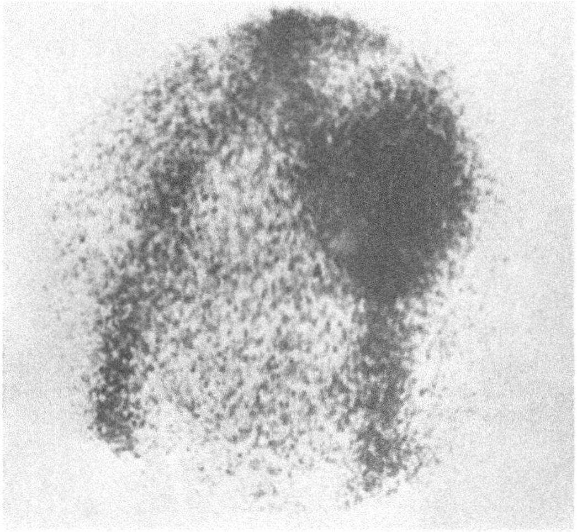


Fig. 16. Radioisotope scan of the transplanted kidney with technicium$^{99}$ and the gamma camera (anger camera). The bifurcation of the aorta, iliac vessels and nephrogram are shown

50—100 microcuries of radiohippuran $I^{131}$ given intravenously will produce a satisfactory scan with the gamma camera (e.g. Anger camera). The isotope is concentrated in the kidney in the absence of measurable urine volumes. The scan can be used to differentiate between an obstructive uropathy and tubular necrosis. Resolution of acute tubular necrosis in a cadaveric renal transplant can be followed with this isotopic method.

10 microcuries of technetium ($Te^{99}$) given intravenously will provide an arteriogram and nephrogram with the gamma camera. This study verifies the viability of an anuric kidney. Cortical necrosis can be distinguished from tubular necrosis by these isotopic methods. We have found it advantageous to obtain double isotopic studies 24—48 hours postoperative on all recipients of cadaveric organs to determine viability (Awad [14]; Figueroa [63]).

When renal function returns, these patients may be managed similarly to those with early graft function.

## C. Subsequent Hospital Care

### 1. Nursing

Two or three days following surgery the patient will usually be on oral feeding and ambulating well. Regular ward care is adequate in most cases. Many patients enjoy a marked increase in the feeling of well-being after successful transplantation, with the "veil" of chronic uremia often being lifted in hours. This is the most gratifying experience for the surgeon.

## 2. Urethral Catheter

The urethral catheter is placed at surgery in those patients with immediate function to allow accurate measurement of fluid balance. The catheter should be removed as soon as diuresis subsides to reduce the risk of infection (see Chapter VIII).

## 3. Wound Drains

We prefer the closed system of wound drainage to reduce the hazard of infection. Several hundred milliliters of lymph, serum and blood frequently drain the first day or two after surgery. The drain tube is removed as soon as drainage ceases, usually in 3—4 days.

## 4. Renal Function — Graft Rejection

Of principal concern in all homografts is the development of the host vs. graft immunological reaction. This process may be manifest by systemic as well as local signs.

1. Systemic signs of graft reaction (rejection). The systemic signs are those of an acute inflammatory process:

(1) fever,
(2) malaise,
(3) anorexia,
(4) leucocytosis.

One or all of these may be masked by large doses of corticosteroids.

2. Local signs of graft reaction (rejection). The local signs, due to inflammation and swelling of the graft, are:

(1) pain,
(2) tenderness,
(3) swelling.

It is of interest that the recipient experiences pain at the site of the denervated kidney. This pain is due to swelling and inflammation in surrounding tissues.

3. Altered renal function. A great many signs tests have been employed to detect the homograft reaction in the transplanted kidney, including:

(1) oliguria,
(2) lymphocyturia (Kauffman, 1964 [103]),
(3) reduced urinary sodium (Ogden [177]),
(4) increased urinary LDH,
(5) increased urinary B-glucuronidase (Ballantyne [21]; Shapiro [209]),
(6) increased urinary histamine (Moore, 1968 [157]),
(7) reduced blood clearance of hippuran (Awad [13]; Blaufox, 1967 [29]; Kountz, 1965 [118]),
(8) increased urinary fibrinogen fragments (Braun [31]).

The hallmark of a graft rejection crisis is reduced renal function. To detect this reaction early and institute appropriate treatment, one must monitor renal function frequently. We determine serum creatinine and endogenous creatinine clearance daily. Since the initial attack appears to be on blood vessels, the effective renal blood flow is reduced early in graft rejection. We have used the blood

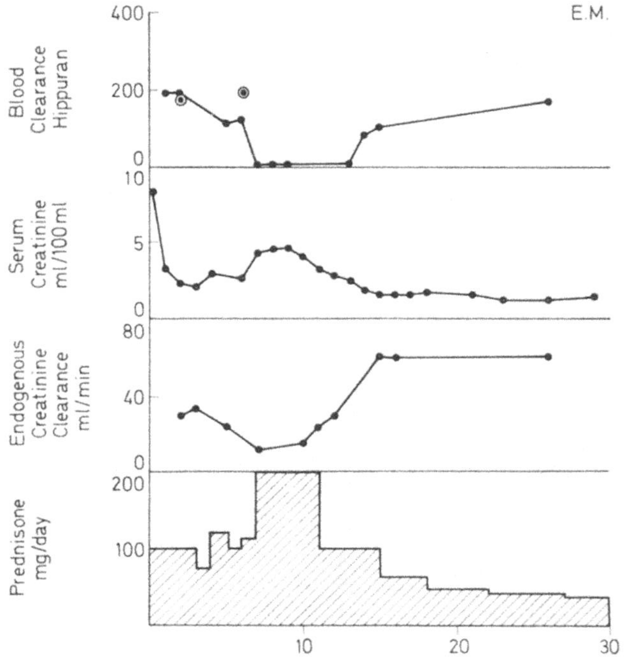


Fig. 17. Blood clearance of radiohippuran following transplantation. Renal blood flow is markedly decreased in homograft rejection reaction but returns following appropriate therapy. The circles with a dark center are the blood clearance values in the donor

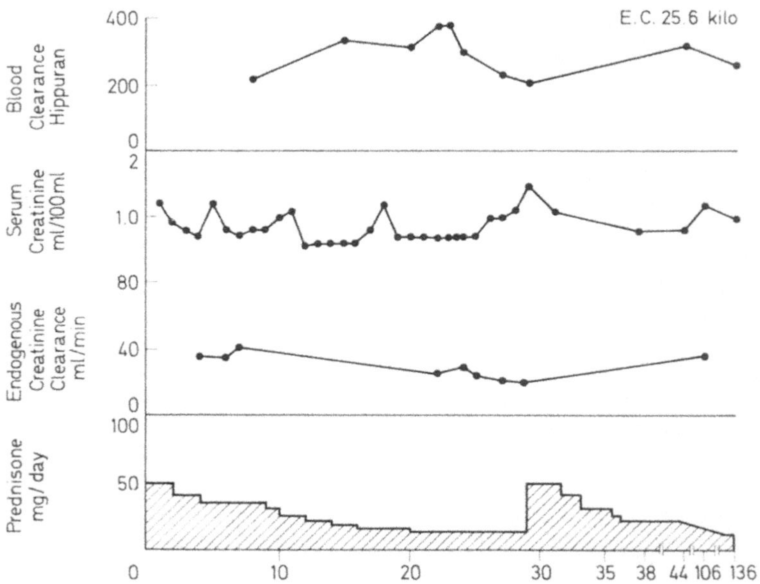


Fig. 18. Blood clearance of radiohippuran following renal transplantation. The blood clearance (flow) falls prior to the detected rise in serum creatinine. This is the earliest functional change for detection of the rejection crisis

clearance of radiohippuran following a single injection with external counters to monitor this parameter of renal function. The pattern of daily determinations is the guide to altered function by this qualitative test (AWAD [13]; BLAUFOX [28]). The blood clearance of hippuran falls 1—2 days before there is a detectable rise in the serum creatinine. As graft rejection is destructive early treatment should provide the best means of maintaining function.

## 5. Laboratory Studies

The parameters of renal function are of paramount importance in the early post transplantation interval. A number of additional studies are indicated:

(1) Bacteriological cultures of the urine are made during and after the interval of catheter drainage. Bacteriuria is treated vigorously to avoid pyelonephritis in the graft.

(2) Urinalysis and urine protein determinations are made at regular intervals once or twice a week.

(3) Hematocrit and white blood count are determined daily. The hematocrit should rise slowly several weeks after transplantation. A falling hematocrit suggests Azathioprine toxicity or gastrointestinal bleeding.

(4) Serum electrolytes, calcium, phosphorus and uric acid are determined weekly. Alterations in serum calcium metabolism are interesting. The hyperparathyroidism of chronic renal failure has been observed to persist after successful transplantation in a number of cases. This may be followed with expectant treatment early in the postoperative interval. Persistence may require subtotal parathyroidectomy.

(5) Blood sugar. The corticosteroids employed for immunosuppression can result in hyperglycemia. This may resolve as the dose of steroid is decreased or it may require dietary and pharmacologic management.

## 6. Radiographic Studies

It is advisable to obtain an excretory urogram when renal function maximal following transplantation to establish baseline architecture of the graft. Any evidence of obstructive uropathy must be followed by further studies.

Micturition cystourethrography is indicated when persistent urinary infection is observed.

Routine chest X-rays will frequently show a reduction in heart size with normalization of blood pressure and blood volume. Chest X-rays are indicated with any febrile illness or respiratory infection as frank pneumonitis may be masked by steroid therapy.

Gastrointestinal X-rays are indicated in patients with symptoms or with falling hematocrit and occult blood in the stools. Peptic ulcer disease as a consequence of the gastric hyperacidity caused by corticosteroids is not infrequent.

Renal arteriography may be advisable in patients with hypertension and a bruit over the graft (SMELLIE [215]). The vascular changes of graft rejection may be characteristic (O'CONNOR [176]).

## 7. Pharmacology

### a) Immunosuppressive Drugs

a) Azathioprine is given empirically in a dose of 1—2 mg/kg body weight. White blood count depression is a toxic side effect and calls for a reduced dose. We prefer to give azathioprine daily in reduced doses even with a low white blood count as the graft can undergo rejection reaction even in the presence of a peripheral leucopenia. The dose must be regulated in relation to the white blood count and the rate of fall.

b) Prednisone. The dose of prednisone is empirical. We prefer to start with 100 mg/day and gradually reduce this as long as renal function is stable. As most graft rejection crises occur in the first three months, it is advisable to maintain a daily dose of not less than 30 mg during this time. Subsequent reduction must be slow and cautious with careful monitor of renal function. When a graft rejection crisis is detected, the dose of prednisone should be markedly increased (at least 2× prior dose). Some patients require 200—400 mg/day to reverse the acute reaction. When renal function improves, the dose can be gradually reduced. The immunosuppressive effect of prednisone is maintained on an alternate day regimen. We have utilized this treatment schedule in many patients in the U.C.L.A. series with good results. Whether an alternate day regimen reduces the undesirable side effects is not proven. There is some evidence to suggest an intermittent or alternate day regimen does not impair the release of growth-hormone by the pituitary (MARTIN, 1968 [136]; MORRIS [158]). We have observed excellent growth patterns in several patients in the 9—13 year age group on alternate day prednisone following renal transplantation.

It has been shown that alternate day steroid does not produce adrenocortical atrophy. This should protect patients from acute adrenal insufficiency.

c) Actinomycin C. This antibiotic which inhibits transfer RNA, has been shown to inhibit the rejection of canine renal grafts (ALEXANDRE, 1963 [8]). It has been used in a large number of clinical cases as an adjuvant agent to inhibit rejection (MURRAY, 1963 [164]). Unfortunately, it is no longer available in the United States. Given intravenously in graft rejection crises, it is used in a daily dose of 200—400 μg for 5—10 doses.

The administration of immunosuppressive drugs directly into the renal artery has been advocated by KOUNTZ (KOUNTZ, 1969 [117]). He places a small plastic catheter in the renal artery at the implantation for administration of azathioprine, decadron, actinomycin C and heparin postoperative. The results of this technique appear excellent (KOUNTZ, 1969 [117]).

### b) Antihypertensives

Many patients with severe hypertension prior to transplantation will require weeks or months before the return of normal blood pressure levels. Increased blood pressure frequently accompanies rejection crises. In these situations, antihypertensive medications are given. A thiazide diuretic is useful as it also reduces edema due to the steroids. Some patients will develop such hyperuricemia that this group of drugs cannot be used. Alpha methyl dopa (Aldomet) has been the most effective antihypertensive drug for most cases. Occasionally it may be necessary to employ hydralazine (Apresoline), guanethadine (Ismelin), or other agents.

### c) Antacid

Increased gastric acidity is directly proportional to the dose of corticosteroids. A vigorous program of antacid therapy is necessary in the early postoperative interval when the risk of peptic ulcer is high. Antacids containing calcium carbonate may occasionally aggravate a pre-existing or latent hypercalcemia.

### D. Post Hospitalization Care

In uncomplicated cases, the recipient of a renal transplant may be ready to leave the hospital in 2—3 weeks. When the patient is released from the hospital, it is necessary to arrange for regular medical evaluations, including determination of hematocrit, white blood count and renal function. These are best obtained two or three times a week initially. The intervals between visits and laboratory tests are increased only when the condition of the patient is good and all parameters are stable. The serum calcium should be determined monthly for the first year postoperative as we have observed the development of hypercalcemia many months after transplantation.

## VI. Urological Complications and Urinary Infections

### A. Urological Complications

The urological complications of renal transplantation are important as they contribute significantly to morbidity and mortality. Urological surgeons should be well informed of the causes and corrective measures needed. The complications may be considered as those due to obstruction, fistula formation and infection.

#### 1. Obstruction

Ureteral obstruction is not a frequent complication, but it may occur early or late following transplantation due to intrinsic or extrinsic factor. Figs. 19 and 20 outline the U.C.L.A. experience with 142 renal transplants from living and cadaveric donors (MARTIN [136]).

Complete ureteral occlusion by a blood clot has been observed during profuse diuresis postoperative. In two such cases in the U.C.L.A. experience the obstructing clot passed spontaneously and diuresis resumed. Another patient at U.C.L.A.

*Type of primary anastomosis*

| | |
|---|---|
| Ureterocutaneous | 4 |
| Ureterovesical | 127 |
| Ureteroureteral | 6 |
| Ureteropelvic | 2 |
| Pyelopelvic | 2 |
| Ureteroileal | 1 |
| | 142 |

Fig. 19. Primary ureteral anastomosis in 142 renal transplants of the U.C.L.A. series

*Complications*

| | |
|---|---|
| A. Obstruction | |
| Ureterovesical anastomosis | |
| Early | 5 |
| Late | 2 |
| B. Fistula | |
| Ureterovesical anastomosis | 10 |
| Ureteroureteral anastomosis | 3 |
| Ureteropelvic anastomosis | 0 |
| Pyelopelvic anastomosis | 1 |
| C. Vesicocutaneous fistula | 3 |

Fig. 20. Urological complications in a series of 142 renal transplants of the U.C.L.A. series

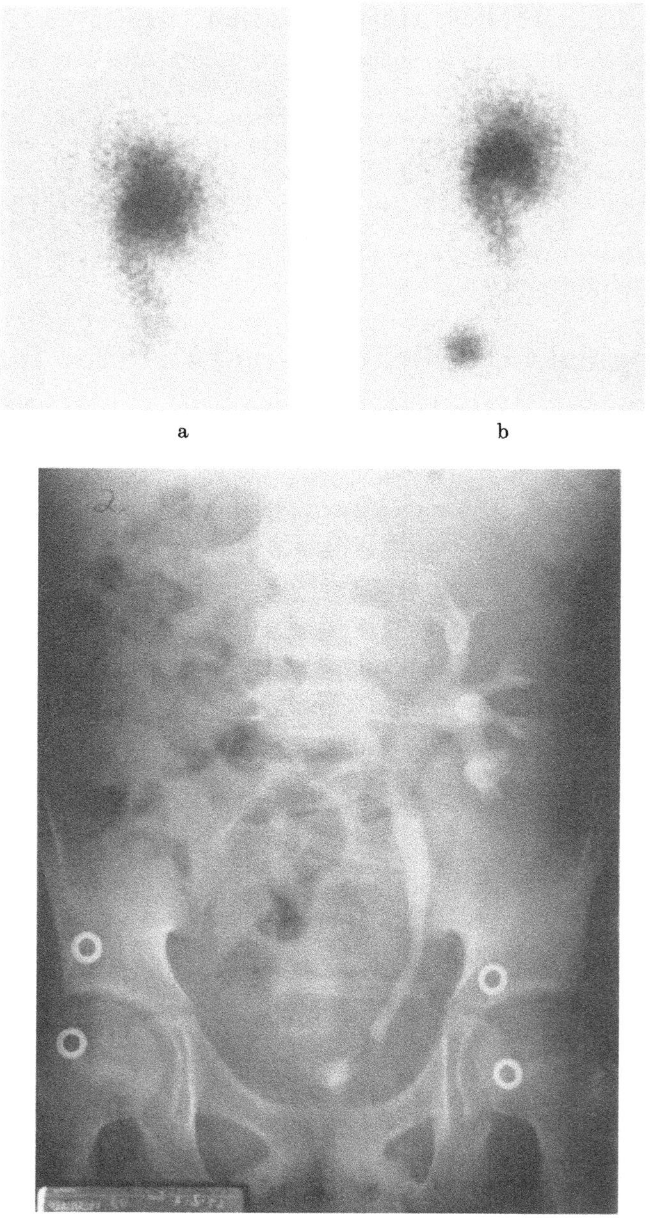

Fig. 21 a—c. Radiohippuran renal scan 48 hours following renal transplantation from a father to his 11 year old son reveals good function with ureteral obstruction (a, b). Excretory urogram confirms the findings of isotope scan (c)

developed ureteral obstruction due to traction on the ureter; this was relieved by implanting the ureter higher in the bladder. Although traction more frequently dislodges the ureter to produce a fistula, it may also cause obstruction. Mild ureteral obstruction occurring shortly after surgery may be treated expectantly.

We have seen ureteral obstruction late following transplantation in two of 142 cases. One was due to ureterovesical stenosis, and the other to a perivesical abscess. When the abscess was drained, the obstruction was relieved (MARTIN [136]).

MURRAY and HARRISON reported five cases of ureteral obstruction in 50 patients (MURRAY [162]). Two were the result of pressure by the spermatic cord,

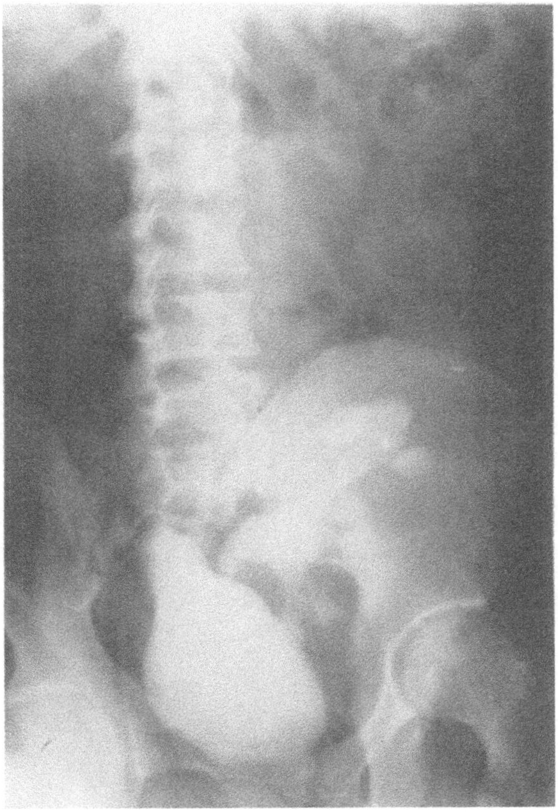

Fig. 22. Excretory urogram 3 months following transplantation reveals moderate obstruction. The patient was asymptomatic with good renal function

two due to torsion of the ureter, and one to a blood clot. PROUT observed only one case of transient hydronephrosis following ureterovesical anastomosis in 92 transplants (PROUT [193]): this resolved spontaneously in two months. STARZL reported four cases of late ureteral stricture in 33 patients followed for four months in the early experience at Denver (STARZL [227]). KISER reported one case of late ureteral obstruction in 121 transplants at Cleveland (KISER [111]).

Two female recipients in the U.C.L.A. series have completed successful pregnancy and delivered vaginally. One patient had no evidence of obstruction prior to delivery (KAUFFMAN [104]); the other had definite hydronephrosis late in pregnancy which resolved after delivery.

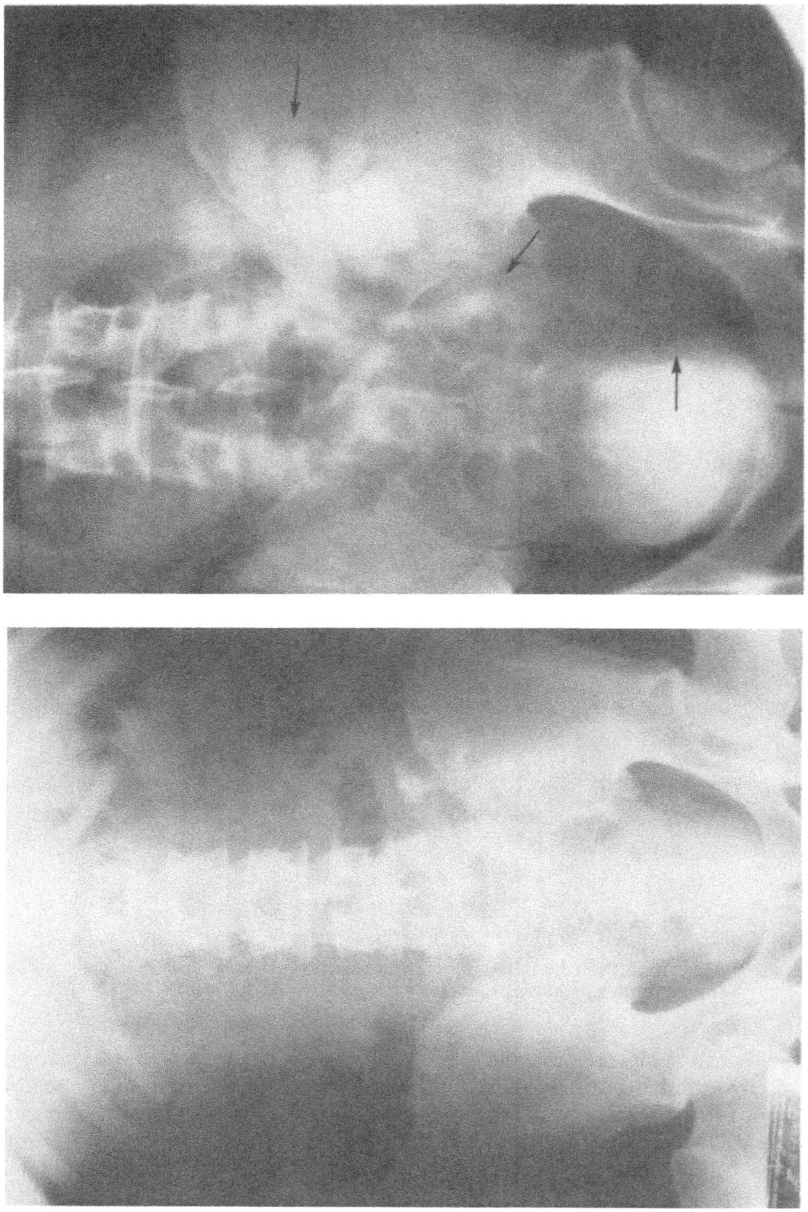

a b

Fig. 23a and b. Excretory urograms following transplantation; ureteral obstruction due to perivesical abscess (b). Drainage of the abscess relieved the obstruction as shown in (a)

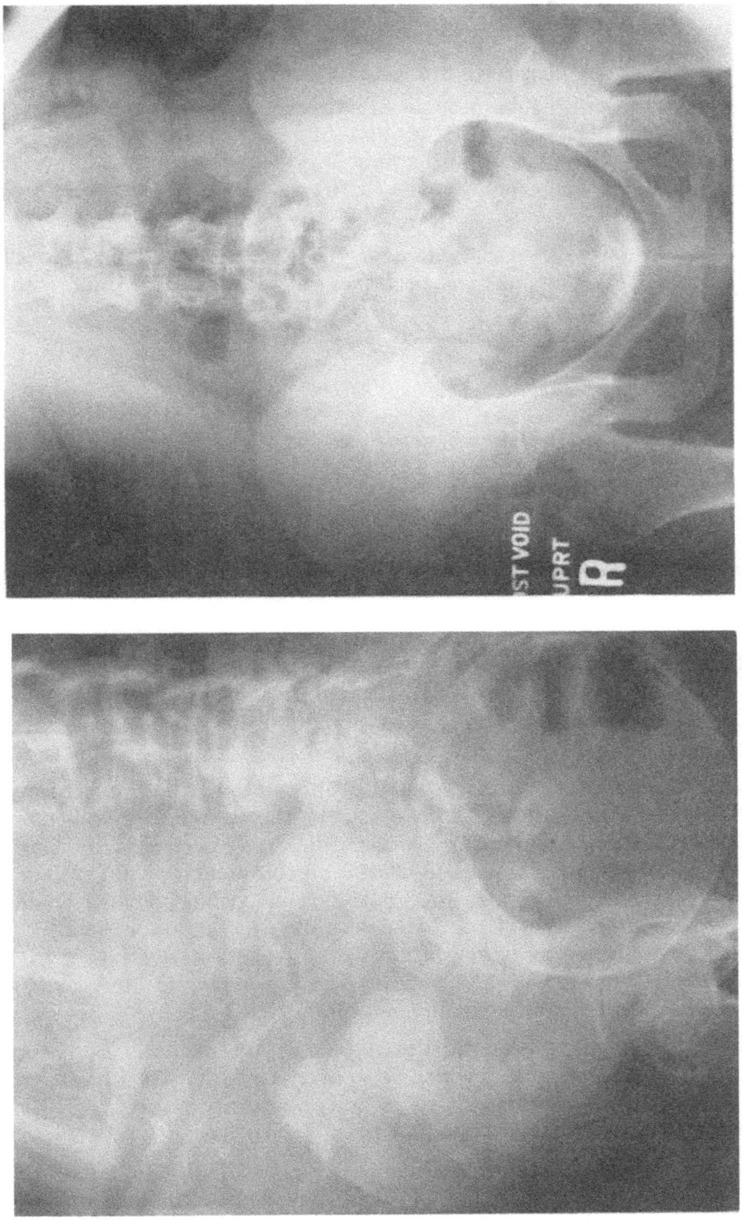


a b

Fig. 24a and b. Excretory urogram late in the third trimester of pregnancy. This patient received a kidney from her mother 18 months prior. Hydronephrosis in the transplanted kidney (a) is seen to resolve post partum (b)

We have not seen ureteral obstruction following ureteroureterostomy or ureteropyelostomy. A recent experience with pyelopyelostomy resulted in a persistent ureterocutaneous fistula due to obstruction of the angulated recipient ureter.

## 2. Fistulae

### a) Ureterocutaneous Fistulae

*a) Etiology.* Ureterocutaneous fistulae are the most frequent and important urological complications (Kiser [111]; Marshall [133]; Martin [137]; Palmer [180]). They invariably give rise to infection and usually require surgical correction. Unresolved, the ureterocutaneous fistula will usually lead to loss of the graft or of the patient's life.

The causes of ureterovesical fistulae in the U.C.L.A. experience are shown in Fig. 25 (Martin [137]). The most frequent cause is withdrawal of the ureter from

*Ureterovesical fistulae*

| | | |
|---|---|---|
| A. Etiology | | |
| Tension | 6 | |
| Intubation → ureteral necrosis | 1 | |
| Inflammation → ureteral necrosis | 3 | |
| B. Treatment | | Successful |
| Reanastomosis to bladder | 4 | 2 |
| Ureteroureteral anastomosis | 4 | 1 |
| Bladder flap | 2 | 1 |

Fig. 25. Urological complications in 142 cases of the U.C.L.A. series. Causes and treatment of ureterovesical fistulae

the bladder. Such fistulae present immediately postoperative or in the first 1—2 weeks. They can be prevented by the creation of a tension-free anastomosis and should occur infrequently with increased experience.

Another important cause of ureterocutaneous fistulae is necrosis of the transplant ureter due to inadequate primary blood supply or to the homograft rejection reaction. Laboratory and clinical studies indicate the ureter is involved in the rejection process (Robertshaw [203]). These fistulae may occur at any time after transplantation: we have seen them 21—27 days postoperative, and others have reported even later necrosis of the ureter and renal pelvis. The only defense is to ensure preservation of ureteral blood supply at the donor nephrectomy. Necrosis of the graft ureter in homograft rejection reaction is a factor in favor of using the recipient ureter in ureteropyelostomy where only the graft renal pelvis can be involved in the homograft reaction.

We continue to favor ureterovesical anastomosis, as it should be associated with the least incidence of primary urinary leak. Anastomoses involving only the ureteral or pelvis wall are difficult to make consistently water-tight. Urinary fistulae greatly increase the hazards of infection.

*b) Treatment.* Ureterocutaneous drainage may occasionally be transient, but in our experience most cases required surgical correction. For this reason, and because of the severe infections of the wound which accompany continued urinary leakage, we recommend early surgical intervention when a fistula is proven. The procedures employed are determined by the length of remaining viable graft ureter. Simple distraction of the ureter from the bladder has been treated by reimplant into the bladder. If the graft ureter was initially short or a portion has been lost, several alternatives may be considered: ureteroureterostomy; ureteropyelostomy, employing the recipient ureter if available; or bladder flap (Boari flap).

We prefer to use the recipient ipsilateral ureter whenever the graft ureter is of questionable length or viability. Fig. 26 shows the pyelogram of a patient two years after repair of ureterocutaneous fistula by ureteroureterostomy. Nephrostomy drainage might be considered in such cases; however, we prefer

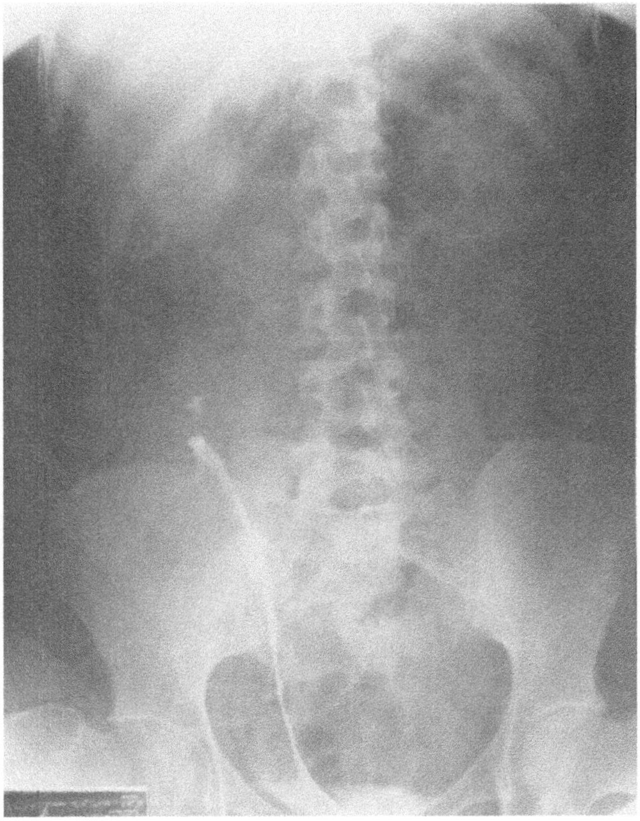

Fig. 26. Retrograde pyelogram 3 years after uretero-ureterostomy to correct a primary ureterovesical fistula. This patient died with chronic rejection $3^1/_2$ years following transplantation from her brother

not to employ it in the transplanted kidney. A ureteral stent might be placed in some cases to reduce the risks of obstruction and leakage. The contralateral ureter has been mobilized and brought across the midline for anastomosis to the graft ureter in a few cases where the ipsilateral ureter was absent.

A bladder flap can be made to reach the graft renal pelvis in many instances, but we do not favor this procedure as it has been associated with delayed healing and infection in our experience. The graft is susceptible to bladder pressure in the presence of a short ureteral segment.

## b) Ureteroureteral Fistulae

These have been transient and have resolved spontaneously without subsequent problems in most cases at U.C.L.A. Those which did not heal spontaneously resulted in severe infection and loss of the graft. Placement of a ureteral catheter by cystoscopy may promote drainage away from the fistula. One of

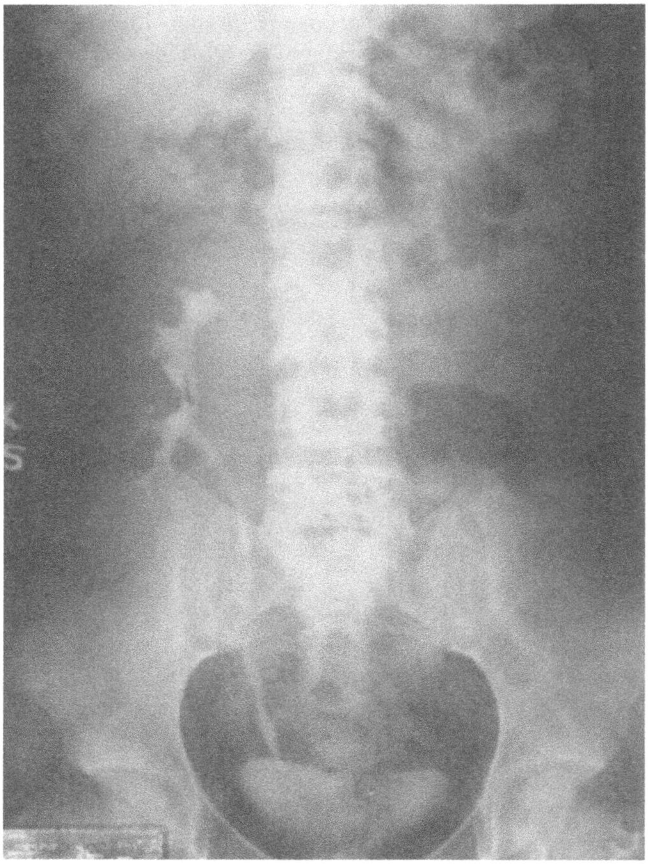

Fig. 27. Excretory urogram 4 years after renal transplantation from mother to daughter. This patient remains well despite a temporary urinary fistula following primary anastomosis of graft ureter to recipient ureter

the advantages of using the recipient's own ureters is the facility with which they can be subsequently catheterized by cystoscopy.

## c) Pyelopelvic Fistulae

*a) Etiology.* We have previously described the technique of pyelopyelostomy employed by Dr. GIL VERNET of Barcelona (GIL VERNET [67]). Our experience is limited and not favorable. Two of three patients developed persistent fistulae, one caused by necrosis of the recipient pelvis and the other by ureteral obstruction.

*b) Treatment.* Both of these cases were resolved by ureteropyelostomy. Fig. 28 shows the pyelograms of the recipient with a pyelocutaneous fistula which required

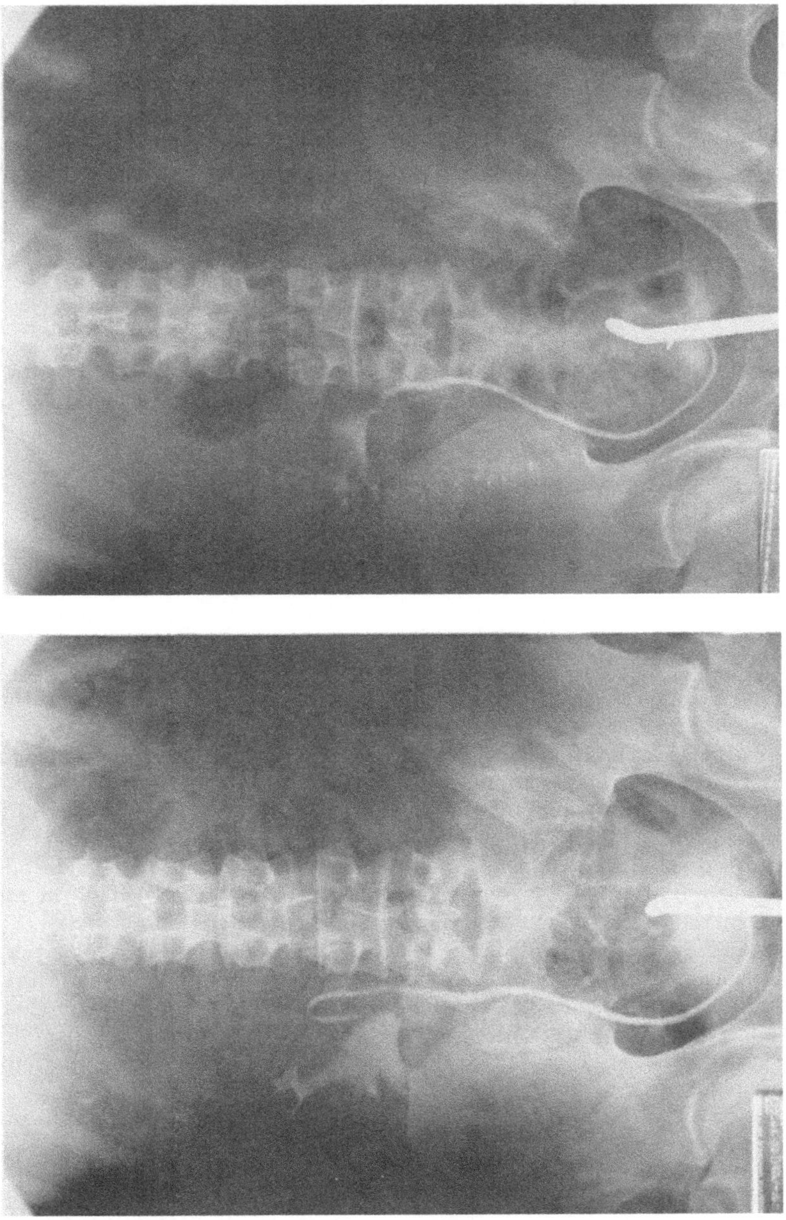

a b

Fig. 28a and b. Retrograde pyeloureterograms following renal transplantation by the technique of Dr. Gil Vernet. A persistent pyelocutaneous fistula (a) required pyeloureteral anastomosis for correction (b) ureteropyelostomy. The long term result have been satisfactory, although a perinephric abscess was found and drained more than six months after closure of this fistula.

Greater experience with this technique would probably reduce the instance of complications. It is apparent, however, that the procedure is fraught with technical difficulties.

### d) Vesicocutaneous Fistulae

These should be rare when bladder closure is carefully made in three layers. Occasionally a patient will develop necrosis of a portion of the bladder wall as a result of vascular embarrassment, infection, or both. Two such patients in our experience followed a course of delayed wound healing but ultimately recovered. Maintenance of adequate surgical drainage was important.

## B. Urinary Infections

The role of clinical urinary infections in the fate of renal transplants has not been extensively evaluated. RIFKIND reported bacteriuria in 15 of 30 recipients at Denver (RIFKIND, [201]). Six of the 15 patients had urosepsis prior to transplantation,

| *Primary diagnosis* | |
|---|---|
| Chronic glomerulonephritis | 46 |
| Chronic pyelonephritis | 22 |
| Polycystic disease | 2 |
| Unclassified renal disease | 2 |
| | 72 |

Fig. 29. Primary diagnosis in 72 recipients of the U.C.L.A. series studied for incidence of urinary infections

while bacteriuria followed the surgery in the other nine. Eleven infections were ultimately cured, two were suppressed and two were not cured.

PROUT observed a significant bacteriuria in 21 of 24 cadaveric transplant recipients and in 34 of 48 related donor recipients (PROUT [193]). Antibiotic treatment cleared the infection in 11 of the 21 cadaveric organ recipients and in 20 of the 34 related donor recipients.

MACKINNON in Montreal reported that 31% of 59 recipients had bacteriuria six months postoperative (MACKINNON [144]). He also observed calculi in four patients with mixed infections.

A survey of 72 renal transplants in the U.C.L.A. series disclosed that 30 patients never had a positive urine culture in a follow-up of at least three months. Thirty-five had significant bacteriuria on the hospitalization for transplantation, and an additional seven had bacteriuria subsequent to the hospitalization. The primary diagnosis in these 72 patients is shown in Fig. 29. In this group of patients, 50 were transplanted from living donors and 22 from cadaveric donors.

The duration of catheter drainage relative to urinary infection is shown in Fig. 30.

Included in the group of 35 patients with infections during the hospitalization for transplantation are 13 who had active infection in the bladder at surgery. This was not suspected nor planned, but occurred despite efforts to sterilize the lower urinary tract pretransplantation.

Twenty of those 35 with infection were subsequently cleared with appropriate antibiotics. In some cases several courses of antibacterial therapy were necessary.

Even patients with Pseudomonas and Klebsiella organisms can be cleared of urinary infections.

Fifteen patients went on to chronic, usually asymptomatic, bacteriuria. The relation of the primary pathologic diagnosis to the development of chronic infection is shown in Fig. 31. As might be anticipated, chronic pyelonephritis was associated with a higher percentage of chronic infection. The 72 patients in this study were followed from three months to seven years. Fifty-one were alive and 21 were dead on analysis. The urinary infection contributed to death in eight patients.

The role of urinary complications following transplantation in the genesis of urinary infections cannot be overemphasized. As stated previously, every

*Urinary infections duration of catheter drainage*

| Days | 0 | 1 | 2 | 3 | 4 | 5 | 6 | 7 | >7 |
|---|---|---|---|---|---|---|---|---|---|
| Infections | 2 | 2 | 4 | 6 | 2 | 2 | 0 | 1 | 16 |
| Cases at risk | 10 | 2 | 18 | 14 | 5 | 2 | 0 | 1 | 20 |

Fig. 30. Relation of catheter drainage to the incidence of urinary infections in 72 renal transplants of the U.C.L.A. series

*Chronic urinary infection relation to primary diagnosis*

| Glomerolonephritis | Pyelonephritis | Polycystic | Unclassified |
|---|---|---|---|
| $\frac{7}{46}$ | $\frac{6}{22}$ | $\frac{1}{2}$ | $\frac{1}{2}$ |

Fig. 31. Relation of primary pathological diagnosis to the incidence of chronic urinary infection in 72 renal transplants of the U.C.L.A. series

patient with a major urological complication developed urosepsis in the U.C.L.A. series. Seven of 18 patients with urological complications fell into the chronic infections group, as compared with eight of 51 patients without urological complications.

Antibacterial agents with potential nephrotoxic properties may be used in recipients of renal grafts when allowances are made for patient size and renal function. When all tubes and drains are removed, persistent bacteriuria should be treated aggressively. We obtain excretory urography and micturition cysto-urethrography on all patients with persistent infection. Obstructive uropathy and reflux into ureteral stumps can be seen and must be corrected before therapy with potent antibacterial agents is instituted.

In view of the significant role urosepsis plays in patient mortality, all steps must be taken to maintain a sterile urinary tract. The shorter the time (consistent with patient security and comfort) urinary catheters are maintained, the smaller the risk of urinary infection by this route.

Recipients of cadaveric kidneys where oliguria or anuria is anticipated during the phase of tubular necrosis do not require catheters, and we find these patients get along well without them.

Recipients with urinary infection present a problem in rendering the bladder sterile prior to transplantation. Bilateral nephrectomy and bladder irrigations have been employed. HINMAN studied the incidence of bladder bacteria in 65 anephric patients. 72% of those initially sterile remained so during the anephric phase. 48% previously infected were rendered sterile by nephrectomy and bladder irrigations with 500 mg neomycin. Urine cultures after transplantation and removal of the catheter showed the same per centage of bacterial growth in irrigated and non irrigated patients. The initial organism was found in half the cases. Bladder irrigations with neomycin reduce the incidence of positive urine cultures at the time of transplantation but not in later follow-up (Hinman [84, 85]).

# VII. Other Complications Following Transplantation

## A. Surgical Complications

The general surgical complications of renal transplantation are infrequent but require consideration (Cohn [47]). They are mentioned briefly in several reports of large series.

### 1. Peptic Ulceration

The administration of large doses of corticosteroids to patients who may have suffered from uremic gastritis can be anticipated to cause clinical peptic ulceration. That it does not occur more frequently is remarkable. We recommend a vigorous program of oral antacid therapy in all patients receiving corticosteroids. This is begun as soon after surgery as oral feeding and is increased when larger doses of steroids are necessary during rejection episodes. We start patients on 30 ml of antacid every two hours and increase to 30 ml every hour when the prednisone dose is increased above 50—100 mg/24 hours. The incidence of occult bleeding from the gastrointestinal tract is unknown. Several patients in the U.C.L.A. series have had massive gastrointestinal hemorrhage requiring transfusions. Only two of more than 150 recipients have required gastric surgery, indicating that most patients are satisfactorily managed medically.

### 2. Pancreatitis

Another complication of corticosteroid therapy is pancreatitis. This is recognized infrequently, but when it does occur it can be recurrent and disabling. We have not confirmed all suspected cases, but two patients at U.C.L.A. came to autopsy with severe pancreatitis and other complications. We suspect it may frequently be due to a posterior peptic ulcer, but both cases seen at autopsy were primary pancreatitis of the type seen in patients on corticosteroids.

Treatment in the transplant recipient is similar to that for other patients; gastric suction, intravenous fluids and anticholinergic drugs. The dose of corticosteroid should be reduced if possible, although these severe complications often occur in the patient who requires large doses of steroid to maintain function in the graft.

### 3. Aseptic Necrosis of the Femoral Head

This is a well recognized complication of corticosteroid therapy. It occurs at least as frequently in other patients on steroids as it does in graft recipients. Cruess reported osseous changes in 10 of 27 renal graft recipients surviving six months in Montreal (Cruess [51]). Nine had aseptic necrosis of the femoral head, five had involvement of the hips alone, others had involvement of the knee joint and/or humeral heads. Symptoms occurred an average of seven months following transplantation. Roentgen changes appeared two months after symptoms.

We have three cases in the U.C.L.A. series. One patient developed this complication within a year of transplantation. He did not require unusual doses of prednisone and had been on 15 mg/day for several months when pain first occurred. Radiographic changes were not seen for two months. This patient had Legge-Perthes disease of the contralateral femoral head, suggesting a congenital predisposition. We followed this patient conservatively for three years, during which time he became slowly and progressively disabled.

Another patient had bilateral disease which was more rapidly disabling. We have no personal experience with orthopedic procedures, but Dr. RALPH STRAFFON of Cleveland states that several patients in their group have benefited substantially from arthroplasty.

The third patient in our experience died of other complications. Femoral head necrosis appeared after a third renal graft with a transplantation-dialysis course of three years.

Orthopedic surgery in patients on immunosuppressive drugs is not enthusiastically recommended.

### 4. Hyperparathyroidism

Persistence of secondary hyperparathyroidism following successful renal transplantation with normal renal function is a "new disease" created by the transplant surgeon. It was first reported by McPHAUL and has since been seen in most centers (McPHAUL [145]). Even more remarkable than persistence of this parathyroid hyperfunction is the development of clinical signs months after transplantation. ALFREY studied the Denver series carefully and concluded that surgical parathyroidectomy is rarely necessary (ALFREY [10]). He observed transient hypercalcemia after transplantation. Corticosteroids, antacids and the status of total body phosphates may play a role in the manifestation of hypercalcemia.

At present one cannot predict which recipients will develop this interesting phenomenon, thus it must be looked for in all patients on follow-up. It may not be detected until months after transplantation.

We have observed four patients with hypercalcemia many months following renal transplantation. In two of these subtotal parathyroidectomy corrected the biochemical findings and reduced metastatic calcifications.

One patient in the U.C.L.A. series developed peptic ulceration, metastatic vascular calcification and necrosis of the terminal portions of her digits with hypercalcemia. Subtotal parathyroidectomy was followed by healing of the digits and slight reduction in the vascular calcification.

## B. Medical Complications

### 1. Hypercorticoid State (Iatrogenic Cushing's Syndrome)

To maintain immune suppression and optimum graft function, recipients of renal grafts with rare exception require corticosteroids in doses sufficient to produce the hypercorticoid state. The larger doses required postoperative produce moon facies, acne and striae in many. Osteoporosis, hypertension, edema, hirsutism and altered glucose tolerance are seen only in patients who require maintenance of larger doses. Many patients tolerate the reduction of steroid doses to levels which are compatible with regression of all or almost all of the above changes.

1. Diabetes mellitus. We observed seven patients with steroid-induced diabetes mellitus in 150 recipients. Most were readily managed by diet and oral hypoglycemic agents; however, one patient had uncontrolled glucose metabolism and rapidly progressive rejection of the graft leading to death in seven months. Reduced doses of corticosteroids assist in medical management and are possible

when the diabetic state occurs with the large doses used for rejection crises. As steroids are reduced, the diabetes becomes amenable to dietary control.

2. Fat embolism. Systemic hypertriglyceridemia and fat embolism with changes in steroid doses have been reported by Jones et al. (Jones [99]).

3. Obesity. Many patients become excessively obese following successful transplantation. Restoration of renal function with steroids contributes to a great appetite. This has been associated with hypertension in several patients.

4. Cataracts. One young patient developed cataracts over the course of three years. He received three grafts and was on large doses of prednisone for many months. This same patient had bilateral aseptic necrosis of the femoral head prior to death.

## 2. Hepatitis

The metabolism of azathioprine appears to be influenced by hepatic and renal function, and toxicity may occur in hepatic or renal insufficiency. Transplantation recipients receive blood transfusions and renal tissue and are exposed to serum hepatitis. The incidence of hepatitis is noted in most reports of major series. Hume reported six cases in recipients and five in personnel caring for them (Hume [89]). One patient died of hepatitis. Another with recurrent hepatitis had azathioprine stopped for 10 months; prednisone 15 mg/day was sufficient immunosuppression to maintain function in the graft. A patient in the Brigham series (Boston) had azathioprine withheld for several months during a bout of hepatitis and renal function was stable initially (Glassock [68]).

Six patients in the U.C.L.A. series had hepatitis. In these patients azathioprine doses were reduced but not discontinued (Reeve [194]). Renal function is usually stable when even small doses of azathioprine are maintained.

Anatomical pathologic changes have been described at autopsy in patients manifesting hepatic dysfunction following dialysis and transplantation. Liver enlargement with areas of irregular color have been seen. The microscopic changes include liver-cell necrosis, bile duct proliferation and increase in portal tract connective tissue (Evans [61]).

1. Unexplained fever. There is a syndrome in renal transplant recipients characterized by intermittent high fever with no other symptoms. This is accompanied by alterations in liver chemistry, primarily elevated serum glutamic oxalacetic transaminase (SGOT), serum glutamic pyruvic transaminase (SGPT) and alkaline phosphatase with normal bilirubin and proteins. The fever is very marked, 38—40° C once or twice every 24 hours, with euthermia between elevations. An illustrative case follows:

B.F. U.C.L.A. 028-03-54. This 19-year old girl was in terminal uremia from glomerulonephritis on November 11, 1963, when she received a kidney from her mother. Initial function of the graft was good. Steroids were not given until December 23, 1963, when all the classical signs of a homograft rejection were observed and the diagnosis confirmed with a renal biopsy. Renal function remained good and the patient's steroids were reduced to 15 mg/day in March, 1964. At this time she developed recurrent spiking fevers to 40° C daily, with normal temperature between. This persisted for three weeks. There were no other symptoms. Liver chemistries showed a slight elevation of alkaline phosphatase and SGPT. Serum bilirubin was normal. Bacteriologic culture of blood, urine, and sputum was repeatedly negative. Occult infection appeared so likely that the patient underwent exploration of the graft site. No abscess was found. Renal biopsy showed a moderate round cell interstitial nephritis reduced from December, 1963. Liver biopsy revealed non-specific changes compatible with toxic hepatitis.

The daily dose of azathioprine was reduced from 150 mg to 75 mg. Two weeks later the patient became afebrile. She survives $5^1/_2$ years after transplantation with a serum creatinine of 2.4 mg-% and an endogenous creatinine clearance of 33 ml/min.

Many other investigators have observed this syndrome, although little is found in the literature. It has been considered due to azathioprine hepatoxicity, but precise definition is lacking.

### 3. Arthritis, Neuritis

Protracted chronic renal disease may be associated with muscle wasting and neuropathy (DINAPOLI [56)], although the severity of these changes may be masked by other prominent features of the illness. Following restoration of renal function, the state of muscle, joint, and nerve change may be evident. In addition to the sequelae of chronic uremia, it is evident that certain changes occur as a consequence of organ transplantation and immunosuppression. There are no clearly defined entities, but there are reports of muscle and joint pain as well as neurological changes. WALLER found positive slide latex tests in 66% of patients studied at Richmond (WALLER [254]). Antinuclear antibodies were detected in the sera of 33% of patients in a study in Denver (BRAVO [32]). Symptoms of peripheral neuropathy are reported, and central nervous system changes have been recorded (SCHNECK [210]).

We have seen representative examples of all of these conditions at U.C.L.A. One of our early cadaveric kidney recipients developed a rapidly progressive ascending peripheral neuropathy two months following transplantation. Prior to and shortly after surgery he had numbness of the soles of his feet but no other disability. Following discharge from the hospital he developed a rapid and progressive loss of motor and sensory function which ascended from the feet to the lower abdomen. He lost sensation during voiding. The hands and forearms were involved, followed by the tip of the tongue and nose. No definitive diagnosis could be made. The renal graft functioned well. A reduction in prednisone seemed to accelerate the neuropathy, and prednisone was empirically increased to 60 mg/day. This was followed by a slow regression of symptoms and signs. He has been fully rehabilitated and remains well $4^1/_2$ years after transplantation.

# VIII. Infections

## A. Introduction

### 1. Surgical Wound Infections

Infections of various types account for at least 75% of the mortality in most reported series of renal homotransplantation (RIFKIND, 1964 [201]; REEVE [194]).

Wound infections are likely to occur in patients with collections of blood, serum or urine in the operative site. Careful hemostasis and adequate drainage should minimize these risks. If the acute inflammation involves the major renal vessels or is adjacent to the vascular anastomosis, the integrity of the vessel wall can be compromised with necrosis and massive hemorrhage. We have observed this sequence of events in three patients when pyogenic infection occurred in the operative site following urinary fistula (in two of the patients) and hemorrhage (in the other) (MARTIN [137]). Removal of functioning renal grafts was necessary to control the bleeding. When infection is recognized to involve the main renal vessels it is safer for the patient to have the graft removed prior to life-threatening hemorrhage.

More superficial wound infections or those involving the area of the bladder may heal by secondary intention. Healing is often slow, and the usual surgical measures of maintaining adequate drainage apply. All patients with a chronic urinary fistula have wound sepsis. Prompt correction of the fistula should minimize the effects of this infection.

### 2. Other Pyogenic Infections

Pyogenic and other infections are not frequent in patients who recover from the surgical procedure with good renal function. When corticosteroids can be progressively reduced to small doses (15—25 mg/day), the danger from an infection is greatly lessened. We rarely see pneumonia or similar infections in ambulatory patients on long-term follow-ups.

Graft recipients who suffer repeated rejection crises necessitating large doses of corticosteroids are particularly prone to the opportunistic infections to be described below. Pyogenic pneumonia may occur with minimal clinical signs in patients on large doses of immunosuppressive agents, and chest roentgenograms are advised for all patients with fever of undetermined origin. We have observed a fulminant pneumonitis develop in two days in an ambulatory patient on large doses of prednisone.

Infections in the skin, teeth, and throat should be treated vigorously by surgical and medical means. Tooth extractions have been necessary in several patients. One patient required surgical drainage of an infection involving the mandible. Aggressive treatment with conventional modalities produced a good result.

### 3. Urinary Infections

See Chapter VI.

## B. Opportunistic Infections

### 1. Introduction

The long-term use of immunosuppressive drugs has exposed patients to the virulence of infectious agents which rarely produce symptoms or disease in intact patients. Large doses of corticosteroids increase the risks; these are often necessitated by poor or failing function in the graft, which further predisposes the patient to infection.

The use of broad spectrum antibiotics for specific pyogenic infections may disturb the normal flora sufficiently to favor growth of these opportunistic organisms. For this reason, we do not use antibiotics routinely in renal transplant recipients but reserve them for specific indications.

### 2. Fungi

Systemic fungal infections have been reported in 23 of 51 patients autopsied following renal transplantation (RIFKIND, 1967 [200]). Males were involved more often than females. Pulmonary infections predominated, but the gastrointestinal tract, central nervous system and urinary tract were also involved frequently.

We have observed two cases of disseminated coccidioidomycosis, one of which was successfully treated with Amphoteracin B. One patient in the U.C.L.A. series died with a disseminated infection (including the central nervous system) of

Candida albicans. Another developed rhino-ocular mucormycosis which was ultimately fatal as a result of other complications (pancreatitis and chronic rejection).

Definitive diagnosis is essential, as renal transplant recipients can be treated with appropriate doses of Amphoteracin B, despite the potential nephrotoxicity of this drug. We have been able to give it to one patient for several months. This patient received a cadaveric kidney in 1965 but never had good renal function. The lowest serum creatinine was approximately 3.0 mg-%. In autumn of 1967, more than two years after transplantation, renal function was stable when a disseminated pulmonary infection due to coccidioidomycosis immitus

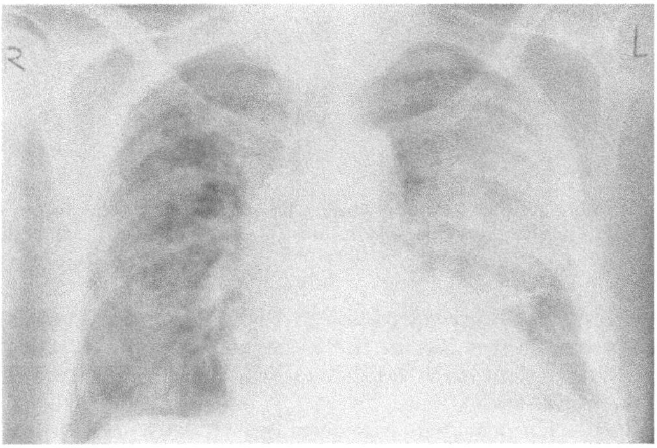


Fig. 32. Chest roentgenogram of a man who received three renal grafts over a 3 year period. Pneumonitis due to Nocardia

was identified. The patient received small doses of Amphoteracin B and responded well with little or no change in renal function. He remains well four years after transplantation.

Pulmonary infections due to fungi may be recognized from appropriate sputum cultures. Patients with even minimal central nervous system signs must be suspect and investigated with spinal tap. The central nervous system involvement may initially produce minimal signs and symptoms, and eradication may depend upon early recognition and treatment.

## 3. Viruses

1. Cytomegalovirus. Infection with cytomegalovirus is thought to be frequent in the general population, but overt clinical disease is rare. The cytomegalovirus may produce serious pathology in renal transplant recipients. Cytomegalic cells were identified in the lungs of 27 of 51 autopsied patients at Denver (Rifkind, 1967 [197]); the lungs only were involved in 19 of these cases, other origins in eight, but the kidney in only one. This virus has been cultured from the urine of many surviving patients. No significant pathology has been attributed to the presence of virus in the urine of well patients (Kanich [100]).

Cytomegalovirus may produce a fulminant pneumonitis with fever, dyspnea, tachypnea, leucocytosis and diffuse nodular infiltrates on chest X-ray. Roentgenographic changes were seen in only seven of 26 cases with nodular densities at autopsy. The diagnosis may be suspected from examination and culture of the sputum, but lung biopsy may be necessary for a definitive diagnosis.

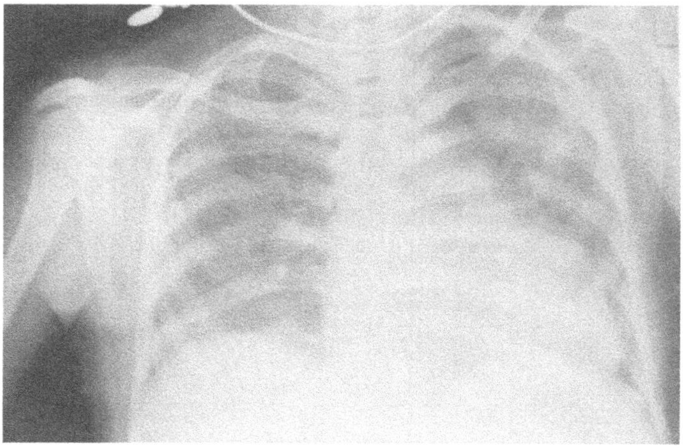

Fig. 33. Chest roentgenogram of a young woman who died $4^1/_2$ months following renal transplantation in 1961. Cytomegalovirus was found at autopsy shortly after this picture was obtained

Therapy with 5-fluoro-dexoxyuridine (5-FUDR) can be life saving.

We have observed the virus in the pancreas at autopsy, and this has also been reported in a patient with fatal hemorrhagic pancreatitis following transplantation (TILNEY [241]).

2. Herpes virus. Herpes virus has been reported to produce infection of the central nervous system in a renal graft recipient.

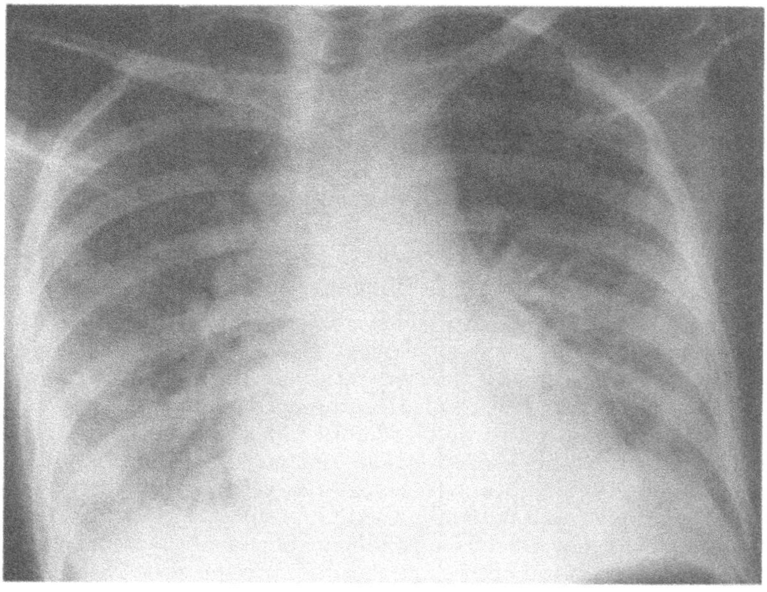

Fig. 34. Chest roentgenogram of pneumonitis due to pneumocystitis carinii several months following renal transplantation. Pathological examination revealed hyalin proteinosis and intraalveolar hemorrhage

### 4. Protozoan

1. Pneumocystitis carinii. This organism produces pneumonia in debilitated patients, those who have immunological defects or are immunosuppressed. The epidemiology of the agent is unknown. Pneumocystis was found in 10 of 41 renal transplant recipients autopsied at Denver following a fatal pneumonia (RIFKIND, 1966 [198]). This protozoan may produce a fulminant pneumonitis with dyspnea, fever and radiographic changes on chest X-ray. The organisms are frequently seen in the lungs at autopsy in patients who have died with multiple complications and infections. The infection may be suspected from examination of stained tracheal aspirates, but definitive diagnosis antemortem is made by lung biopsy (KOPPEL [114]; DE VITA [55]). This is important as specific chemotherapy is now available; Pentamidine isethionate is reported to produce good results despite potential nephrotoxicity (KOPPLE [114]; DE VITA [55]).

### 5. Autoimmune Pneumonitis

It has been suggested for some time that a pneumonitis in renal graft recipients may be due to an immunological reaction (HUME [89]). Some of the patients so classified in the past may well have suffered from one of the opportunistic infections described above. Patients with unexplained pneumonitis characterized by dyspnea, tachypnea, fever, leucocytosis and diffuse changes on chest roentgenogram should have a lung biopsy before this condition is attributed to an autoimmune reaction. One cannot rule out an infectious process short of lung biopsy A marked alveolar-capillary block is a characteristic of all these conditions (KOPPEL [114]).

## C. Specific Infections

### Tuberculosis

Patients with a history of tuberculosis may be considered as high risk for renal transplantation in view of the immunosuppressive regimen required. We have attempted to avoid transplantation in these cases. However, HUME has reported satisfactory progress in patients with arrested tuberculosis who were also kept on antituberculous therapy after transplantation (HUME [89]). STARZL had a recipient develop diffuse tuberculosis in a renal graft; and it was never clear whether the renal infection occurred before or after transplantation.

# IX. Pathology

Our present understanding of the pathological processes involved in the renal homograft rejection is derived from laboratory models and clinical experience. Much of the data from laboratory work concerns the untreated or unmodified host, whereas the clinical recipients are treated with various immunosuppressive agents. The laboratory data may not be directly transferable to the clinical situation, but there appear to be many similarities.

## A. Unmodified Host

The canine renal homograft has served as a most satisfactory model for evaluation of pathological and functional changes. Serial biopsy and frequent determinations of function indicate that host factors affect the anatomy of the graft in 24—72 hours.

## 1. Anatomy

The initial attack on the vascular endothelium of small intertubular vessels is made by mononuclear cells. Progressive involvement of vessels results in ischemic damage and changes in the tubular cells going on to tubular necrosis. There is an associated edema and accumulation of polymorphonuclear and mononuclear leucocytes in the interstitium. The glomeruli are relatively uninvolved until advanced vascular injury occurs.

## 2. Physiology

Studies on the intrarenal distribution of blood flow in laboratory animals using $Xenon^{133}$ indicate there is cortical ischemia early in rejection. The rapid reversibility of this disturbance suggests a functional (vasoconstrictive) rather than anatomical cause (TRUNIGER [244]; RETIK, 1967 [195]; RETIK, 1969 [196]).

Another early physiological change is a reduction in renal blood flow. This occurs shortly after the above anatomical changes, usually by 72 hours. One can detect a fall in creatinine clearance 24—48 hours after the fall in renal blood flow; this progresses to oliguria and increasing azotemia (KOUNTZ [118]).

Knowledge of these early anatomical and physiological changes has been applied to the control of clinical grafts.

These changes are seen in the first set graft rejection. A second graft from the same donor will pass through similar phases at a more rapid rate; where the first graft may be non-functioning after 7—9 days, the second will reach this phase in 4—5 days. The degree of edema and cellular infiltrate is more severe, so that the second graft swells in excess of the first. Accelerated rejection of the second graft is dependent upon the initial viability of the first. If the first graft is a technical failure with resultant necrosis, the second graft from the same donor will reject in the pattern of a first transplant.

# B. Modified Host

The data for this section are derived from personal experience and reports in the literature concerning human renal grafts. Many of the features observed in laboratory animals will be seen in human material. The rate at which these pathological processes occur is variable and no doubt depends on many factors, e.g., histocompatibility antigens, immunosuppressive drugs, and prior sensitization by leucocytes or organ grafts. In our early clinical experience, when corticosteroids were withheld until clinical evidence of graft rejection appeared, biopsy material of patients most closely resembled the described laboratory data. The current practice of giving large doses of corticosteroids immediately with the graft will modify the clinical and pathological findings. The pathology primarily involves the vessels, tubules and interstitium. The glomeruli show few changes early but may become devascularized as a result of progressive changes.

## 1. Interstitium

Cellular infiltration with mononuclears is common but varies greatly in degree. This may be associated with edema and may progress to fibrosis in cases where the process cannot be arrested.

## 2. Tubules

Tubular necrosis is usually seen only in a severe acute rejection. Atrophy following vascular injury, edema and interstitial fibrosis is more frequent in advanced rejection.

## 3. Glomeruli

As previously mentioned, the glomeruli are spared in the early attack; however, basement membrane thickening and inflammatory cells may be seen in a few cases. The late glomerular changes related to ischemia and the vascular disease are fibrosis of the tufts and periglomerular fibrosis. Fibrinoid necrosis of the afferent arteriole may extend into the glomerular capillaries. Hyperplasia and increased granularity of the juxtaglomerular body are rare.

## 4. Vessels

We have emphasized the early vascular changes, endothelial swelling and perivascular cuffing with mononuclear cells. Cellular, fibrin and platelet deposition

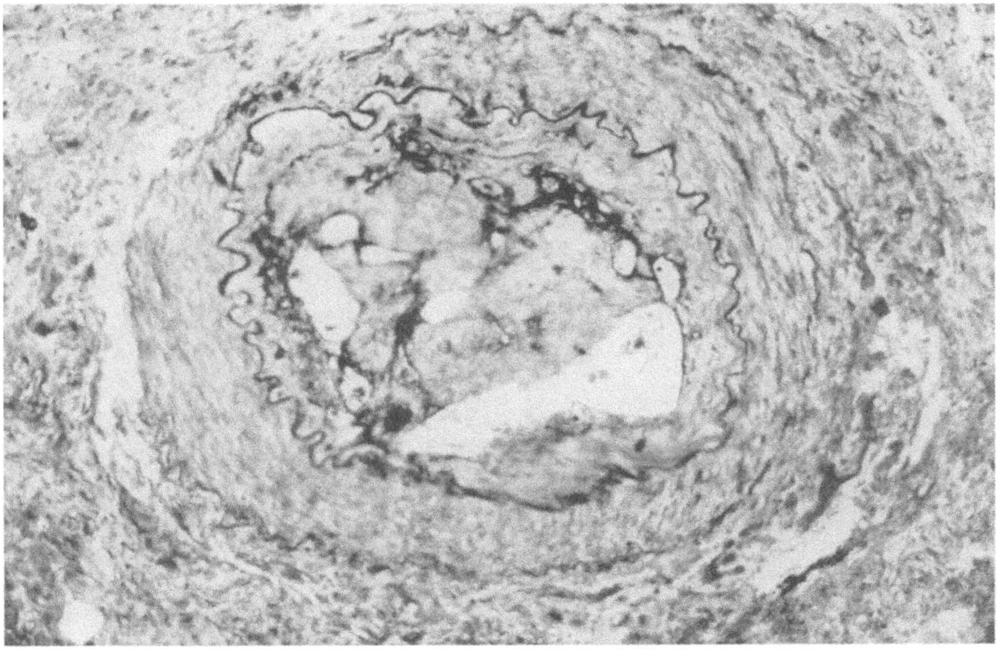

Fig. 35. Photomicrograph of a cadaver renal graft 56 days following transplantation. ×10. Phosphotungstic acid hematoxylin stain. Despite initial good function in the graft, the homograft rejection progressed to renal failure in 56 days. Vascular occlusion by fibrin and platelet thrombii was prominent

on the intima of arcuate and interlobar arteries progresses to fibrosis and progressive obliteration of the lumen. Many patients with relatively good function 1—2 years following transplantation are found to have marked narrowing of the vessels by intimal fibrosis. This is interpreted as the residual change of a prior, initially cellular, reaction. When the rejection reaction progresses unrestricted by immunosuppressives, we see large wedge-shaped cortical infarcts.

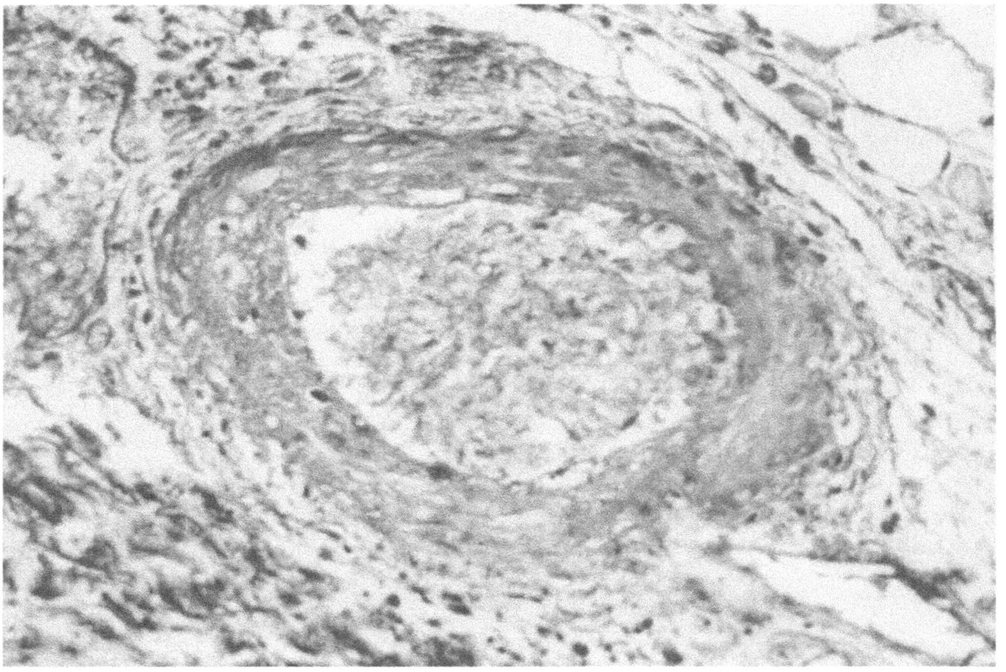

Fig. 36. Photomicrograph of a cadaver renal transplant 56 days post operative. ×10. Eosin von Giemsa stain. The severe vascular changes in this rapidly progressive rejection process include occlusion of the lumen and damage to the vessel wall

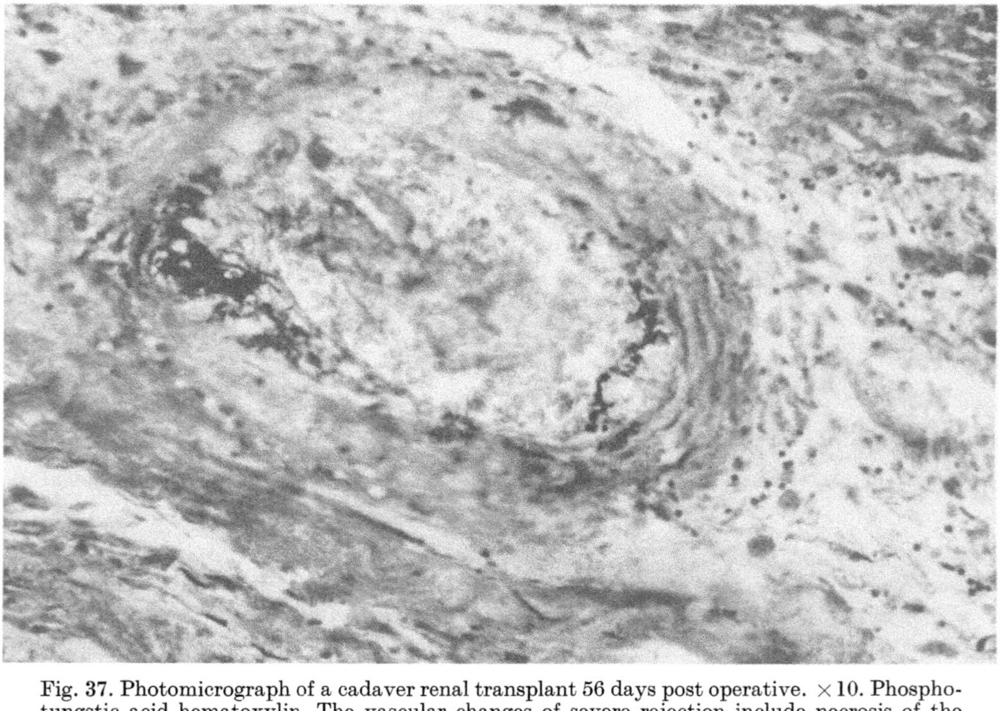

Fig. 37. Photomicrograph of a cadaver renal transplant 56 days post operative. ×10. Phosphotungstic acid hematoxylin. The vascular changes of severe rejection include necrosis of the vessel wall as illustrated here

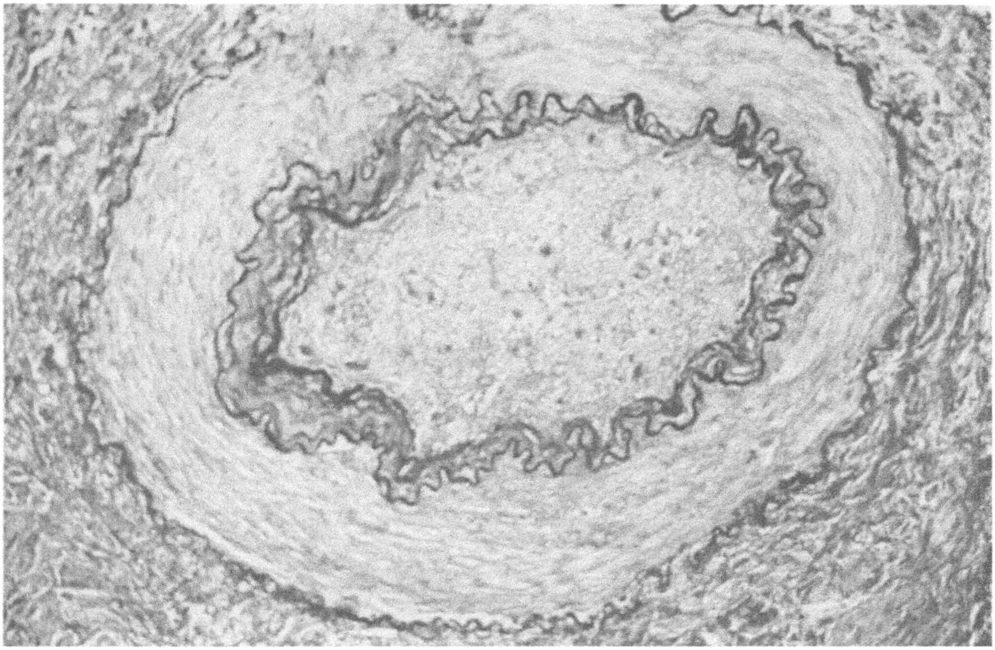

Fig. 38. Photomicrograph of a cadaver renal transplant 56 days post operative. ×10. Eosin von Giemsa. The most prominent vascular changes of the rejection process are vessel occlusion by fibrin and platelets. Duplication of the internal elastic lamina may occur as illustrated here

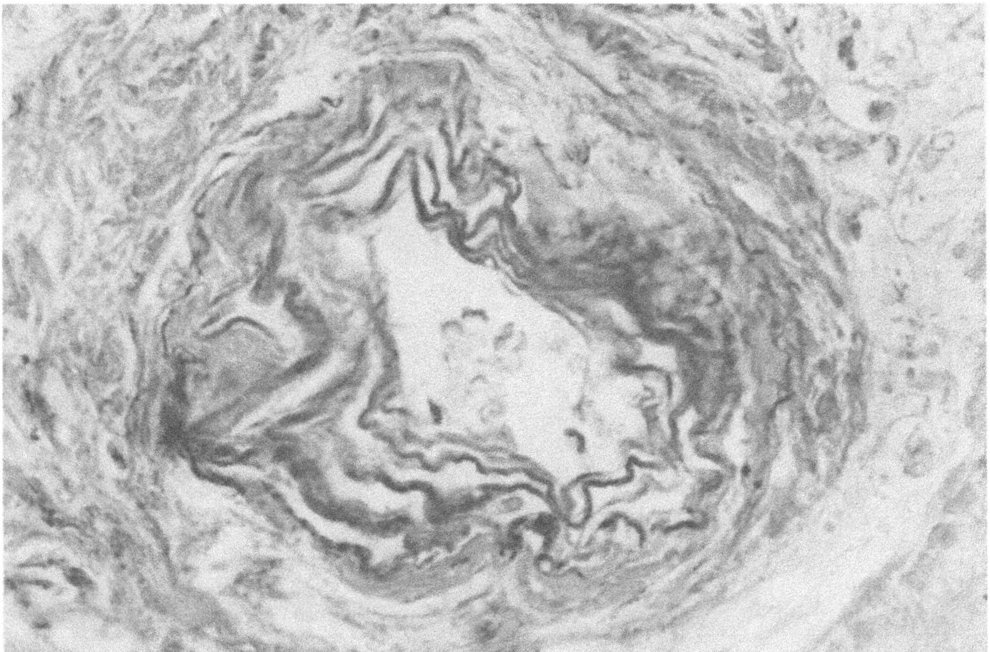

Fig. 39. Photomicrograph of a cadaver renal graft 56 days following transplantation. ×40. Eosin von Giemsa. The vascular changes of graft rejection include marked alteration of the elastic lamina as illustrated here

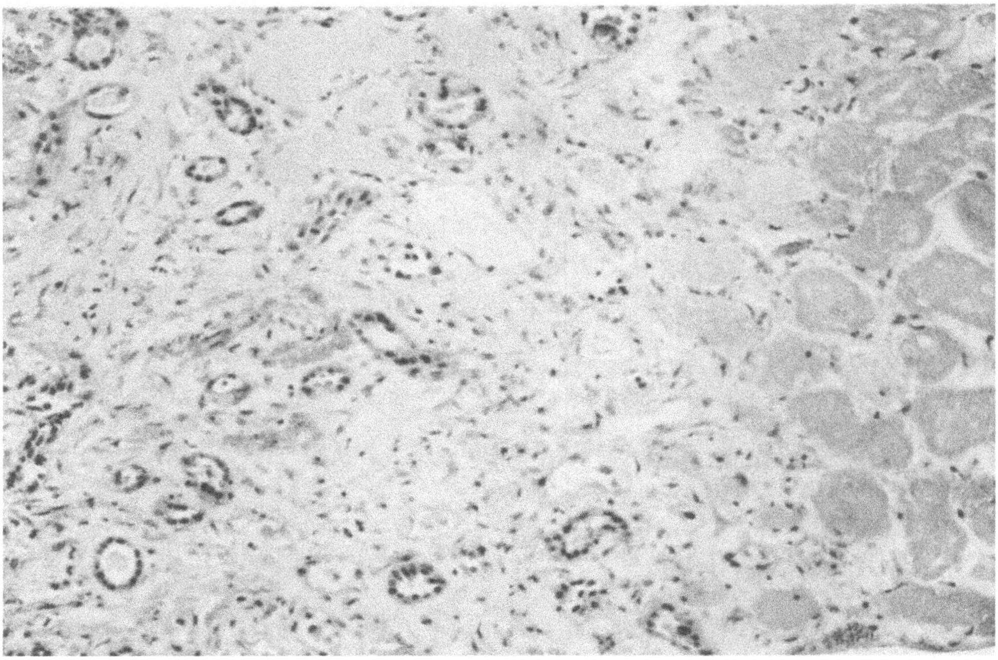

Fig. 40. Photomocrigraph of a cadaver renal transplant 56 days post-operative. ×10. Hematoxylin and eosin stain. The severe vascular changes result in tubular atrophy, interstitial fibrosis and frank cortical necrosis shown in this photo

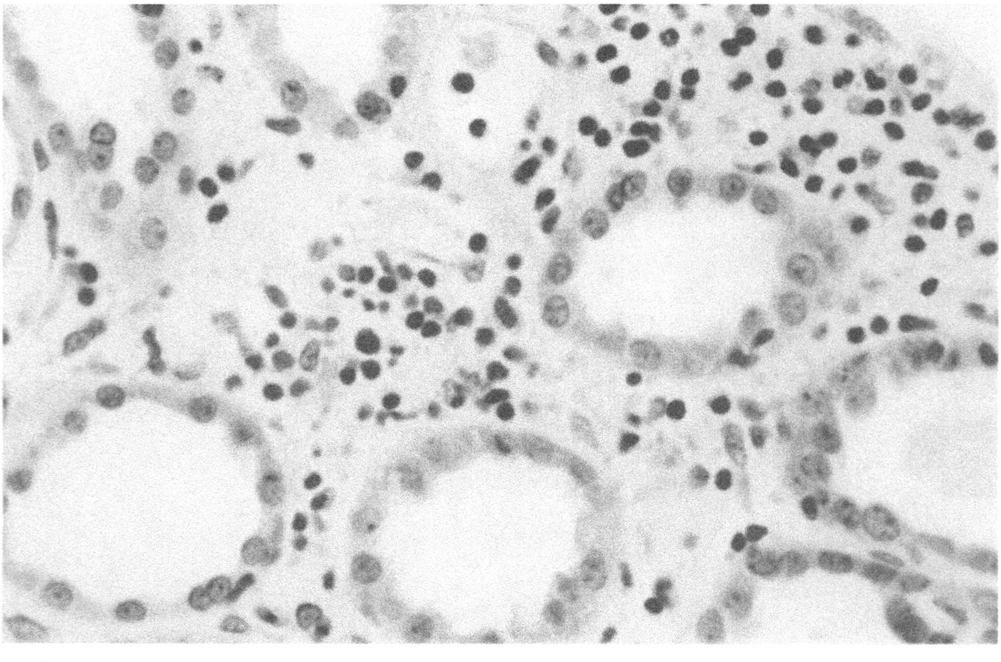

Fig. 41. Photomicrograph of a cadaver renal graft 56 days post operative. ×40. Hematoxylin and eosin stain. The severe vascular changes of rejection result in tubular epithelial injury. There is an accompanying interstitial cellular infiltrate

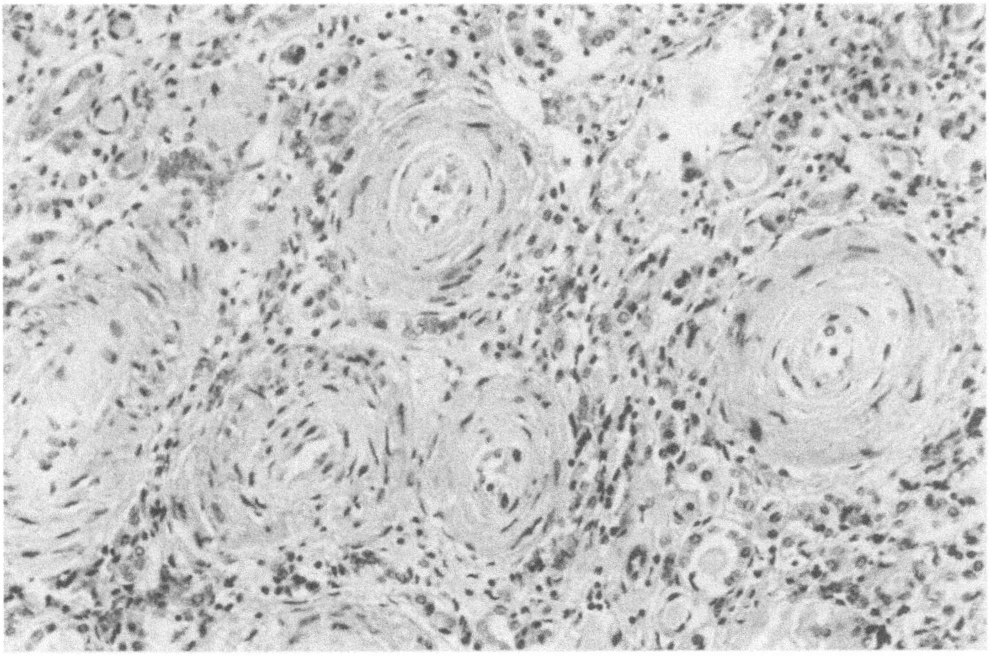

Fig. 42. Photomicrograph of a cadaver renal graft at necropsy 75 days post transplantation. ×10. Hematoxylin and eosin. The graft rejection is characterized by severe vascular intimal proliferation. Renal function deteriorated despite intensive immunosuppression

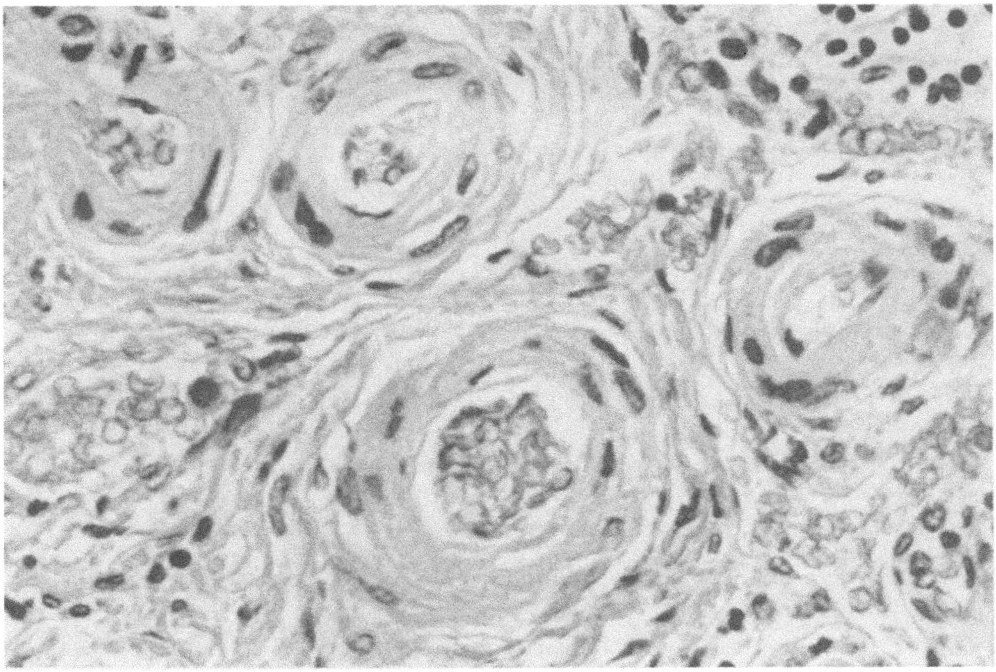

Fig. 43. Photomicrograph of a cadaver renal graft 75 days post transplantation. ×25. Hematoxylin and eosin. Progressive graft rejection despite vigorous immunosuppression was accompanied by vascular endothelial proliferation

Fibrinoid necrosis of the walls of the afferent arterioles is seen in patients with a progressive rejection reaction. These vascular changes are often accompanied by hypertension, raising the question as to which is primary — hypertension or vascular disorder. In view of the protean nature of the immunological attack on organ grafts, we believe the hypertension is secondary to anatomical pathology.

### 5. Ureter and Pelvis

The vessels of the ureter and renal pelvis are also involved in the pathological process. These changes are accompanied by interstitial edema and cellular infiltrates. It is not surprising that ureteral or pelvic necrosis with urinary extravasation may occur at any time after renal transplantation. In view of the slender ureteral blood supply, it is a wonder this complication does not occur more often.

The histology and function of renal grafts 2 or more years following transplantation has been correlated with lymphocyte antigen matching. Several reports suggest more compatible donor-recipient pairs have less anatomic pathology and better renal function (STARZL, 1965 [228]; OGDEN [178]).

## C. Circulating Antibodies

Patients exposed to leucocyte or tissue antigens (multiple transfusions, pregnancy, abortion, prior organ grafts) may develop circulating antibodies detectable by cytotoxicity or leucoagglutination (BERAH [27]; WILLIAMS [257]; WALFORD [252];

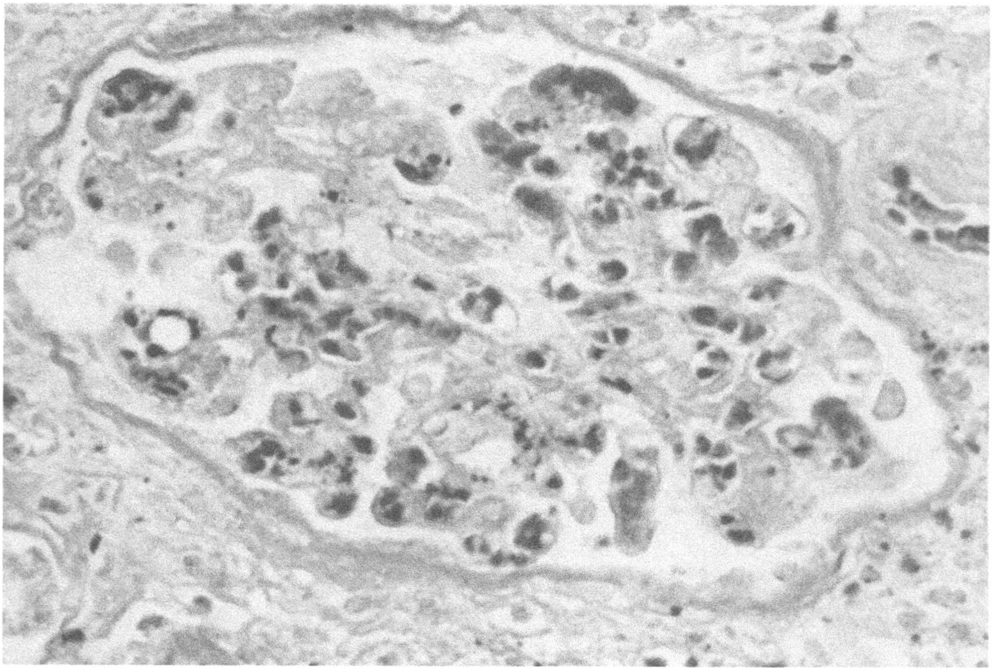

Fig. 44. Photomicrograph of a renal transplant 3 days postoperative. ×25. Phosphotungstic acid hematoxylin stain. This patient with circulating antibodies to lymphocyte antigens of the donor has fibrin and platelet thrombii in the glomerular loops. The rapidly progressive vascular lesions halt circulation through the kidney

LOSTUMBO [128]). When a renal graft is made from a donor with antigens to which a recipient has circulating antibodies, the pathological processes may proceed at a rapid rate. Kidneys have been observed to undergo a progressive loss of circulation in the cortex within minutes after completion of the vascular anastomosis. The organs become mottled, black and soft, despite widely patent primary anastomoses. This is similar to the pathology seen in transplantation between AB0 mismatched patients (e.g., A→0, B→A). The histopathology is similar to

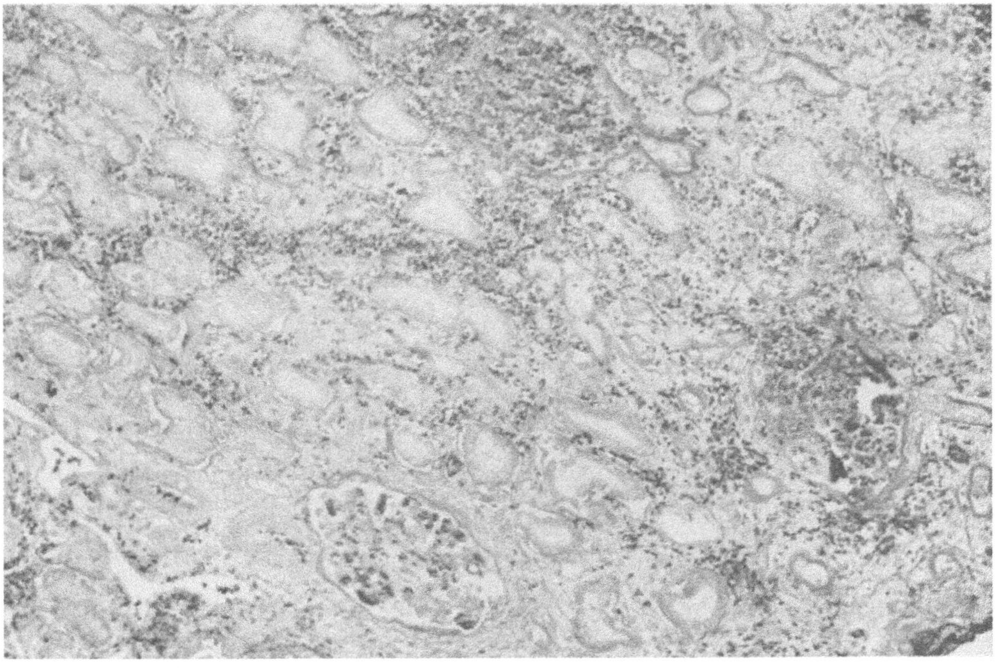

Fig. 45. Photomicrograph of a renal transplant 3 days postoperative. ×25. Phosphotungstic acid hematoxylin stain. This recipient had circulating antibodies to the lymphocyte antigens of the donor. There is a marked cellular infiltrate and tubular necrosis accompanied by vascular occlusion with fibrin and platelet thrombii. These changes begin minutes after vascularization of the graft

the vascular changes previously described, with cellular and fibrin deposition occluding the lumen. The resultant cortical necrosis may occur in minutes, hours or days (WILLIAMS [257]). The degree of fibrin deposition may be more marked, leading some to suggest an analogy with the Schwartzman reaction (STARZL [222]; KISSMEYER-NIELSEN [112]). The process is likely due in part to the presence of performed antibodies which immediately attack the graft and accelerate the pathological changes.

In view of the prominence of fibrin deposition and similarity to the Schwartzman reaction, the use of heparin has been recommended (STARZL [222]). This is supported by recent laboratory experiments (DUBERNARD [57]). Patients with known circulating antibodies can be successfully transplanted from donors who do not have antigens to which these antibodies react (STEWART [229]; PATEL [184]).

All recipients should be tested for the presence of circulating antibodies prior to transplantation. Blood transfusions should not contain white blood cells, to minimize this source of sensitization.

### D. Glomerulonephritis

#### 1. Identical Twins

Recurrent glomerulonephritis is a frequent observation in renal transplantation between identical twins. Glassock reviewed the experience at the Brigham Hospital (Boston) and found 11 of 18 recipients with glomerulonephritis had evidence of recurrent disease in the graft. Seven patients had died one month to seven years following discovery of recurrent nephritis. Six deaths were due to renal failure and one to a myocardial infarction (Glassock [69]).

#### 2. Non Twins

As previously emphasized, the glomerulus is spared in the early events of the graft rejection process. A few reports of the primary glomerular disease developing in a homograft are to be found in the literature (Krieg [120]; Zukoski [271]; Hallenbeck [77]; O'Brien [175]); however, this is uncommon. It would appear that recipients with a short history and rapidly progressive course of their disease are more likely to develop glomerulonephritis in a homograft. Circulating antibodies to glomerular basement membranes can be detected in some laboratories. This should be looked for in suspected cases where the pathological process is proliferative glomerulonephritis and is rapidly progressive. One patient in Richmond developed a glomerulonephritis in the graft despite a primary disease of pyelonephritis (O'Brien [175]).

Najarian surveyed many transplantation centers and determined only 10 cases of well documented glomerulonephritis occurred in more than 1,000 recipients (Najarian [167]).

## X. Antigen Identification and "Matching"

### A. Introduction

The identification of those cellular antigens involved in the homograft rejection process has been the goal of many determined investigators. Recognition of these antigens would provide the clinician with a system for selection of donor-recipient pairs ("matching"). Histocompatibility antigens are presently detected only with biological tests. Chemical definition is a rather distant goal at this time.

Clinical organ transplantation has provided both a strong stimulus and a valuable biologic standard for data regarding antigens and matching. The parenchymal organ transplant with its gross vascular attachments behaves in a different manner from skin grafts, and suppression or reversal of the homograft reaction process in organ grafts provides data not advailable from skin experiment. Red and white cell antigens appear to be involved in the organ graft rejection process.

### B. Red Blood Cell Antigens

In the early clinical experience, renal transplants between individuals with incompatible red blood cell types appeared to be successful (Starzl [223]). Further clinical experience revealed that many grafts between such pairs would undergo an intravascular red cell agglutination resulting in immediate failure. This process usually occurred within a matter of minutes after restoration of circulation; however, it was occasionally seen one to two days later. The cortex of the kidney became progressively cyanotic and black in these patients, with the gross pathology progressing to total cortical necrosis. The danger of such a disaster made AB0 incompatible transplants inadvisable. Subsequent investigations with human skin grafts indicate that red cell antigens also play a role in graft survival (CEPPELLINI, 1966 [43]; DAUSSET [52]). Renal transplant donor and recipient should be of the same AB0 blood type to eliminate the risk of immediate intravascular agglutination and to reduce the histocompatibility differences.

## C. Leucocyte Antigens

The identification of leucocyte antigens by serologic methods is one of many developments from the effort to achieve successful organ transplantation. There are six antigens recognized by investigators all over the world. These are designated by a new nomenclature: HL-A 1,2,3,5,7,8. The HL stands for "human leucocyte", and A designates the first locus identified. All six antigens are at one locus of one chromosome.

### 1. Lymphocyte Cytotoxicity

Several immunological techniques (cytotoxicity, agglutination, immune adherence) can be utilized to identify these antigens, but cytotoxicity is probably in widest use. This test is made by isolating lymphocytes from the blood by hemolysis

*Terasaki criteria for matching grades*

A = Occasional mismatch with isolated sera
B = Several mismatches with isolated sera
C = Definite mismatch in 1 recognized group
D = Definite mismatch in 2 or more recognized groups

Fig. 46. Terasaki criteria for matching donor and recipient on the basis of in vitro lymphocyte cytotoxicity

of red cells and selective adherence of granulocytes to plastic mesh. The lymphocytes are incubated with antisera and rabbit complement for 1—4 hours. Cell death is determined by morphology in phase microscopy; Trypan blue exclusion may be used if desired to separate living from dead cells. The percentage of killing determines whether the reaction is positive or negative.

The sera initially employed contained polyvalent antibodies occuring in women after multiple pregnancies or abortions (TERASAKI, 1964 [234]). They can be developed by skin and organ grafts or by injection of lymphocytes (WALFORD, 1965 [253]). The leucocyte antigens appear to be shared by all nucleated cells. The existence of organ specific antigens has not been proved, although they may occur as, for example, tumor specific antigens do (PREHN [192]).

Early efforts to relate the success of kidney transplants to the "match" of lymphocyte antigens were encouraging (TERASAKI, 1965 [235]). These studies were retrospective and involved primarily living related donors. A prospective study of living unrelated renal donors was undertaken in Denver, where prisoners in the state penitentiary volunteered, and the results supported the concept of antigen matching for selection of donor-recipient pairs (TERASAKI, 1966 [237]). The survival of human skin grafts has been observed to correlate with the match of lymphocyte antigens (WALFORD [253]). Several major transplantation centers have since pooled their resources to utilize matching in cadaver renal transplantation (Patel, 1968 [182]; van Rood [247]; Morris [160]). The data are scant, but there is a consistent trend to better graft function in matched pairs.

The heterogenous distribution of antigens makes it difficult to obtain the most favorable match in many cases. In the greater Los Angeles area, with a population well in excess of seven million, only 34% of the cadaver kidneys transplanted in eight cooperating hospitals were compatible. This is caused in part by the donor institution utilizing one kidney and sending the second to the best match at another hospital. If all kidneys were "pooled", the ratio of matched kidneys could be increased to 80%. To evaluate the potential benefit of antigen matching, a large number of recipients should be available for a given kidney. This involves regional or national cooperative studies; adequate preservation of the graft must be available for transportation to a remote recipient.

## 2. Other Tests of Leucocyte Antigens

1. Mixed lymphocyte culture. Lymphocytes of two individuals with different antigenic compositions proliferate in an accelerated manner in vitro, and in vitro incubation has been proposed as a method of detecting antigenic differences for organ grafting (Hirschhorn [86]). It has the advantage of not requiring a number of different antisera which may not represent all antigens involved; it has the distinct disadvantage for clinical application of requiring 1—2 days. In mixed culture one cannot determine the direction of incompatibility. Attempts have been made to identify this direction by inactivation of one antigen with nitrogen mustard, which adds further to the complexity of the test but appears to provide the desired information (Ceppelini, 1965 [44]).

2. Normal lymphocyte transfer. Brent and Medawar observed varying degrees of cutaneous reaction from intradermal injection of lymphocytes in guinea pigs and found that these reactions were related to the antigenic differences of the animals and could be correlated with survival of skin grafts (Brent [33]). They believe the intradermal reaction which produces erythema and edema results from the immunologically competent cells reacting to host antigens. Clinical application of this test in Boston has not been entirely satisfactory (Gray [74]; Carpenter [40]). Carpenter found that the lymphocytes of uremic individuals produced a poor reaction. This observation was controlled by testing with cells from identical twins. He believes the reaction is more likely host versus lymphocyte graft. Clinical experience with the normal leucocyte transfer test indicated it had predictive value for those patients who would do well clinically after grafting (Carpenter [40]). However, a strong reaction does not always mean a poor prognosis. This is analogous to lymphocyte cytotoxicity tests, where many "mismatched" patients appear to do well clinically, at least for 1—2 years.

3. Irradiated hamster. The lethally irradiated hamster has been employed as an immunologically indifferent milieu for histocompatibility testing. Lymphocytes from pairs of test individuals injected intradermally produce a skin reaction related to the degree of compatibility. In comparison with skin grafts, the pair of test subjects with the longest skin graft survivals had the least reaction in the hamster. This complicated biological technique involves mixed cells, so the direction of incompatibility is not determined. The test has not achieved widespread acceptance.

4. Leucocyte agglutination. Agglutination of leucocytes (granulocytes and lymphocytes) by sera originally obtained from multiparous women has been widely applied in the identification and elucidation of leucocyte antigens concerned with organ grafting (Payne, 1964 [186)]. A retrospective analysis of leuco-

agglutination testing with clinical renal transplants has indicated a favorable correlation. Fourteen of 23 related donor grafts were found to be compatible, but not identical, with seven antigens tested. The clinical course of the kidney graft correlated with the laboratory findings of antigen compatibility (Payne, 1967 [185]).

5. Immune adherence. The complex of antibodies on cellular antigens can be detected with indicator red blood cells in the immune adherence technique described by Melief (Melief [147]). This test has several advantages over other serologic tests. The quality of test cells is less critical, as dead cells do not result in a false positive reaction, and the technique can be applied to skin fibroblasts and renal cells as well as lymphocytes. A preliminary report of immune adherence tests with renal cells in monolayer culture using 20 antisera revealed a greater number of reactions with renal cells than with lymphocytes (Williams [259]), which suggests this technique may detect antigens on renal cells which are either not present or less reactive on lymphocytes.

### D. Direct Cross-Match of Recipient Serum and Donor Leucocytes

In addition to providing valuable information for selection of donor-recipient pairs, serologic methods can alert the surgeon to the danger of immediate graft failure due to preformed antibodies. As previously mentioned, these antibodies can develop as a result of prior pregnancy, abortion, transfusion or organ grafts, and they must be looked for in all prospective organ recipients. In an analysis of 681 prospective recipients, Patel found 15% of the males and 25% of the females had preformed cytotoxic antibodies. In 80% of the cases where the antibodies of the recipient killed the lymphocytes of the donor in vitro, immediate failure of the renal graft was observed (Patel, 1969 [184]).

A direct cross match with incubation of donor cells, recipient serum and complement for evidence of cytotoxic activity is indicated before all organ transplants to avoid immediate failure.

The pathological changes in the grafts of recipients with preformed antibodies have been described in Chapter IX.

### Summary

The application of our knowledge of the leucocyte antigens to selection of renal donors offers great promise for improved results in organ transplants. The early results (3—6 months) do not correlate as well as do the long-term results (1—3 years).

# XI. Thymectomy and Splenectomy

## A. Thymectomy

### 1. Introduction

The use of ablative surgery to modify the lymphatic (immunologic) system in the human involves a complex problem. A great deal of data has accumulated from efforts to elucidate the role of lymphocytes in graft rejection. Alteration of the lymphatic system by irradiation, extirpation, thoracic duct drainage, antimetabolites, alkylating agents, corticosteroids, and antilymphocyte sera will depress the host reaction to tissue and organ transplants. However, all of these modalities have a gross effect on many cell types, so the mechanism of action remains unclear. Studies on the evolution of the lymphatic system suggest more than one anatomical origin, with initially separate and well defined functions. The thymus, first seen in the lamprey, can be shown to play a major role in delayed hypersensitivity and homograft rejection reaction. The ability to produce circulating antibody develops with the appearance of the thymus and, more importantly, with the development of spleen and lymph structures in the gut. The anatomical separation of the two action mechanisms, cellular and humoral, of the immunological system is most distinct in the chicken, which has a discrete lymphatic organ in relation to the hindgut, the bursa of Fabricius (Cooper [48]). Ablation of this bursa in the chick allows the animal to reject skin grafts, but no antibody will be formed (Glick [70]). The clinical syndrome analogous to this laboratory experiment is the sex-linked congenital agammaglobulinemia of the Bruton type. Children with this condition reject skin grafts but never form antibodies (Bruton, 1952 [36]). The thymus is of normal size and architecture; blood lymphocytes are normal, but no plasma cells form.

Ablation of the thymus in the chick interferes with graft rejection primarily and with antibody production to a lesser extent. A clinical syndrome comparable to the loss of both organs is the Swiss type of lymphopenic agammaglobulinemia, in which both cellular and humoral components are lacking due to deficiency of the early primordia. Children with this condition accept skin grafts and do not form antibodies. Death from infection usually occurs at an early age.

Thymectomy in the neonatal mouse has a profound effect upon the immunological response to tissue grafts (Miller, 1962 [152]). The removal of the thymus in an adult rodent has a less striking effect (Miller [153]; Monaco [155]).

Adult thymectomy in man might be expected to play a minor role in immunological reactivity. Cells with the same function as thymocytes in the neonatal mouse are likely distributed to the bone marrow and other organs in man (Nossal [174]; Murray [166]). Evidence for this theory comes from the distinctive differences in life span. In contrast to the long-lived small lymphocyte, thymus and bone marrow lymphocytes in rodents have a rapid rate of replacement and short life span (Craddock, 1965 [50]). In a clinical experiment, thymectomy in children undergoing thoracotomy did not immediately alter their ability to reject skin grafts (Zollinger [270]). However, the effect of adult thymectomy on immunological reaction may not be observed for years. In rodents the immunological deficit following adult thymectomy is not apparent for weeks or years, occurring as a progressive "decay" of the immunological responses (Taylor [233]; Metcalf [150]).

## 2. Clinical Renal Transplantation

A group of renal graft recipients were subjected to thymectomy in the early cases at Denver (Starzl [227]). A number of these patients fared extremely well, with many years of stable renal function and minimal pathological damage of the graft, on small doses of immunosuppressive drugs. The role of thymectomy in the favorable immunological course of these grafts is open for speculation, since a control study is not available and many other patients in Denver and elsewhere have followed a comparable course without thymectomy.

Adult thymectomy was used briefly in Cleveland but abandoned when incomplete removal of the thymus by the transcervical route was observed. No morbidity or mortality was observed due to this procedure (Kiser [111]).

At the present time it seems reasonable to conclude there is no proven advantage of thymectomy in adults undergoing organ transplants. Thymectomy may not result in changes in the immunological reaction for a number of years; thus a controlled study of long-term cases is needed for better evaluation.

## B. Splenectomy

### 1. Introduction

While thymectomy has been used infrequently in the recipients of clinical renal transplants, splenectomy has often been employed in a number of centers. This is due in part to accessibility of the spleen during the removal of the recipient's diseased kidneys.

### 2. Laboratory Data

In adult mice, splenectomy will be associated with prolongation of skin graft survival (WERDER [255]). Splenectomy with canine renal homotransplantation has not prolonged function in the graft (KOUNTZ [115]; VEITH [248, 249]).

### 3. Clinical Data

Splenectomy may be performed prior to or at the time of renal transplantation.

Favorable reports from Denver were a significant factor in the widespread use of splenectomy in renal transplant recipients. Renal graft success in Denver was associated with the use of large doses of azathioprine and prednisone, and it appeared the patients in the Denver series tolerated larger doses of the antimetabolite. This was considered possibly due to splenectomy, which will produce peripheral leucocytosis. Subsequent reviews of large numbers of patients and other laboratory data indicate that splenectomy does not increase tolerance to azathioprine.

Statistical data to indicate the beneficial role of splenectomy in the renal graft recipient has not accumulated. From laboratory experiments with dogs and clinical data at the Brigham hospital, VEITH concluded splenectomy did not allow the use of increased doses of azathioprine nor did it mitigate graft rejection crises. In two small parallel series he observed more frequent rejection episodes in splenectomized patients (VEITH [249]). KISER reported that three patients with severe leucopenia tolerated larger doses of azathioprine following removal of the spleen. Two patients with persistent leucocytosis tolerated increased immunosuppressive drug therapy, which reversed the graft rejection; the third patient died of sepsis with recurrent leucopenia (KISER [111]).

HUME compared 31 splenectomized renal recipients with 51 non-splenectomized recipients. He observed a four-fold increase in thromboembolic phenomena and a two-fold increase in infections in the splenectomized patients. There was no overall difference in patient survival (HUME [89]; PIERCE [188]).

Platelets were increased in most patients undergoing splenectomy. In view of the role of the clotting factors fibrin and platelets in the vascular aspects of the homograft rejection, one can speculate that increased circulatory platelets may be deleterious.

In summary it is possible to conclude that thymectomy and splenectomy play a minor role, if any, in the immunological fate of whole organ transplants in man. Laboratory results from small animals were not reproduced in canine experiments. Controlled series with a long period of observation may be necessary to fully evaluate the role of thymectomy.

# XII. Renal Preservation

## A. Introduction

In all transplantation there is an interval of variable duration when the organ is deprived of its normal circulation. If this interval is short (20—30 min), there is little detectable alteration in function. This is usually the case in renal transplantation from a living donor where the two procedures of nephrectomy and implantation are coordinated to reduce ischemic time to the minimum.

From our laboratory work with dogs we have found that the kidney suffers no detectable injury with 15 min of euthermic ischemia. A slight, transient depression of renal function occurs with 30 min of ischemia at 37° C. When animals are sustained by only the test organs after one hour of ischemia, there will be moderate alteration in renal function with transient azotemia, but all survive. One half of the animals sustained by test organs after 90 min of ischemia at 37° C will survive, and the other half will die. Transplantation of organs after 120 min of renal ischemia will be fatal to most experimental animals. These are the results of experiments in our laboratory and set the guidelines for work on renal preservation.

Laboratory experiments with renal preservation consist primarily of those using canine renal autotransplant models. Many early experiments were concerned with animal survival only, and a normal contralateral organ was frequently left in situ for 2—3 weeks to maintain the animal while the test organ recovered from injury, often acute tubular necrosis. These experiments are of general interest, but they are not of great practical concern as the surgeon does not wish to subject the kidney to injury during the time it is ex vivo.

These early experiments are to be contrasted with those more recent ones in which we attempted to determine the limits of preservation of the kidney without detectable functional or anatomical injury from storage. In these latter experiments total renal function is provided by the experimental organ.

Preservation of the kidney may be approached with either of two goals: 1. Maximum protection of the organ for short-term storage, 2. Maintenance of the organ from limited storage or, 3. Permanent preservation. The former are available today and have great clinical application; the latter is not available, and the means of achieving permanent preservation are complex.

## B. Short-Term Storage

In our laboratory we have found the canine renal autograft maintains excellent function after eight hours of ex vivo storage at 5—7° C. Surface cooling is as efficacious as any perfusion technique we have employed and has the advantage of simplicity, eliminating the complications of perfusion, most notably that of injury or obstruction of the vascular tree resulting in infarction. Cooling to 5—7° C by perfusion or surface cooling alone for eight hours can preserve the canine kidney so that there is no detectable difference in renal function when compared with a kidney autotransplanted without storage.

These observations support previous reports (KISER [109]). FISHER et al., found canine kidneys supported life when cooled for 12 hours (FISHER [65]). In a careful study of the histology by light and electron microscopy, FISHER and his coworkers found minimal alteration of the ultrastructure after 12 hours. Survival precipitously decreased when kidneys were maintained at 1—5° C outside the body for 15 hours or more. These organs exhibited more pronounced changes in subcellular organization.

It appears from the laboratory experiments that the canine kidney can be well preserved for 12 hours by surface cooling to 1—5° C alone. These organs support life and demonstrate excellent function immediately. Cold storage for 15 hours or more will result in some mortality and definite alterations in function and structure. Some dogs can survive on kidneys maintained cold ex vivo for

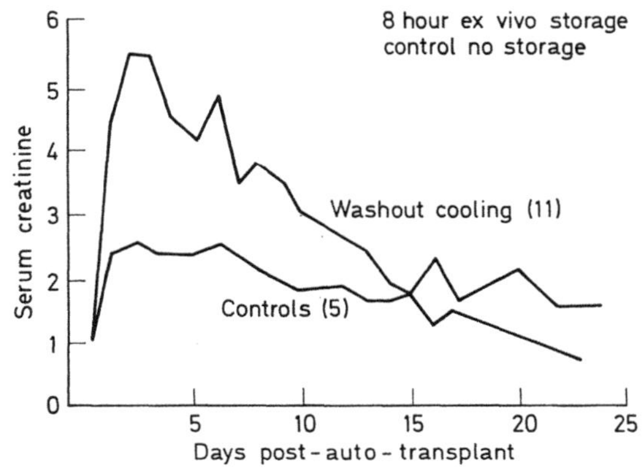


Fig. 47. Renal preservation — canine experiments. Control animals had renal autotransplantation and contralateral nephrectomy. The mean of daily serum creatinine determination is plotted to demonstrate the quality of renal function. Experimental animals had renal autotransplantation following 8 hours of cold storage and immediate contralateral nephrectomy. The kidneys were cooled by intra arterial infusion of cold salt solution

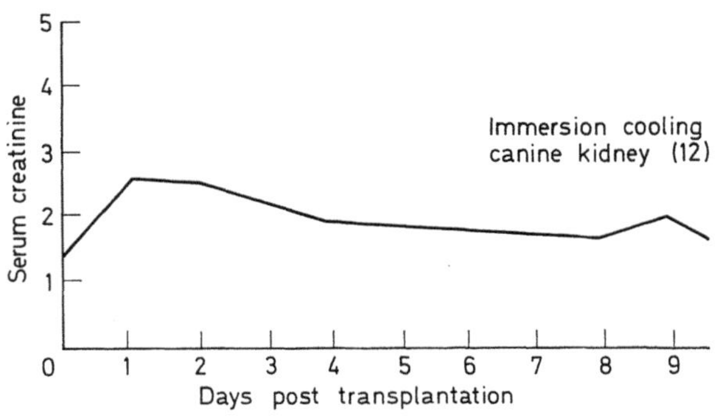


Fig. 48. Renal preservation — canine experiments. The mean of daily serum creatinine is plotted to demonstrate excellent renal function after 8 hours of cold storage without perfusion. The contralateral kidney was removed at reimplantation

24 hours, but in most reports in the literature a contralateral normal organ was left in situ for three weeks to maintain the dog over the interval of impaired renal function in the graft (Hendry [81]).

Hyperbaric oxygen has no proven beneficial role in kidneys preserved by cooling (Manax [130]; Makin [129]).

## C. Long-Term Preservation

To maintain homeostasis in the preserved organ beyond 12 hours, it is necessary to provide an artificial circulation. This problem has an interesting history, going back to the experiments of CARREL and LINDBERG (HUMPHRIES [93]). Early attempts to support the canine kidney with an extracorporeal pump and whole blood were singularly unsuccessful. The kidneys soon swelled, vascular resistance increased, and renal function ceased. The major difficulties were overcome by use of non-cellular perfusate with careful regulation of pressure, pH, and temperature. The canine kidney has been maintained on perfusion for 72 hours (BELZER [25]) and 120 hours (HUMPHRIES [94]) with life sustaining function on re-implantation. These dogs have a transient azotemia, but survive. Although they exhibit renal damage, it is reversible.

This technique has been applied to human cadaveric renal transplantation with success after 17 hours of storage (BELZER, 1968 [26]). The apparatus is relatively complex. The perfusate is homologous plasma which has fibrin and lipids removed by filtration after cooling. These steps are extremely important as lipids and fibrin precipitate out of cooled plasma and will plug arterioles and glomeruli during cold perfusion. A simplified system of low flow, low pressure, single pass perfusion has been suggested by HERRMANN and TURCOTTE (HERRMANN [82]). While this may extend preservation beyond cold storage alone, it is associated with renal injury.

We have found no advantage to a low flow (100 ml/hour) perfusion at 5—7° C for eight-hour storage.

## D. Permanent Preservation

Cellular homogenates are preserved indefinitely by freezing to −180° C with liquid nitrogen. These cells are protected from the destructive effects of freezing by suspension in glycerol or dimethyl sulfoxide, which hold cellular water in solution to reduce crystal formation. Permanent storage of the kidney awaits the application of these principles to whole organs.

## E. Tests of Renal Injury

In the clinical setting there is frequently an interval of warm ischemia prior to or after death which results in renal injury before preserving techniques can be established. This injury is difficult to evaluate in clinical cases. MANAX et al., found that profound hypothermia (28° C) prior to death conveyed a significant protective effect to canine kidneys (MANAX [131]). We have attempted to determine the extent of renal injury prior to nephrectomy in the cadaver by evaluation of metabolism in the tubular cells of the renal cortex with a tetrazolium dye. The dehydrogenase enzymes produce a color change in the dye on the surface of the cells. The time required for a color change is related to the renal injury; the longer the ischemia time, the slower the color change (TERASAKI [236]; SMITH [218]). Clinical application of this tetrazolium test to a small biopsy of cadaveric kidneys has allowed the transplantation of organs of questionable viability prior to testing (SMITH [217]).

The effects of the agonal events on renal architecture and function are difficult to evaluate. Fig. 49 shows the physiological parameters in a cadaveric renal donor just prior to death. Despite a warm ischemic time after death of 35 min, and a total of 215 min without circulation, this kidney resumed function after recovering from acute tubular necrosis. We have documented the acute tubular necrosis in several cadaveric organs. It appears no different histologically from that due to other forms of ischemia or toxicity. The recovery may be complete and of long duration. Although acute tubular necrosis is a significant renal injury

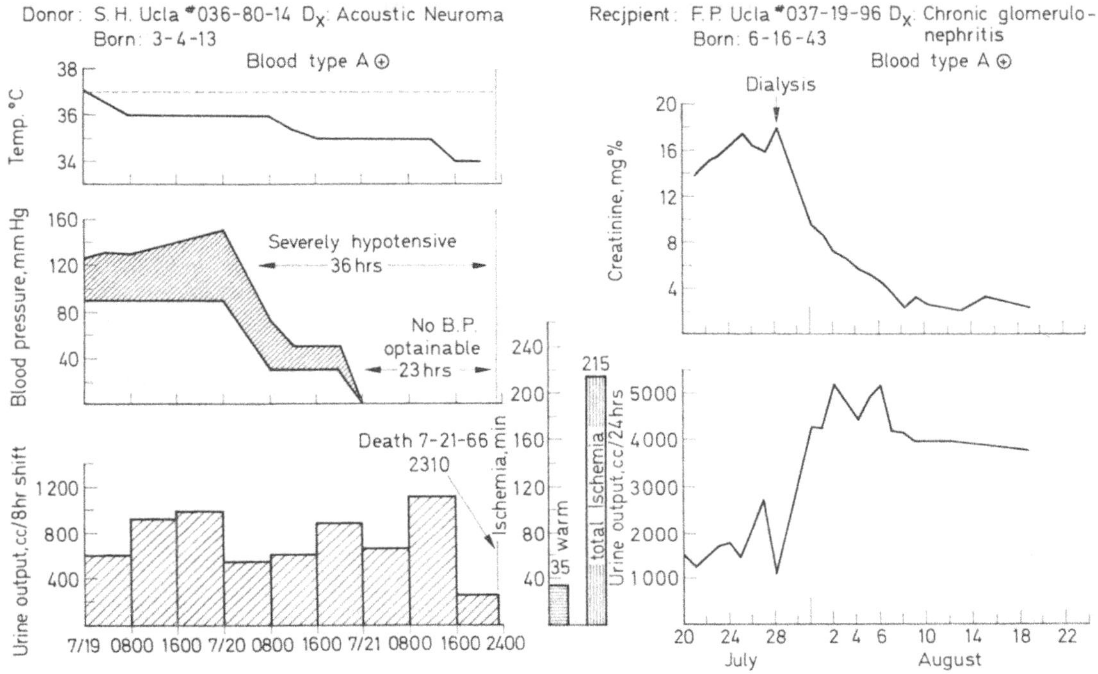


Fig. 49. Chart of the physiological parameters of an organ donor prior to death and subsequent course of the recipient

and complicates the post transplantation management of cadaveric renal recipients, it is compatible with recovery of excellent renal function and long-term survival.

## F. Biochemical Methods of Enhancing Organ Tolerance to Ischemia

As described previously, cold and/or maintenance of an "artificial" circulation are established methods of preserving organs out of the body. The application of biochemical and pharmacologic agents to increase cellular tolerance to ischemia has been little explored. Corticosteroids have been suggested to stabilize cellular membranes (YAMADA [268]). Phenothiazines may inhibit cellular metabolism and prevent intracellular disruption (EYAL [62]). A mercurial diuretic may alter cellular metabolism of renal tubular cells to increase tolerance to ischemia (CLUNEY [45]).

These may prove areas of promise for investigation in the future.

# XIII. Unusual Cases

## A. Introduction

All the backache and heartbreak of working in the field of renal dialysis and transplantation is relieved by the rewards of seeing a chronically ill patient restored to full rehabilitation. Many interesting and unusual events occur to intrigue the surgeon and stimulate scientific curiosity. The prolongation of life by dialysis and/or transplantation has led to the development of new disease or the revelation of pathology previously masked by renal failure. Neuropathy and hyperparathyroidism of renal failure were minor problems until the life of these patients was greatly prolonged.

## B. Erythremia

Anemia is responsible for many of the symptoms in chronic renal failure, and spontaneous recovery from anemia is one of the remarkable benefits of successful renal transplantation. The return to normal hemoglobin and red

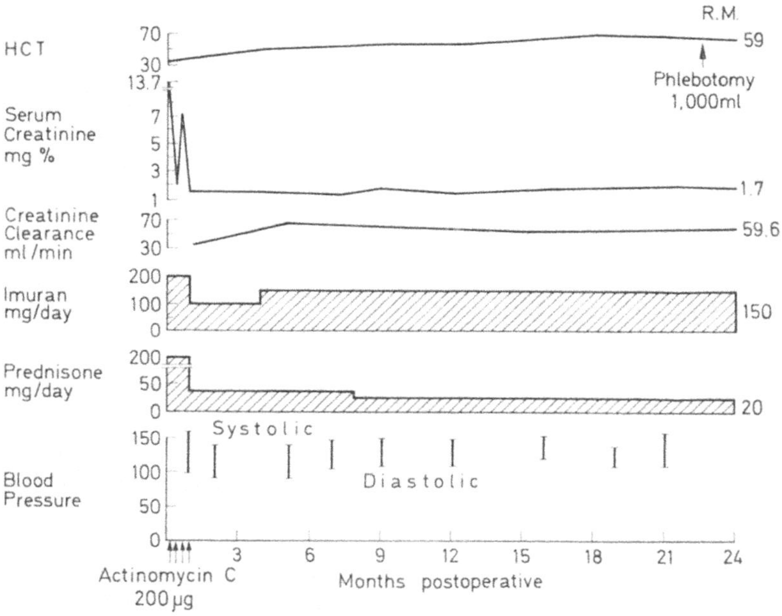


Fig. 50. Clinical course of a 37 year old male with polycystic renal disease whe received a kidney from his mother July 5, 1964. Persistent erythremia was treated with monthly phlebotomy. This patient recently recovered from myocardial infarction with stable renal function

blood cell levels is likely a major reason transplant recipients feel better than chronic dialysis patients do. Several studies point to the grafted kidney as the source of erythropoietin responsible for the cure of anemia (DENNY [54]; ABBRECHT [2]). It is of interest that this mechanism can "overshoot" the normal level to produce erythremia (NIES [172]; MARTIN, 1967 [135]; SWALES [232]). We have observed several patients develop a hematocrit level above 50% following successful transplantation. In most cases this will gradually resolve to normal levels, although two patients in the U.C.L.A. series have required repeated phlebotomy to maintain the hematocrit below 60% (MARTIN, 1967 [135]; REEVE [194]). Renal ischemia due to immunological reaction has been suggested as a pathological cause for excessive erythropoietin release from the kidney. However, both of our patients at U.C.L.A. had good, stable renal function for months and years following transplantation, casting doubt on this theory of the cause of erythremia.

## C. Renovascular Hypertension

Hypertension following renal transplantation is usually accompanied by signs of a homograft rejection process and may be due to renal ischemia, as the vascular tree is a center of the graft rejection process. Decreased renal blood flow is a characteristic of this event. Stenosis at the arterial anastomosis can also produce renal ischemia and hypertension (NEWTON [171]). The transplanted kidney behaves like any other in response to severe arterial stenosis and its relief (SMELLIE [215]).

## D. Pregnancy

The return of health in renal graft recipients is clearly documented by the ability to pass through pregnancy successfully. There are several reports in the literature of successful childbirth following transplantation. The first occurred in identical twin transplants, but others have been reported following homotransplantation (KAUFMAN [104]; HUME [89]; MURRAY [165]). Two females in the U.C.L.A. series have delivered healthy sons by the vaginal route; two male recipients have sired two sons (we have a new formula to produce male heirs!). The potential teratogenic effects of azathioprine have not been seen.

## E. Transplantation of Disease

### 1. Carcinomas

Not all of the unusual observations following renal transplantation are favorable. Carcinoma cells transplanted with the kidney can proliferate rapidly and

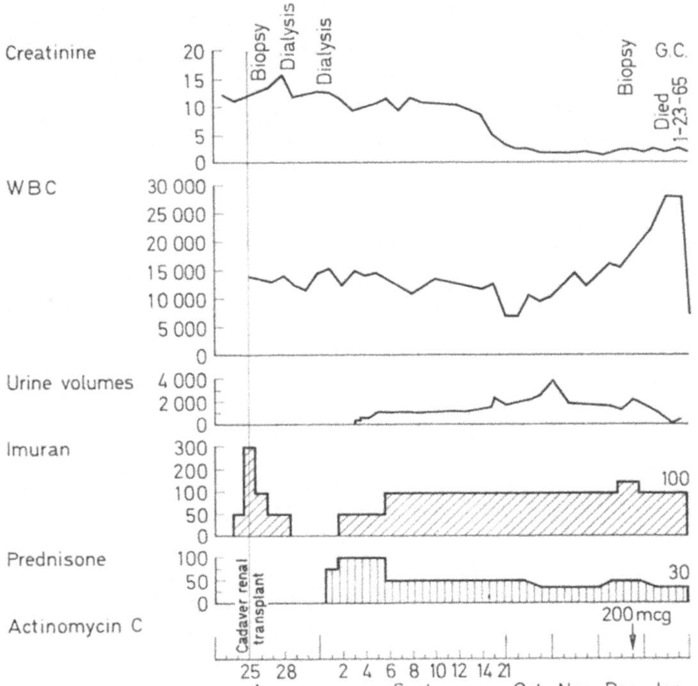


Fig. 51. Clinical course of a 46 year old man who received a cadaveric kidney in August, 1964. The donor had a bronchogenic carcinoma with cerebral metastasis. The kidney contained microscopic tumor cells which proliferated and disseminated resulting in demise

disseminate in the recipient (MARTIN, 1965 [138]; MCPAUL [146]). Cadaveric donors with carcinoma which can involve the graft must not be used. The antimetabolite azathioprine might be considered a potential antitumor agent, but its immuno-suppressive actions favors the growth of the tumor in the recipient. Withdrawal of immunosuppression can allow the recipient to reject the tumor as any other homograft (WILSON [261]).

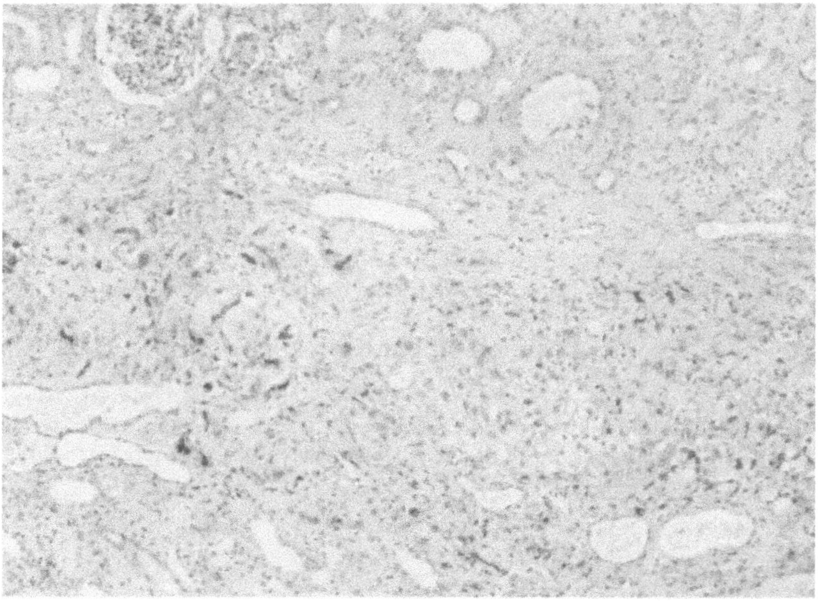

Fig. 52. Photomicrograph of the renal transplant containing metastatic (donor) tumor

### 2. Infectious Diseases

Histoplasmosis has been reported to have been transmitted by the graft (HOOD [88]). Serum hepatitis occurred in both recipients of a cadaveric renal donor, suggesting the viral agent was transplanted (HUME [89]).

## F. Hyperparathyroidism

Persistence or development of hyperparathyroidism following successful renal transplantation with normal renal function is a curious development. In many patients the hyperparathyroidism is transient (ALFREY [10]). One can understand how a previously "overactive" gland could continue to oversecrete following transplantation. However, many other patients develop the hyperparathyroidism months following transplantation subsequent to an interval of normal serum calciums (REEVE [194]).

An explanation for this sequence of events is lacking. All renal graft recipients must be observed for alteration in calcium and phosphorus metabolism for months and years following transplantation.

# XIV. Results of Clinical Renal Transplantation

## A. Introduction

The results of clinical renal transplantation fall short of the desired goal, although many individuals do survive with excellent function and no disability. The clinical experience with whole organ grafts has been far more successful than was anticipated from the results of experimental work with skin grafts. Rejection of skin grafts is largely an all-or-none phenomenon, but the vascularized parenchymal organ is able to survive an acute inflammatory reaction (immunological) and even recover lost function.

The fate of individual renal grafts is impossible to predict. Several clinical patterns are seen:

1. Acute immunological destruction of the graft in minutes, hours, or days.
2. Persistent acute rejection after an interval of good function, with resultant necrosis in 2—6 weeks.
3. Repeated episodes of acute rejection, with loss of function not recovered despite continued use of intensive immunosuppression.
4. Slowly progressive loss of graft function over months or years, with no other clinical symptoms or signs and no response to increased immune suppression.
5. Continued excellent, stable renal function for years with reduced immunosuppressive drug doses.

Fortunately, the majority of patients fall into the latter two categories.

The total functional life of renal grafts cannot be estimated at the present time. A modest number of patients have been found to have little or no histological change in the graft, a situation compatible with lengthy survival; however, most of the long-term (2—4 years) survivors have moderately severe changes in the graft as a result of prior immunological reactions.

## B. Monozygotic Twins

The excellent results of renal transplantation between identical twins was a great stimulus to homotransplantation (Merrill [149]). Observation of twin re-

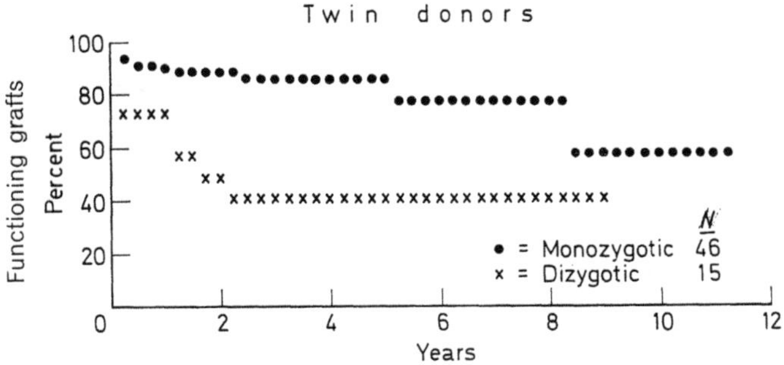


Fig. 53

Figs. 53—57. Results of renal transplants reported to the Boston Registry, December 31, 1968

cipients for several years has shown those patients are not free of their disease. Eleven of 18 recipients with glomerulonephritis have been observed to develop the original disease in the grafted kidney (Glassock [69]). Seven of these have died one month to seven years after discovery of the current nephritis; six of the deaths were due to renal failure and one to myocardial infarction (with recurrent disease). There was a tendency for the glomerulonephritis to develop more frequently in the grafts of patients with a short history of renal disease prior to transplantation. Proliferative glomerulonephritis is most likely to be associated with recurrent disease in the renal transplant.

A total of 46 identical twin renal transplants have been reported to the registry in Boston. There have been two technical failures: one due to vascular thrombosis, and one due to ureteral necrosis and subsequent calculus formation (Murray [162]). Fig. 53 shows the fraction surviving to December 31, 1968.

## C. Dizygotic Twins

Dizygotic twins are genetically the same as siblings. They may have the opportunity to exchange cells (antigens) during intrauterine development and thus become chimera. It is known that twin calves tolerate exchange skin grafts; this is presumably due to the fact they are chimera and share a common placenta in utero.

Two dizygotic twin recipients of renal grafts are surviving with good renal function since transplantation in 1959. These are the longest surviving non-identical twin recipients (Merrill, 1960 [148]; Hamburger [80]). Both received total body radiation prior to transplantation. It is impossible to say whether this provided immune suppression or whether they were in fact chimera and thus able to tolerate tissues from one another.

A total of 15 dizygotic twin renal grafts have been recorded, with survival comparable to that of other sibling transplants.

## D. Related Donors

### 1. Sibling Donors

Siblings receive half their genetic material from each parent and have an equal opportunity to share or not share antigens with one another. As they are

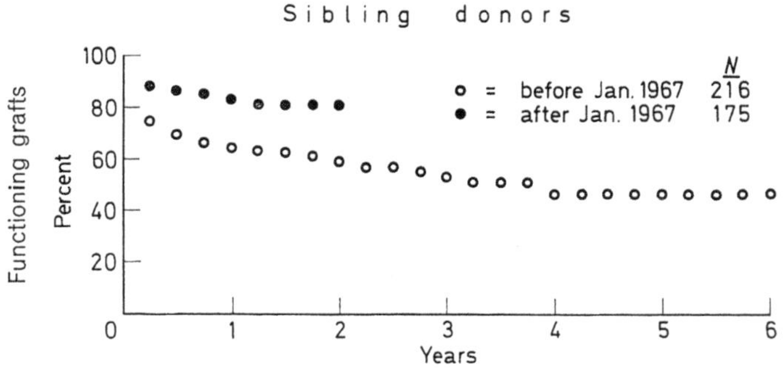


Fig. 54

of the same generation, transplantation from a sibling usually involves a younger donor (organ); this may have some bearing on the ultimate fate of the transplant. A total of 391 sibling grafts have been recorded with survival curves as illustrated in Fig. 54.

## 2. Parent Donors

The child receives genetic material from each parent, and thus always shares some antigens with each parent. This favors a compatible combination in renal transplantation from parent to offspring. The donor is necessarily many years older than the recipient. The age of an organ may affect its functional potential, although we have no statistics to establish this possibility. Fig. 55 shows the results of parent donor transplants recorded in the Boston registry to December 31, 1968.

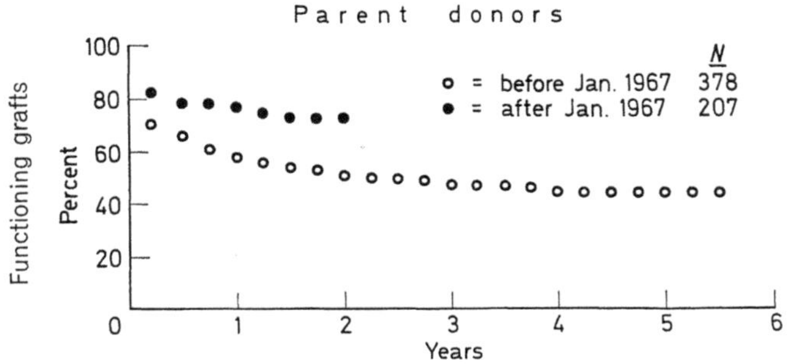


Fig. 55

## 3. Other Blood Relative Donors

Because of the genetic transmission of antigens, blood relatives are statistically more favorable donors than unrelated persons. Obviously, the closer the relationship, the more likely it is that the pair will share antigens. The small number of such pairs makes statistical analysis difficult.

# E. Cadaveric Donors

The human population is a heterogeneous group with regard to genetic material, and random organ transplants are more likely to result in mismatching

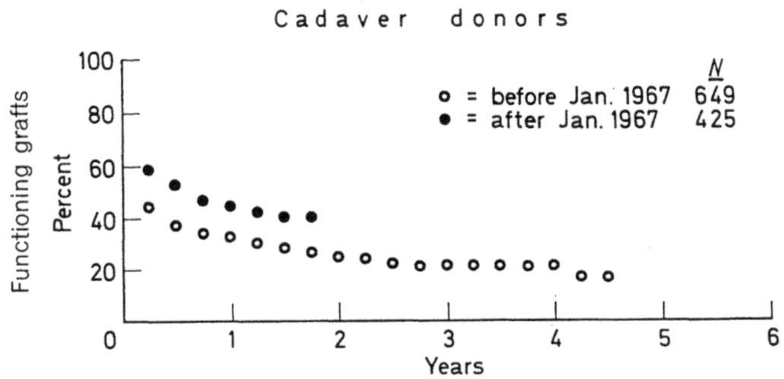


Fig. 56

of histocompatibility antigens than in matching. Clinical results reflect this; the failure rate of transplants from cadaveric donors is much higher than with related donors. Fig. 56 gives the results accumulated in the registry. The outcome of attempts to match histocompatibility antigens is discussed in Chapter X.

In addition to the greater immunological barrier, there are the problems of obtaining healthy organs from cadavers. Many factors are active in the rather poor results with cadaveric kidneys.

## F. Living Unrelated Donors

There has been limited experience with living unrelated donor renal transplants. Unless a prospective matching plan is used, the results might be expected to be only a little better than those of cadaver transplantation. The accumulated results in the transplantation registry bear this out. The past record indicates

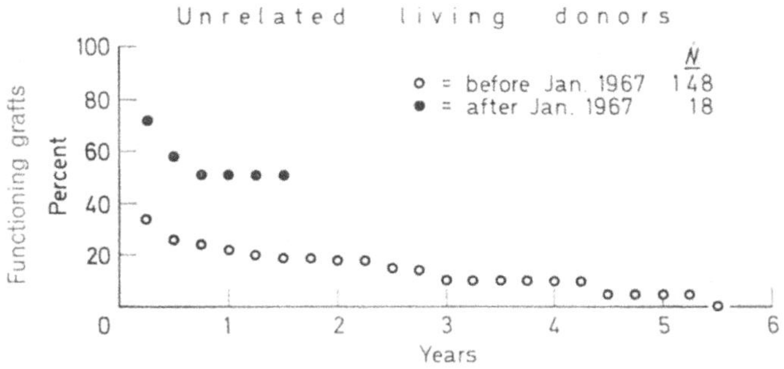


Fig. 57

living unrelated donor kidneys did not function as well as kidneys from cadavers, for reasons which are not apparent. This might be overcome with careful matching of transplantation antigens.

## Summary

The accumulated statistics in the transplantation registry offer some help for prognostication in general, but the outcome in individual cases cannot be predicted. It is important to recognize that the results in the registry refer to

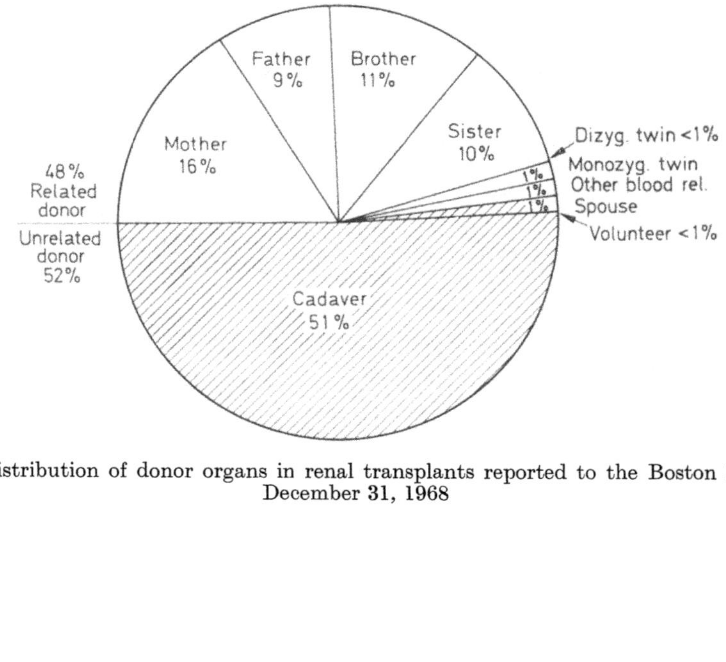


Fig. 58. Distribution of donor organs in renal transplants reported to the Boston Registry, December 31, 1968

graft, not patient, survival. Patient survival should include 10—20% of the failure groups, as many patients return to dialysis or receive a second transplant. The causes of failure are multiple, including all forms of surgical complication as well as immunological factors.

*Estimated transplant survival at one year*

| Donor | Percent | S.E. |
|---|---|---|
| Monozygotic twin | 91 | 4 |
| Sibling | 91 | 3 |
| Parent | 83 | 4 |
| Other blood relative | 67 | 7 |
| Cadaver | 42 | 5 |
| Unrelated living | 58 | 20 |

Fig. 59. Estimated survival based upon results reported to the Boston Registry, December 31, 1968. These calculations are based upon graft survival, not patient survival (which should be higher, as many patients return to dialysis following graft failure)

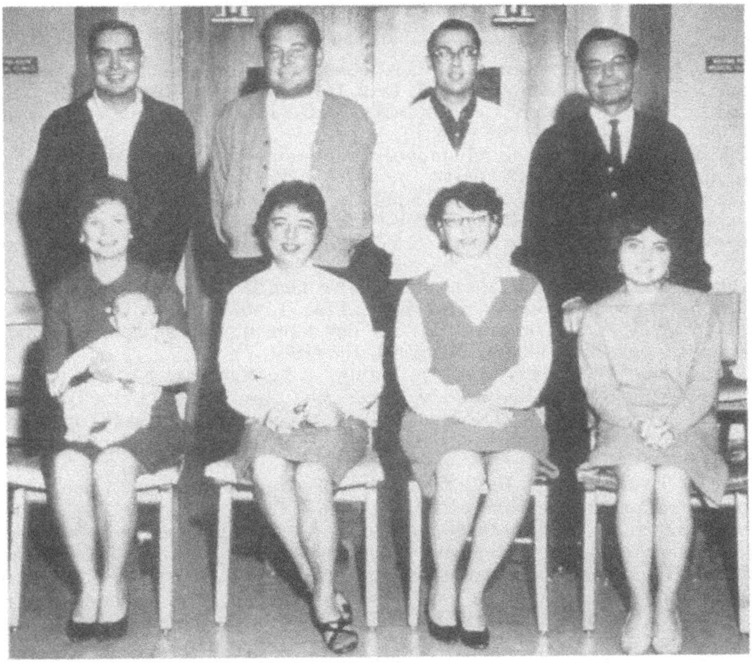

Fig. 60. Eight happy recipients of renal grafts from living donor and cadaveric sources. The woman on the extreme left gave birth to a healthy son 15 months following renal transplantation as did the woman second from the right. Three of the four men received a cadaveric organ 3—$4^1/_2$ years earlier

## References

1. Abbott, W. M., Otherson, H. B., Monaco, A. P., Simmons, R. L., Wood, M. L., Russell, P. S.: Prolonged survival of renal allografts in dogs treated with anti-lymphocyte serum. Surg. Forum **17**, 228 (1966).
2. Abbrecht, P. H., Greene, J. A., Jr.: Serum erythropoietin after renal homotransplantation. Ann. intern. Med. **65**, 908 (1966).

3. Ackerman, J. R., Hopkinson, W. I., Murphy, D. M. G., Kenyon, J. R.: Successful 24—48 hour canine kidney preservation. In: Advance in transplantation, p. 743. Copenhagen: Munksgaard 1967.
4. — Snell, M. E.: Cadaveric renal transplantation: A technique for donor kidney removal. Brit. J. Urol. **40**, 515 (1968).
5. Ackerman, J. R. W., Fisher, A. J. G., Barnard, C. N.: Live storage of kidneys: a preliminary communication. Surgery **60**, 720 (1966).
6. Ackman, C. F. C., Atkinson, J. C., Barnes, B. A., et al.: Sixth report of the human kidney transplant registry. Transplantation **6**, 944 (1968).
7. Adler, S., Lindeman, R. D., Yiengst, M. J., Beard, E.: Effect of acute acid loading on urinary acid excretion by the aging human kidney. J. Lab. clin. Med. **72**, 278 (1968).
8. Alexandre, G. P., Murray, J. E.: Further studies on renal homotransplantation in dogs treated by combined imuran therapy. Surg. Forum **13**, 64 (1962).
9. Alexandre, G. P. J., Murray, J. E., Dammin, G. K., Nolan, B.: Immunosuppressive drug therapy in renal homografts. Transplantation **1**, 432 (1963).
10. Alfrey, A. C., Jenkins, D., Groth, C. G., Schorr, W. S., Gecelter, L., Ogden, D. A.: Resolution of hyperparathyroidism, renal osteodystrophy and metastatic calcification after renal homotransplantation. New Engl. J. Med. **279**, 1349 (1968).
11. Altman, B.: Tissue transplantation; circulating antibodies in homotransplantation of kidney and skin. Ann. Roy. Coll. Surg. Engl. **33**, 79 (1963).
12. Attai, L. A., Veith, F. J., Furman, S., Denize, A., Boley, S. J., Robinson, G., Gliedmen, M. L.: Intracorporeal cadaver organ preservation by mechanical ventricular assistance. Surg. Forum **19**, 202 (1968).
13. Awad, W., Bennett, L., Martin, D. C.: Detection of renal homograft rejection reaction with a single dose of radiohuppuran. J. Urol. (Baltimore) **100**, 223 (1968a).
14. — Boake, R. C., Bennett, L. R., Martin, D. C.: Double isotope scan in kidney transplantation. Amer. Surg. **34**, 768 (1968b).
15. Bach, F. H., Hirschhorn, K.: Lymphocyte interaction: a potential histocompatibility test in vitro. Science **143**, 813 (1964).
16. — Kisken, W. A.: Predictive value of results of mixed leukocyte cultures for skin allograft survival in man. Transplantation **5**, 1046 (1967).
17. — Voynow, N. K.: One-way stimulation in mixed leukocyte cultures. Science **153**, 545 (1966).
18. Bach, J. F., Dardenne, M., Dormont, J., Antoine, B.: A new in vitro test evaluating anti-lymphocyte serum potency. Transplant. Proc. **1**, 403 (1969).
19. Bain, B., Vas, M. R., Lowenstein, L.: The development of large immature mononuclear cells in mixed leucocyte cultures. Blood **23**, 108 (1964).
20. Balakrishman, S. L., Armstrong, D., Rubin, A. L., Stenzel, K. H.: Cytomegalovirus infection after renal transplantation. J. Amer. Med. Ass. **207**, 1712 (1969).
21. Ballantyne, B., Wood, W. G., Meffan, P. M.: Sequential analyses of urinary enzymes in early diagnosis of parenchymal damage after renal homotransplantation. Brit. med. J. **1968 II**, 667.
22. Balner, H., Eysvoogel, V. P., Cleton, F. J.: Testing of anti-human lymphocyte serum in chimpanzees and lower primates. Lancet **1968 I**, 19.
23. Basso, A., Lotti, T., Laurenti, C., D'Amore, A.: Twenty-four-hour renal preservation using perfusion cooling by autologous arterial blood. Brit. J. Urol. **50**, 522 (1968).
24. Bauer, K. H.: Homoiotransplantation von Epidermis bei eineiigen Zwillingen. Brun's Beitr. klin. Chir. **141**, 442 (1927).
25. Belzer, F. O., Ashby, B. S., Dunphy, J. E.: 24-hour and 72-hour preservation of canine kidneys. Lancet **1967 II**, 536.
26. — — Gulyassy, P. F.: Successful seventeen-hour preservation and transplantation of human-cadaver kidney. New Engl. J. Med. **278**, 608 (1968).
27. Berah, M., Makabowicz, R., Graydon, J. J.: Leuco-agglutinins in normal and abnormal pregnancy. Med. J. Aust. **2**, 1030 (1966).
28. Blaufox, M. D., Merrill, J. P.: Evaluation of renal transplant function by iodohippurate sodium $I^{131}$. J. Amer. med. Ass. **202**, 575 (1967a).
29. — Potchen, E. J., Merrill, J. P.: Measurement of effective renal plasma flow in man by external counting methods. J. nucl. Med. **8**, 77 (1967b).
30. Board, J. A., Lee, H. M., Draper, D. A., Hume, D. M.: Pregnancy following kidney homotransplantation from a non-twin: report of a case with current administration of azathioprine and prednisone. Obstet. and Gynec. **29**, 318 (1967).
31. Braun, W. E., Merrill, J. P.: Urine fibrinogen fragments in human renal allografts. New Engl. J. Med. **278**, 1366 (1968).
32. Bravo, J. F., Herman, J. H. Smyth, C. J.: Musculoskeletal disorders after renal homotransplantation. Ann. intern. Med. **66**, 87 (1967).

33. BRENT, L., MEDAWAR, P. B.: Tissue transplantation: a new approach to the "typing" problem. Brit. med. J. **1963 II**, 269.
34. BROSIG, W., NAGEL, R.: Nierentransplantation. Berlin: Walter de Gruyter 1965.
35. BROWN, J. B.: Homografting of skin: with report of success in identical twins. Surgery **1**, 558 (1937).
36. BRUTON, O. C.: Agammaglobulinemia. Pediatrics **9**, 722 (1952).
37. BUSSEY, J. G., SABISTON, F., JR., PFAFF, W. W.: Humoral cytotoxic antibodies in allograft rejection. Surg. Forum **18**, 223 (1967).
38. CALNE, R. Y.: Renal transplantation, second edit. London: Arnold 1967.
39. — MURRAY, J. E.: Inhibition of the rejection of renal homografts in dogs by Burroughs Wellcome, 57—322. Surg. Forum **12**, 118 (1961).
40. CARPENTER, C. B., GLASSOCK, R. J., GLEASON, R., CORSON, J. M., MERRILL, J. P.: The application of the normal lymphocyte transfer reaction to histocompatibility testing in man. J. clin. Invest. **45**, 1452 (1966).
41. CARREL, A.: Remote results of the replantation of the kidney and spleen. J. exp. Med. **12**, 146 (1910).
42. — GUTHRIE, C. C.: Anastomosis of blood vessels by the patching method and transplantation of the kidney. J. Amer. med. Ass. **47**, 1648 (1906).
43. CEPPELLINI, R., CURTONI, E. S., MATTIUZ, P. L., LEIGHEB, G., VISETTI, M., COLOMBI, A.: Survival of test skin grafts in man: Effects of genetic relationship and of blood groups incompatibility. Ann. N.Y. Acad. Sci. **129**, 421 (1966).
44. — FRANCESCHINI, P., MIGGIANO, V. C., TRIDENTE, G.: Directional activation of mixed lymphocyte cultures. In: Histocompatibility testing, p. 225. Copenhagen: Munksgaard 1965.
45. CLUNIE, G. J. A., LINDSEY, E. S., REEMTSMA, K.: Mercurial diuretic protection of the ischemic kidney in the rat. Surg. Forum **17**, 239 (1966).
46. COHEN, H. E., MOSES, M.: The critical interval in cadaver kidney transplantation. Function of canine renal autotransplants after variable periods of ischemia. Surgery **60**, 750 (1966).
47. COHN, R., KOUNTZ, S., SWENSON, R.: General surgical complications associated with renal allotransplantation using related donors. Amer. J. Surg. **114**, 274 (1967).
48. COOPER, M. D.: Division of the lymphoid tissues of chickens into two distinct functional and morphological components. Fed. Proc. **24**, 490 (1965).
49. — PETERSON, R. D. A., GOOD, R. A.: Delineation of the thymic and bursal lymphoid systems in the chicken. Nature (Lond.) **205**, 143 (1965).
50. CRADDOCK, C. G.: Bone marrow lymphocytes of the rat as studied by autoradiography. Acta haemat. (Basel) **33**, 19 (1965).
51. CRUESS, R. L.: Aseptic necrosis following renal transplantation. J. Bone Jt Surg. **50**, 1577 (1968).
52. DAUSSET, J., RAPAPORT, F. T.: Role of AB0 erythrocyte groups in human histocompatibility reactions. Nature (Lond.) **209**, 209 (1966).
53. DEALY, J. B., DAMMIN, G. J., MURRAY, J. E., MERRILL, J. P.: Total body irradiation in man: Tissue patterns observed in attempts to increase receptivity of renal homografts. Ann. N.Y. Acad. Sci. **87**, 572 (1960).
54. DENNEY, W. F., FLANIGAN, W. T., ZUKOSKI, C. F.: Serial erythropoietin studies in patients undergoing renal homotransplantation. J. Lab. clin. Med. **67**, 386 (1966).
55. DE VITA, V. T., EMMER, M., LEVINE, A., JACOBS, B., BERARD, C.: Pneumocystis carinii pneumonia. New Engl. J. Med. **280**, 287 (1969).
56. DINAPOLI, R. P., JOHNSON, W. J., LAMBERT, E. H.: Experience with a combined hemodialysis — renal transplantation program: neurological aspects. Proc. Mayo Clin. **41**, 809 (1966).
57. DUBERNARD, J. M., CARPENTER, C. B., BUSCH, G. J., DIETHELM, A. G., MURRAY, J. E.: Rejection of canine renal allografts by passive transfer of sensitized serum. Surgery **64**, 752 (1968).
58. DUKEMINIER, J., JR., SANDERS, D.: Organ transplantation: A proposal for routine salvaging of cadaver organs. New Engl. J. Med. **279**, 413 (1968).
59. ENDE, N., ZUKOSKI, C. F.: Emergency autopsy for the selection of donor kidneys. J. Amer. med. Ass. **191**, 902 (1965).
60. ENGELFRIET, C. P., MELIEF, C. J. M., VAN DER HART, M., VAN LOGHEM, J. J.: The importance of the immune adherence assay for the demonstration of leucocyte iso-antigens on leucocytes and cells of other tissues. In: Histocompatibility testing, p. 407. Baltimore: Williams & Wilkins 1967.
61. EVANS, D. B., MILLARD, P. R., HERBERTSON, B. M.: Hepatic dysfunction associated with renal transplantation. Lancet **1968 II**, 929.

62. Eyal, A., Manax, W. G., Block, J. H., Lillihei, R. C.: Successful in vitro preservation of the small bowel, including maintenance of mucosal integrity with chlorpromazine, hypothermia, and hyperboric oxygenation. Surgery **57**, 259 (1965).
63. Figueroa, W. J., Rodriquez-Antimez, A., Nakamoto, S., Kolff, W. J.: The scintigram after renal transplantation in man. New Engl. J. Med. **273**, 1406 (1965).
64. Fish, J. C., Sarles, H. E., Remmers, A. R., Jr., Tyson, K. R. T., Canales, C. O., Beathard, G. A., Fukushima, M., Ritzmann, S. E., Levin, W. C.: Circulating lymphocyte depletion in preparation for renal transplantation. Surg. Gynec. Obstet. **128**, 777 (1969).
65. Fisher, E. R., Copeland, C., Fisher, B.: Correlation of ultrastructure and function following hypothermic preservation of canine kidneys. Lab. Invest. **17**, 99 (1967).
66. Franksson, C., Blomstrand, R.: Drainage of the thoracic lymph duct during homologous kidney transplantation in men. Scand. J. Urol. Nephrol. **1**, 123 (1967).
67. Gil-Vernet, J. M., Caralps, A.: Human renal homotransplantation. New surgical technique. Urol. Int. **23**, 201 (1968).
68. Glassock, R. J.: Personal communication.
69. — Feldman, D., Reynolds, E. S., Dammin, G. J., Merrill, J. P.: Recurrent glomerulonephritis in human renal isograft recipients: a clinical and pathologic study. In: Advance in transplantation, p. 361. Copenhagen: Munksgaard 1967.
70. Glick, B. T., Chang, T. S., Jaap, R. G.: The bursa of Fabricius and antibody production. Poultry Sci. **35**, 224 (1956).
71. Good, R. A., Gabrielsen, A. E., Cooper, M. D., Peterson, R. D. A.: The role of the thymus and bursa of Fabricius in the development of effector mechanisms. Ann. N.Y. Acad. Sci. **129**, 130 (1966).
72. Goodwin, W. E., Kaufman, J. J., Mims, M. M., Turner, R. D., Glassock, R., Goldman, R., Maxwell, M. M.: Human renal transplantation. I. Clinical experiences with six cases of renal transplantation. J. Urol. (Baltimore) **89**, 13 (1963).
73. — Martin, D. C.: Renal transplantation, chap. 56. In: Campbell's urology, third edit. Philadelphia: Saunders 1969.
74. Gray, J. G., Russell, P. S.: The lymphocyte transfer test in man. Nat. Acad. Sci. Histocompatibility testing **1229**, 105 (1965).
75. Greaves, M. F., Tursi, A., Playfair, J. H. L., Torrigiani, G., Zamir, R., Roitt, I. M.: Immunosuppressive potency and in vitro activity of antilymphocyte globulin. Lancet **1969 I**, 68.
76. Hall, M. C., Elmore, S. M., Bright, R. W., Pierce, J. C., Hume, D. M.: Skeletal complications in a series of human renal allografts. Amer. med. Ass. J. **208**, 1825 (1969).
77. Hallenbeck, G. A., Shorter, R. G., Titus, J. L., Thomford, N. R., Johnson, W. J., De Weerd, J. H.: Apparent glomerulonephritis in a homotransplant. Surgery **59**, 522 (1966).
78. Hamburger, J., Crosnier, J., Dormont, J.: Experience with 45 renal homotransplantations in man. Lancet **1965 I**, 985.
79. — Vaysse, J., Crosnier, J., Auvert, J., La Lanne, A. M., Hopper, J., Jr.: Renal homotransplantation in man after irradiation of the recipient. Amer. J. Med. **32**, 854 (1962).
80. — — — Tubiana, M., La Lanne, C. M., Antoine, J., Auvert, J., Soulier, J. P., Dormont, J., Salmon, C., Maisonnet, M., Amiel, J. L.: Transplantation d'un rein entre jumeaux non monozygotes apres irradiation du receveur. Presse méd. **67**, 1771 (1959).
81. Hendry, W. F., Struthers, N. W., Duguid, W. P., Hopkinson, W. I.: Twenty-four-hour storage of kidneys. Lancet **1968 I**, 1221.
82. Herrmann, T. J., Turcotte, J. G.: Preservation of canine kidneys. Arch. Surg. **98**, 121 (1969).
83. Hill, R. B., Jr., Rowlands, D. T., Jr., Rifkind, D.: Infectious pulmonary disease in patients receiving immunosuppressive therapy for organ transplantation. New Engl. J. Med. **271**, 1021 (1964).
84. Hinman, F., Jr., Belzer, F. O.: Urinary tract infection and renal homotransplantation: I. Effect of antibacterial irrigations on defences of the defunctionalized bladder. J. Urol. (Baltimore) **101**, 477 (1969a).
85. — Schmaelzle, J. F., Belzer, F. O.: Urinary tract infection and renal homotransplantation: II. Post-transplantation bacterial invasion. J. Urol. (Baltimore) **101**, 673 (1969b).
86. Hirschhorn, K., Firschein, I. L., Bach, F. H.: Histocompatibility monograph. p. 131, Washington, D.C., 1965a.
87. — — — Immune response of human peripheral blood lymphocytes in vitro. Nat. Acad. Sci. Histocompatibility testing **1229**, 131 (1965b).
88. Hood, A. B., Inglis, F. G., Lowenstein, L.: Histoplasmosis and thrombocytopenic purpura; transmission by renal homotransplantation. Canad. med. Ass. J. **93**, 587 (1965).

89. Hume, D. M., Lee, H. M., Williams, G. M., White, H. J. O., Ferré, J., Wolf, J. S., Prout, G. R., Jr., Slapak, M., O'Brien, J., Kilpatriek, S. J., Kauffman, H. M., Jr., Cleveland, R. J.: Comparative results of cadaver and related donor renal homografts in men, and immunologic implications of outcome of second and paired transplants. Ann. Surg. **164**, 352 (1966).
90. — Merrill, J. P., Miller, B. F., Thorn, G. W.: Experiences with renal homotransplantation in the human: Report of nine cases. J. clin. Invest. **34**, 327 (1955).
91. — Wolf, J. S.: Modification of renal homograft rejection by irradiation. Transplantation **5**, 1174 (1967).
92. Humphries, A., Russell, R., Ostafin, J., Goodrich, S. M. O., Moretz, W. H.: Successful reimplantation of canine kidney after 24-hour storage. Surgery **54**, 136 (1963).
93. Humphries, A. L.: Organ preservation: a review. Transplantation **5**, 1138 (1967).
94. — Russell, R., Stoddard, L. D., Moretz, W. H.: Successful five-day kidney preservation. Invest. Urol. **5**, 609 (1968).
95. Humphries, A. L., Jr., Russell, R., Stoddard, L. D.: Three-day kidney preservation: perfusion of kidneys with hypothermic, diluted blood of plasma. Surgery **63**, 646 (1968).
96. Huntley, R. T., Taylor, P. D., Iwasaki, Y., Marchioro, T. L., Jeejeebho, H., Porter, K. A., Starzl, T. E.: Use of anti-lymphocyte serum to prolong dog homograft survival. Surg. Forum **17**, 230 (1966).
97. Iwasaki, Y., Porter, K. A., Amend, J. R., Marchioro, T. L., Zühlke, V., Starzl, T. E.: The preparation and testing of horse antidog and antihuman antilymphoid plasma or serum and its protein fractions. Surg. Gynec. Obstet. **124**, 1 (1967).
98. Jackson, B. T., Mannick, J. A.: Serial blood flow in first set renal homotransplants undergoing rejection. Surg. Gynec. Obstet. **119**, 1265 (1964).
99. Jones, J. P., Engleman, E. P., Najarian, J. S.: Systemic fat embolism after renal homotransplantation and treatment with corticosteroids. New Engl. J. Med. **273**, 1453 (1965).
100. Kanich, R. E., Craighead, J. E.: Cytomegalovirus infection and cytomegalic inclusion disease in renal homotransplant recipients. Amer. J. Med. **40**, 874 (1966).
101. Kashiwagi, N., Groth, C. G., Amend, J. R., Gelcelter, L., Blanchard, H., Starzl, T. E.: Improvements in the preparation of heterologous antilymphocyte globulin with special reference to absorption and diethylaminoethyl cellulose batch production. Surgery **65**, 477 (1969).
102. Kauffman, H. M., Cleveland, R. J., Dwyer, J. J., Lee, H. M., Hume, D. M.: Prolongation of renal homograft function by local graft radiation. Surg. Gynec. Obstet. **120**, 49 (1965).
103. — — Lee, H. M., Hume, D. M.: Significance of lymphocyturia in renal homograft rejection. Surg. Forum **15**, 168 (1964).
104. Kaufman, J. J., Dignam, W., Goodwin, W. E., Martin, D. C., Goldman, R., Maxwell, M. H.: Successful normal childbirth after kidney homotransplantation. J. Amer. med. Ass. **200**, 338 (1967).
105. Kelly, W. D., Merkel, F. K., Markland, C.: Ilial urinary diversion in conjunction with renal homotransplantation. Lancet **1966 I**, 222.
106. Khastagir, B., Montandon, A., Nakamoto, S., Kolff, W. J.: Early and late failures of human cadaveric renal allografts. Arch. intern. Med. **123**, 8 (1969).
107. Kincaid,-Smith, P.: Histological diagnosis of rejection of renal homografts in man. Lancet **1967 II**, 849.
108. — Marshall, V. C., Mathew, T. H., Eremin, T. H., Brown, J., Johnson, R. B., Lovell, N., McLeish, R. R. H., Fairley, K. F., Allcock, E. A., Ewing, M. R.: Cadaveric renal transplantation. Lancet **1967 II**, 59.
109. Kiser, J. C., Farley, H. H., Mueller, G. F., Strobel, C. J., Hitchcock, C. R.: Successful renal autografts in the dog after 7-hour selective renal refrigeration. Surg. Forum **11**, 26 (1960).
110. — Telander, R. L., Peterson, T. A., Coe, J. L., Hitchcock, C. R.: Canine renal autografts. Arch. Surg. **83**, 502 (1961).
111. Kiser, W. S., Straffon, R. A., Hewitt, C. B., Stewart, B. H., Nakamoto, S., Kolff, W. J.: Clinical experience with one hundred twenty-one human kidney transplants. Amer. Surg. **33**, 304 (1967).
112. Kissmeyer-Nielsen, F., Olsen, S., Petersen, V. P., Fjeldborg, O.: Hyperacute rejection of kidney allografts, associated with pre-existing humoral antibodies against donor cells. Lancet **1966 II**, 662
113. Knight, P. R., Tomkiewicz, Z. M., Couch, N. P.: Evaluation of functioning canine renal autografts after 6-hour storage. Surg. Forum **14**, 171 (1963).
114. Koppel, M. H., Coburn, J. W., Rosen, V. J., Davis, A., Rubini, M. E.: Transplantation pneumonia: the importance of early open lung biopsy for etiologic diagnosis. Clin. Res. **17**, 120 (1969).

115. KOUNTZ, S. L., COHN, R.: Prolonged survival of a renal homograft by simultaneous splenectomy and splenic homotransplantation. Surg. Forum **13**, 59 (1962).
116. — — The pathophysiology of renal allotransplants in subjects on immunosuppressive therapy. In: Advance in transplantation, p. 617. Copenhagen: Munksgaard 1967.
117. — — Initial treatment of renal allografts with large intrarenal doses of immunosuppresive drugs. Lancet **1969 I**, 338.
118. — LAMB, D. R., COHN, R.: Detecting and treating early renal homotransplant rejection. J. Amer. med. Ass. **191**, 996 (1965).
119. — WILLIAMS, M. A., WILLIAMS, P. L., KAPROS, C., DEMPSTER, W. J.: Mechanism of rejection of homotransplanted kidneys. Nature (Lond.) **199**, 257 (1963).
120. KRIEG, A. F., BOLANDE, R. P., HOLDEN, W. D., HUBAY, C. A., PERSKY, L.: Membranous glomerulonephritis occurring in a human renal homograft: Report of a case. Amer. J. clin. Path. **34**, 155 (1960).
121. KÜSS, R., TEINTURIER, J., MILLIEZ, P.: Quelques essais de greffe de rein chez l'homme. Mem. Acad. Chir. **77**, 755 (1951).
122. LANNON, S. G., TUKARAM, K. T., OLIVER, J. A., MCKINNON, K. J., DOSSETOR, J. B.: Preservation of kidneys assessed bya biochemical parameter. Surg. Gynec. Obstet. **124**, 999 (1967).
123. LAWLER, R. H., WEST, J. W., MCNULTY, P. H., CLANCY, E. J., MURPHY, R. P.: Homotransplantation of the kidney in the human, a preliminary report. J. Amer. med. Ass. **144**, 844 (1950).
124. LAWSON, R. K., ELLIS, L. R., HODGES, C. V.: Anti-lymphocyte serum in prolongation of dog renal homografts. Surg. Forum **17**, 515 (1966).
125. LEADBETTER, G. W., MONACO, A. P., RUSSELL, P. S.: A technique for reconstruction of the urinary tract in renal transplantation. Surg. Gynec. Obstet. **123**, 839 (1966).
126. LERNER, R. A., GLACCOCK, R. J.: DIXON, F. J.: The role of anti-glomerular basement membrane antibody in the pathogenesis of human glomerulonephritis. J. exp. Med. **126**, 989 (1967).
127. LEVEY, R. H., MEDAWAR, P. B.: Mechanism of action of antilymphoid antisera. Surg. Forum **17**, 247 (1966).
128. LOSTUMBO, M. M., HOLLAND, P. V., SCHMIDT, P. J.: Isoimmunization after multiple transfusions. New Engl. J. Med. **275**, 141 (1966).
129. MAKIN, G. S., HOWARD, J. M.: Hyperbaric oxygenation and profound hypothermia to preserve canine kidneys. Arch. Surg. **91**, 568 (1965).
130. MANAX, W. G., BLOCK, J. H., LILLEHEI, R. C.: Successful 24-hour in vitro preservation of canine kidneys by combined use of hyperbaric oxygen and hypothermia. Surgery **56**, 275 (1964).
131. — HIDALGO, F., LYONS, G. W., DIETZMAN, R.,LILLEHEI, R. C.: Canine "cadaver" kidneys. J. Amer. med. Ass. **195**, 1010 (1966).
132. MARCHIORO, T. L., WADDELL, W. R., STARZL, T. E.: Use of extracorporeal cadaver perfusion for preparation of organ homografts. Surg. Forum **14**, 174 (1963).
133. MARSHALL, V., KINCAID-SMITH, P., MORRIS, P. J., SAKER, B., EVERMIN, J.: Cadaveric renal transplantation. Lancet **1968 II**, 927.
134. MARTIN, D. C.: Urinary tract infection in clinical transplantation. Arch. Surg. **99**, 474 (1969).
135. — GOODWIN, W. E.: Renal transplantation in polycystic renal disease with decrease in size of the cystic kidneys and erythremia. J. Amer. med. Ass. **201**, 1044 (1967).
136. — — KAUFMAN, J. J., MIMS, M. M., GOLDMAN, R., RUBINI, M., GONICK, H.: 92 kidney transplants: Results, lessons learned, future prospects. J. Urol. (Baltimore) **100**, 227 (1968).
137. — MIMS, M. M., KAUFMAN, J. J., GOODWIN, W. E.: The ureter in renal transplantation. J. Urol. (Baltimore) **101**, 680 (1969).
138. — RUBINI, M., ROSEN, V. J.: Cadaveric renal homotransplantation with inadvertent transplantation of carcinoma. J. Amer. med. Ass. **192**, 752 (1965).
139. — VAN DE WATER, J., RANDEL, D. E., LEE, D.: Prolonged survival of canine renal grafts with local radiation. Surg. Forum **15**, 156 (1964).
140. MARTIN, M. M., GABOARDI, F., PODOLSKY, S., RAITI, S., CALCAGNO, P. L.: Intermittent steroid therapy. New Engl. J. Med. **279**, 273 (1968).
141. MAYER, D. J., DUMONT, A. E.: Prolongated survival of skin homografts following diversion of thoracic duct lymph. Surg. Forum **14**, 194 (1963).
142. MCGREGOR, D. D., GOWANS, J. L.: The antibody response of rats depleted of lymphocytes by chronic drainage from the thoracic duct. J. exp. Med. **117**, 303 (1963).
143. MCINTOSH, D. A., PETERSON, E. W., MCPHAUL, J. J.: Autonomy of parathyroid function after renal homotransplantation. Ann. intern. Med. **65**, 900 (1966).
144. MCKINNON, K. J., OLIVER, J. A., MOREHOUSE, D. D., TAGUCHI, Y.: Cadaver renal transplantation: Emphasis on urological aspects. Trans. Amer. Ass. gen.-urin. Surg. **59**, 44 (1967).

145. McPhaul, J. J., McIntosh, D. A., Hammond, W. S., Park, O. K.: Autonomous secondary (renal) parathyroid hyperplasia. New Engl. J. Med. **271**, 1342 (1964).
146. McPhaul, J. J., Jr., McIntosh, D. A.: Tissue transplantation still vexes. New Engl. J. Med. **272**, 105 (1965).
147. Melief, C. J. M., van der Hart, M., Engelfriet, C. P., van Loghem, J. J.: Immune adherence of leucocytes and fibroblasts derived from skin, sensitized by cytotoxic leucocyte iso-antibodies and complement, to the surface of indicator cells. Vox Sang (Basel) **12**, 374 (1967).
148. Merrill, J. P., Murray, J. E., Harrison, J. H., Friedman, E. A., Dealy, J. B., Dammin, G. J.: Successful homotransplantation of kidney between nonidentical twins. New Engl. J. Med. **262**, 1251 (1960).
149. — — — Guild, W. R.: Successful homotransplantation of the human kidney between identical twins. J. Amer. med. Ass. **160**, 227 (1956).
150. Metcalf, D.: Delayed effect of thymectomy in adult life on immunological competence. Nature (Lond.) **208**, 1336 (1965).
151. Milgrom, F., Litvak, B. I., Kano, K., Witebsky, E.: Humoral antibodies in renal homograft. J. Amer. med. Ass. **198**, 226 (1966).
152. Miller, J. F. A. P.: Role of thymus in transplantation immunity. Ann. N.Y. Acad. Sci. **99**, 340 (1962).
153. — Immunological significance of thymus of adult mouse. Nature (Lond.) **195**, 1318 (1962).
154. — Effect of neonatal thymectomy on the immunological responsiveness of the mouse. Proc. roy Soc. B **156**, 415 (1962).
155. Monaco, A. P., Wood, M. L., Russell, P. S.: Adult thymectomy: Effect on recovery from immunologic depression in mice. Science **149**, 432 (1965).
156. — — — Some effects of purified heterologous antihuman lymphocyte serum in man. Transplantation **5**, 1106 (1967).
157. Moore, T. C., Chang, J. K., Hume, D. M.: Urinary excretion of histamine in renal transplant patients. Surg. Gynec. Obstet. **127**, 1023 (1968).
158. Morris, H. G., Jorgensen, J. R., Jenkins, S. A.: Plasma growth hormone concentration in corticosteroid-treated children. J. clin. Invest. **47**, 427 (1968).
159. Morris, P. J., Kincaid-Smith, P., Ting, A., Stocker, J. W., Marshall, V. C.: Prospective leucocyte typing in cadaver renal transplantation. Lancet **1968 II**, 803.
160. — Terasaki, P. I., Williams, G. M., Hume, D. M.: The development of cytotoxic antibodies in renal transplantation. Surg. Forum **18**, 270 (1967).
161. Muether, R. O., Schuessler, W. P., Sommer, A. J.: Laboratory studies on the aging kidney. J. Amer. Geriat. Soc. **15**, 260 (1967).
162. Murray, J. E., Harrison, J. H.: Surgical management of fifty patients with kidney transplants including eighteen pairs of twins. Amer. J. Surg. **105**, 205 (1963a).
163. — Merrill, J. P., Dammin, G. J., Dealy, J. B., Walter, C. W., Brooke, M. S., Wilson, R. E.: Study on transplantation immunity after total body irradiation: Clinical and experimental investigation. Surgery **48**, 272 (1960).
164. — — Harrison, J. H., Dammin, G. J., Wilson, R. E.: Prolonged survival of human kidney homografts by immunosuppressive drug therapy. New Engl. J. Med. **268**, 1315 (1963b).
165. — Reid, D. E., Harrison, J. H., Merrill, J. P.: Successful pregnancies after human renal transplantation. New Engl. J. Med. **269**, 341 (1963c).
166. Murray, R. G., Woods, P. A.: Studies on the fate of lymphocytes. III. The migration and metamorphosis of in situ labeled thymic lymphocytes. Anat. Rec. **150**, 113 (1964).
167. Najarian, J. S.: Personal communication, May 20, 1969.
168. — Gulyassy, P. P., Stoney, R. J., Duffy, G., Braunstein, P.: Protection of the donor kidney during homotransplantation. Ann. Surg. **164**, 398 (1966).
169. — Merkel, F. K., Moore, G. E., Good, R. A., Aust, J. C.: Clinical use of antilymphoblast serum. Transplant. Proc. **1**, 460 (1969).
170. — Perper, R. J.: Participation of humoral antibody in allogenic organ transplantation rejection. Surgery **62**, 213 (1967).
171. Newton, W. T., Keltner, R. M., Shankel, S. W.: Acquired renovascular hypertension in a patient with renal allotransplantation. Amer. J. Surg. **113**, 292 (1967).
172. Nies, B. A., Cohn, R., Schrier, S. L.: Erythremia after renal transplantation. New Engl. J. Med. **273**, 785 (1965).
173. Norman, J. C.: Organ perfusion and preservation. New York: Meredith Corp. 1968.
174. Nossal, G. J. V.: Studies on the rate of seeding of lymphocytes from the intact guinea pig thymus. Ann. N.Y. Acad. Sci. **120**, 171 (1964).
175. O'Brien, J. P., Hume, D. M.: Membranous glomerulonephritis in two human renal homotransplants. Arch. intern. Med. **65**, 504 (1966).

176. O'Connor, J. F., Dealy, J. B., Lindquist, R., Couch, N. P.: Arterial lesions due to rejection in human kidney allografts. Radiology **89**, 614 (1967).
177. Ogden, D. A., Holmes, J. H.: Urinary solute excretion as an index of renal homograft rejection. Ann. intern. Med. **64**, 806 (1966).
178. — Porter, K. A., Terasaki, P. I., Marchioro, T. L., Holmes, J. H., Starzl, T. E.: Chronic renal homograft function. Amer. J. Med. **43**, 837 (1967).
179. Orchardson, R. L.: Renal function and age. J. Coll. gen. Practit. **12**, 287 (1966).
180. Palmer, J. M., Kountz, S. L., Swenson, R. S., Lucas, Z. J., Cohn, R.: Urinary tract morbidity in renal transplantation. Arch. Surg. **98**, 352 (1969).
181. Parsons, F. M., Markland, C., Raper, F. P., Fox, M.: Cadaveric renal transplantation. Brit. med. J. **1963 I**, 930.
182. Patel, R., Glassock, R., Terasaki, P. I.: Serotyping for homotransplantation. XIX. Experience with an interhospital scheme of cadaver kidney sharing and tissue typing. J. Amer. med. Ass. **207**, 1319 (1969a).
183. — Mickey, M. R., Terasaki, P. I.: Serotyping for homotransplantation. XVI. Analysis of kidney transplants from unrelated donors. New Engl. J. Med. **279**, 501 (1968).
184. — Terasaki, P. I.: Significance of the positive crossmatch test in kidney transplantation. New Engl. J. Med. **280**, 735 (1969b).
185. Payne, R., Perkins, H. A., Najarian, J. S.: Compatibility for seven leukocyte antigens in renal homografts: utilization of a micro-agglutination test with few sera. In: Histocompatibility testing, p. 237. Baltimore: Williams & Wilkins 1967.
186. — Tripp, M., Weigle, J., Bodmer, W., Bodmer, J.: A new leukocyte isoantigen system in man. Cold Spr. Harb. Symp. quant. Biol. **29**, 285 (1964).
187. Persky, L., Jacobs, S.: Effect of ACTH and cortisone on homologous kidney transplants. Proc. Soc. exp. Biol. (N.Y.) **77**, 66 (1951).
188. Pierce, J. C., Hume, D. M.: The effects of splenectomy on the survival of first and second renal homografts in man. Surg. Gynec. Obstet. **127**, 1300 (1968).
189. — Varco, R. L.: Induction of tolerance to a canine renal homotransplant with 6-mercaptopurine. Lancet **1962 I**, 781.
190. Porter, K. A., Calne, R. Y., Zukoski, C. F.: Vascular and other changes in 200 canine renal homotransplants treated with immunosuppressive drugs. Lab. Invest. **13**, 810 (1964).
191. Thomson, W. B., Owens, K., Kenyon, J. R., Mowbray, J. F., Peart, W. S.: Obliterative vascular changes in four human kidney homotransplants. Brit. med. J. **1963 I**, 639.
192. Prehn, R. T., Main, J. M.: Immunity to methylcholanthrene-induced sarcomas. J. nat. Cancer Inst. **18**, 769 (1957).
193. Prout, G. R., Hume, D. M., Lee, H. M., Williams, G. M.: Some urological aspects of 93 consecutive renal homotransplants in modified recipients. J. Urol. (Baltimore) **97**, 409 (1967).
194. Reeve, C. E., Martin, D. C., Gonick, H. C., Kaufman, J. J., Rubini, M. E., Mims, M. M., Goodwin, W. E., Koppel, M. H., Kopple, J. O., Goldman, R.: Kidney transplantation: a comparison of results using cadaver and related living donors. Amer. J. Med. (in press).
195. Retik, A. B., Hollenberg, N. K., Rosen, S. M., Merrill, J. P., Murray, J. E.: Cortical ischemia in renal allograft rejection. Surg. Gynec. Obstet. **124**, 989 (1967).
196. — Rosen, S. M., Hollenberg, N. K., Murray, J. E., Harrison, J. H.: Intrarenal distribution of blood flow in canine renal allografts treated with immunosuppressive drugs. J. Urol. (Baltimore) **101**, 482 (1969).
197. Rifkind, D.: Cytomegalovirus infection after renal transplantation. Arch. intern. Med. **116**, 554 (1965).
198. — Faris, T. D., Hills, R. B., Jr.: Pneumocystis carinii pneumonia: studies on the diagnosis and treatment. Ann. intern. Med. **65**, 943 (1966).
199. — Goodman, N., Hills, R. B., Jr.: The clinical significance of cytomegalovirus infection in renal transplant recipients. Ann. intern. Med. **66**, 1116 (1967a).
200. — Marchioro, T. L., Schneck, S. A., Hills, R. B.: Systemic fungal infections complicating renal transplantation and immunosuppressive therapy. Amer. J. Med. **43**, 28 (1967b).
201. — — Waddell, W. R., Starzl, T. E.: Infectious diseases associated with renal homotransplantation. I. Incidence, types, and predisposing factors. J. Amer. med. Ass. **189**, 397 (1964a).
202. — Starzl, T. E., Marchioro, T. L., Waddell, W. R., Rowlands, D. T., Jr., Hills, R. B., Jr.: Transplantation pneumonia. J. Amer. med. Ass. **189**, 808 (1964b).
203. Robertshaw, G. E., Madge, G. E., Kauffman, H. M.: Ureteral pathology in treated and untreated renal homografts. Surg. Forum **17**, 236 (1966).
204. — — Williams, G. M., Hume, D. M.: Nephrotoxic activity of hyperimmune homologous dog immune serum. Surg. Forum **18**, 276 (1967).

205. Rock, R., Rosenau, W., Najarian, J. S.: A clinicopathologic study of human renal homotransplantation. Surg. Gynec. Obstet. **125**, 289 (1967).
206. Rosenau, W., Lee, J. C., Najarian, J. S.: A light fluorescence, and electron microscopic study of functioning human renal transplants. Surg. Gynec. Obstet. **128**, 62 (1969).
207. Russell, P. S., Monaco, A. P.: Heterologous antilymphocyte sera and some of their effects. Transplantation **5**, 1086 (1967).
208. Samuelson, J. S., Fisher, B., Fisher, E. R.: Prolonged survival of skin homografts in dogs with thoracic duct fistula. Surg. Forum **14**, 192 (1963).
209. Schapiro, A., Paul, W., Gonick, H.: Urinary beta-glucuronidase in urologic diseases of the kidneys. J. Urol. (Baltimore) **100**, 146 (1968).
210. Schneck, S. A.: Neuropathological features of human organ transplantation. J. Neuropath. exp. Neurol. **25**, 18 (1966).
211. Schwartz, R., Damashek, W.: Drug-induced immunological tolerance. Nature (Lond.) **183**, 1682 (1959).
212. Shanfield, I., Ladaga, L. G., Wren, S. F. G., Blennerhasset, J. B., MacLean, L. D.: Prolongation of canine renal allograft survival with antilymphoid antisera. Surg. Gynec. Obstet. **127**, 29 (1968).
213. Singal, D. P., Mickey, M. R., Terasaki, P. I.: Serotyping for homotransplantation. XXIII. Analysis of kidney transplants from parental versus sibling donors. Transplantation **7**, 246 (1969).
214. Singh, L. M., Fega, R. E., Makin, G. S., Howard, J. M.: External thoracic duct fistula and canine renal homograft. J. Amer. med. Ass. **191**, 1009 (1965).
215. Smellie, W. A. B., Vinik, M., Hume, D. M.: Angiographic investigation of hypertension complicating human renal transplantation. Surg. Gynec. Obsted **128**, 963 (1969)..
216. Smith, R. B.: Alexis Carrel (1873—1944) Invest. Urol. **5**, 102 (1967a).
217. — Martin, D. C., Terasaki, P. I., Mims, M. M., Kaufman, J. J., Goldman, R., Rubini, M., Goodwin, W. E.: Experience with 47 renal homotransplantations from cadaver donors with emphasis on the donor with marginally acceptable kidneys. Amer. Surg. **35**, 1 (1969).
218. — Terasaki, P. I., Martin, D. C.: A rapid metabolic screening test to evaluate potential cadaveric kidney donors. J. Amer. med. Ass. **201**, 160 (1967b).
219. — — — Clinical use of the tetrazolium test for evaluation of potential cadaveric donors for renal homotransplantation. J. Amer. med. Ass. **100**, 361 (1968).
220. Starzl, T. E.: Experience in renal transplantation. Philadelphia: Saunders 1964a.
221. — Brettschneider, L., Penn, I., Schmidt, R. W., Bell, P., Kashiwagi, N., Townsend, C. M., Putman, C. W.: A trial with heterologous antilymphocyte globulin in man. Transplant. Proc. **1**, 448 (1969).
222. — Lerner, R. A., Dixon, F. J., Groth, C. G., Brettschneider, L., Teaesaki, P. I.: Schwartzman reaction after human renal homotransplantation. New Engl. J. Med. **278**, 642 (1968).
223. — Marchioro, T. L., Holmes, J. H., Hermann, G., Brittain, R. S., Stonington, O. H., Talmage, D. W., Waddell, W. R.: Renal homografts, in patients with major donor-recipient incompatibilities. Surgery **55**, 195 (1964b).
224. — — Hutchison, D. E., Porter, K. A., Cerilli, J., Brettschneider, L.: The clinical use of antilymphocyte globulin in renal homotransplantation. Transplantation **5**, 1100 (1967a).
225. — — Morgan, W. W., Waddell, W. R.: A technique for use of adult renal homografts in children. Surg. Gynec. Obstet. **119**, 106 (1964c).
226. — — Porter, K. A., Iwasaki, Y., Cerilli, G. J.: The use of heterologous antilymphoid agents in canine renal and liver homotransplantation and in human renal homotransplantation. Surg. Gynec. Obstet. **124**, 301 (1967b).
227. — — — Moore, C. A., Rifkind, D., Waddell, W. R.: Renal transplantation: Late function and complications. Ann. intern. Med. **61**, 470 (1964d).
228. — — Terasaki, P. I., Porter, K. A., Faris, T. D., Herrmann, T. J., Vredevoe, D. L., Hutt, M. P., Ogden, D. A., Waddell, W. R.: Chronic survival after human renal homotransplantation. Ann. Surg. **162**, 749 (1965).
229. Stewart, J. H., Sheil, A. G. R., Johnson, J. R., Wyatt, K. M., Sharp, A. M., Johnston, J.: Successful renal allotransplantation in presence of lymphocytotoxic antibodies. Lancet **1969 I**, 176.
230. Straffon, R.: Personal communication.
231. Straffon, R. A., Kiser, W. S., Stewart, B. H., Hewitt, C. B., Gifford, R. W., Nakamoto, S.: Four years clinical experience with 138 kidney transplants. J. Prol. (Baltimore) **99**, 479 (1968).
232. Swales, J. D., Evans, D. B.: Erythremia in renal transplantation. Brit. med. J. **2**, 80 (1969).

233. Taylor, R. B.: Decay of immunological responsiveness after thymectomy in adult life. Nature (Lond.) **208**, 1334 (1965).
234. Terasaki, P. I., Mandell, M., van de Water, J., Edgington, T. S.: Human blood lymphocyte cytotoxicity reactions with allogenic antisera. Ann. N.Y. Acad. Sci. **120**, 332 (1964).
235. — Marchioro, T. L., Starzl, T. E.: Serotyping of human lymphocyte antigens. II. Preliminary trials on long term kidney homograft survivors. Nat. Acad. Sci. Monograph on Histocompatibility testing, Washington, D.C. 1965, p. 83.
236. — Martin, D. C., Smith, R. B.: A rapid metabolism test to screen cadaver kidneys for transplantation. Transplantation **5**, 76 (1967a).
237. — Porter, K. A., Marchioro, T. L., Mickey, M. R., Vredevoe, D. L., Faris, T. D., Starzl, T. E.: Serotyping for homotransplantation. VII. Selection of kidney donors for 32 recipients. N.Y. Acad. Sci. **129**, 500 (1966).
238. — Vredevoe, D. L., Mickey, M. R.: Serotyping for homotransplantation. X. Survival of 196 grafted kidneys subsequent to typing. Transplantation **5**, 1057 (1967b).
239. Thompson, B. W., Denny, W. F.: Erythropoietin after renal autotransplantation. Amer. J. Surg. **116**, 800 (1968).
240. Thompson, J. S., Severson, C. D., Lavender, A. R., Forland, M., Russe, H. P.: Assay of human leukoagglutinins by capillary migration. Transplantation **6**, 728 (1968).
241. Tilney, N. L., Collins, J. J., Wilson, R. E.: Hemorrhagic pancreatitis. A fatal complication of renal transplantation. New Engl. J. Med. **274**, 1051 (1966).
242. — Murray, J. E.: The thoracic duct fistula as an adjunct to immunosuppression in human renal transplantation. Transplantation **5**, 1204 (1967).
243. Traeger, J., Carraz, M., Fries, D., Perrin, J., Saubier, E., Bernhardt, J. P., Revillard, J. P., Bonnet, P., Archimbaud, J. P., Brochier, J.: Studies of antilymphocyte globulins made from thoracic duct lymphocytes. Transplant. Proc. **1**, 455 (1969).
244. Truniger, B., Rosen, S. M., Kriek, H., Merrill, J. P., Murray, J. E.: Intrarenal distribution of blood flow in the rejecting homotransplanted dog kidney. Surg. Forum **16**, 254 (1965).
245. Tunner, W. S., Carbone, P. P., Blaylock, W. K., Irvin III, G. L.: Effect of thoracic duct lymph drainage on the immune response in man. Surg. Gynec. Obstet. **121**, 334 (1965).
246. Ullmann, E.: Experimentelle Nierentransplantation. Wien. klin. Wschr. **15**, 281 (1902).
247. Van Rood, J. J.: A proposal for international cooperation in organ transplantation: Eurotransplant. 1967.
248. Veith, F. J., Luck, J., Murray, J. E.: Splenectomy in immunsuppressive regimens in dog and man. Surg. Forum **15**, 161 (1964).
249. — — — The effects of splenectomy on immunosuppressive regimens in dog and man. Surg. Gynec. Obstet. **121**, 229 (1965).
250. Voronoy, U.: Sobre el bloqueo del aparato reticulo-endotelial de hombre en algunas formas de intoxicacion por el sublimado y sobre la transplantacion del rinon cadaverico como metoda de traitamiento de la anuria consecutiva a aquella intoxicacion. Siglo méd. **97**, 296 (1936).
251. Waksman, B. H., Arbouys, S., Arnason, B. G.: The use of specific "lymphocytic antisera" to inhibit hypersensitive reactions of the delayed type. J. exp. Med. **114**, 997 (1961).
252. Walford, R. L.: The relation of anti-leukocyte antibodies to the homograft reaction: their occurrence in human sera. Transplant. Bull. **5**, 55 (1958).
253. — Martin, D. C., Troup, G. M., Goodwin, W. E.: Skin graft survival times in human donor-recipient pairs selected on the basis of lymphocyte typing. In: Histocompatibility testing, p. 89. Copenhagen: Munksgaard 1965.
254. Waller, M., Irby, R., Mullinax, F., Toone, E. C.: Connective-tissue disease and rheumatoid factors in patients with renal transplants. New Engl. J. Med. **273**, 12 (1965).
255. Werder, A. A., Hardin, C.: Effect of splenectomy on survival rate of homologous skin grafts in C.F.W. mice. Surgery **35**, 405 (1954).
256. Wheeler, J. R., White, W. F., Calne, R. Y.: Selective lymphopenia by use of intralymphatic $^{198}$Au and splenectomy. Brit. med. J. **1965 II**, 339.
257. Williams, G. M., Hume, D. M., Hudson, R. P., Morris, P. J., Kano, K., Milgrom, F.: "Hyperacute" renal-homograft rejection in man. New Engl. J. Med. **279**, 611 (1968a).
258. — — Kano, K., Milgrom, F.: Transplantation antibodies in human recipients of renal grafts. J. Amer. med. Ass. **204**, 119 (1968b).
259. — Rolley, R. T., Hume, D. M.: A comparison of lymphocyte and kidney cell typing in eleven patients. Surg. Forum **19**, 209 (1968c).

260. WILLIAMSON, C. S.: Some observations on the length of survival and function of homologous kidney transplants. Preliminary report. J. Urol. (Baltimore) **10**, 275 (1923).
261. WILSON, R. E., HAGER, E. B., HAMPERS, C. L., CORSON, J. M., MERRILL, J. P., MURRAY, J. E.: Immunologic rejection of human cancer transplanted with a renal allograft. New Engl. J. Med. **278**, 479 (1968).
262. WINKELSTEIN, A., CRADDOCK, C. G., MARTIN, D. C., LIBBY, R. L., NORMAN, A., SASAKI, M. S.: $Sv^{90}$-$Y^{90}$ extracorporal irradiation in goats and men. Radiat. Res. **31**, 215 (1967).
263. WOLF, J. S., HUME, D. M.: Prolongation of renal homograft survival by external radiation of renal arterial blood. Fed. Proc. **24**, 583 (1965).
264. — LEE, H. M., O'FOGHLUDHA, F. T., HUME, D. M.: Effect of circulating blood radiation with an extracorporeal $strontium^{90}$ shunt on transplantation immunity in dogs and man. Surg. Forum **17**, 245 (1966a).
265. — MCGAVIC, J. D., HUME, D. M.: Inhibition of the effector mechanism of transplantation immunity by local graft irradiation. Surg. Gynec. Obstet. **128**, 584 (1969).
266. — O'FOGHLUDHA, F. T., KAUFFMAN, H. M., HUME, D. M.: Prolongation of renal homograft survival by indwelling beta irradiation. Surg. Gynec. Obstet. **122**, 1262 (1966b).
267. WOODRUFF, M. F. A.: The transplantation of tissues and organs. Springfield, Ill.: Thomas 1960.
268. YAMADA, T., BOSHER, L. H., JR., RICHARDSON, G. M.: Observations on the autoperfused heart-lung preparation. Amer. Soc. Art. Int. Organs **11**, 192 (1965).
269. ZMIJEWSKI, C. M.: A critical analysis of the leukocyte agglutination reaction as applied to histocompatibility testing for human renal homotransplantation. In: Histocompatibility testing, p. 193. Copenhagen: Munksgaard 1965.
210. ZOLLINGER, R. M., LINDEM, M. C., FILLER, R. M., CORSON, J. M., WILSON, R. E.: Effect of thymectomy on skin-homograft survival in children. New Engl. J. Med. **270**, 707 (1964).
271. ZUKOSKI, C. F., ENDE, N.: Membraneous glomerulonephritis complicating prolonged survival of a homografted kidney. Transplantation **3**, 118 (1965).
272. — LEE, H. M., HUME, D. M.: The effect of 6-mercaptopurine on renal homograft survival in the dog. Surg. Gynec. Obstet. **112**, 707 (1961).

# Open Surgery of the Prostate

R. F. Gittes

With 15 Figures

## A. Introduction

Today's urologists have inherited from their teachers an understanding of surgical prostatectomy which has relegated such a procedure to a routine performance. This chapter will concern itself with the distillation of the present day practice of open surgical prostatectomy with special attention to the indications, the preoperative preparation and diagnostic evaluation, the established successful surgical techniques, and the management of possible complications. Transurethral prostatectomy, which has rightly become the technique most frequently used by American urologists for routine prostatectomy, will be considered in a separate chapter in deference to its special technical problems.

The triumphs and the earnest failures of our predecessors in the last eighty years are relegated to the chapter on the history of urology. Although not detailed here, they represented a colorful epic of daring perserverance and frequent disillusion. It is a fitting tribute to the accomplishment of the great clinicians of the past that prostatectomy by the suprapubic, retropubic, or perineal route is now a routine procedure.

## B. Indications and Choice of Operation

### I. Benign Prostatic Hypertrophy

It is generally agreed that the presence of prostatic enlargement alone, if there is no suspicion of malignancy, is not a sufficient indication for prostatic surgery. Patients with demonstrable prostatic enlargement who develop urinary retention or have objectively demonstrable urethral obstruction and impaired renal function must of course be advised to have surgery. Between these two extremes, judgment and wisdom must be exercised in advising surgery. Obstructive symptoms must be considered in the light of whether there is or is not infection present. In the absence of demonstrable infection, the presence of frequency, urgency, nocturia, weakening of the stream, or difficulty in initiating the stream may now be considered sufficient indication for corrective surgery and such surgery is likely to lead to gratifying results. In the presence of demonstrated infection, such symptoms may be transient and completely eliminated by specific medical therapy and elimination of the infection. Patients with recurrent infections, particularly if associated with epididymitis and with definite prostatic enlargement, should also undergo elective prostatectomy. The presence of a post-voiding residual is no longer a necessary indication before surgery is recommended, but if present does indicate significant decompensation of the bladder and the need for surgery. Other indications for such elective surgery include the development of bladder calculi, the recurrence of repeated episodes of prostatic bleeding from engorged vessels on the surface of the prostate, and the presence of an inguinal hernia which is aggravated by the patient straining to void.

The presence of a neurogenic bladder disfunction must be considered. It is important to realize that a previous cerebrovascular accident is a frequent cause of bladder spasticity with intact bladder sensation but impaired inhibitory control of reflex bladder contractions. Such patients may have symptoms indistinguishable from those of moderate prostatic obstruction. The rectal examination and cystoscopy will show unexpectedly little prostatic enlargement or bladder neck obstruction and in such cases a careful cystometrogram will unmask the presence of the neurogenic bladder. Such patients are not ideal for prostatectomy because the procedure may increase their urgency incontinence. It is best to treat such patients with anticholinergic medication and to follow them closely for the secondary development of infection or obstruction.

## II. Chronic Prostatitis and Prostatic Calculi

Recurrent chronic prostatitis is to be treated if at all possible only with conservative medical measures which include specific antibiotics, judicious use of prostatic massage, and local heat. In some instances, these cases appear to progress to a bladder neck obstruction, presumably on the basis of the chronic inflammation around the bladder outlet, and usually accompanied by the presence of a small fibrous scarred prostate gland which is not in itself obstructive. Multiple small calculi are frequently present in such glands. Although some authorities advocate open prostatectomy and bladder neck revision for these cases, we prefer the more simple step of performing a transurethral resection of the bladder neck and prostatic tissue as the first choice of therapy. In those cases in which secondary bladder neck obstruction develops after a transurethral resection, then the use of open bladder neck revision becomes a treatment of choice.

There are some cases of active chronic prostatitis in which the symptoms of pain and dysuria seem to be unusually prominent. These are often accentuated in patients who have had a transurethral resection of a gland with prostatitis. A likely mechanism for such difficulty is the presence of occluded inflammatory pockets in the residual prostatic tissue or particularly in the seminal vesicle. The severity and unresponsiveness of such cases justifies the recommendation of open surgery to insure the removal of such chronically inflamed tissue and to provide symptomatic relief. The best procedure in such unusual cases is a perineal or retropubic prostatovesiculectomy, with subtotal resection of the apex of the prostate and the bladder neck to permit a more functional reapproximation of the bladder outlet. Sexual impotence is to be predicted after such a procedure. In fact, most patients in such a special category have already developed impotence as a part of their presenting picture; and if they have not, they are willing to accept it in return for the elimination of their severe symptoms.

Prostatic calculi which are small in size and are seen in plain X-rays of patients afflicted with chronic prostatitis, are in themselves not an indication for prostatectomy. However, if subtotal transurethral resection has been carried out in the past and infection exists in contact with such calculi, such infection is almost impossible to eradicate and open surgery is indicated. Further, prostatic calculi occasionally are large enough to produce outlet obstruction. Rare cases have been noted in which the calculus in itself was as large as a hypertrophied gland. Occasionally such large calculi can be dislodged into the bladder and there crushed and eliminated without open surgery. But as a rule open surgical exposure is necessary and is indicated by the perineal or retropubic routes.

## III. Prostatic Abscess

The advent of powerful antibiotics has not only drastically reduced the incidence of prostatic abscess but has also permitted a more circumspect approach to their therapy (Becker and Harrin, 1964). Rather than immediate drainage, the effect of antibiotics on the condition of the patient and the size of the abscess can be monitored. If progressive shrinkage is not achieved, internal drainage by transurethral unroofing of the abscess cavity should be attempted after the initial control of the symptoms with antibiotic therapy. Rarely a large abscess has formed which has broken through the prostatic capsule and presents primarily as a phlegmon in the perineum or against the rectal wall. In that case, such a collection is best drained through a standard perineal incision. Most commonly an acute prostatitis and abscess formation may lead to urinary retention with bladder outlet occlusion. The abscess in these cases may be relatively inaccessible to a perineal or transurethral approach and presents an indication for a suprapubic exposure with transvesical unroofing of the abscess and diversion with a suprapubic tube. Late complications of prostatic abscess include the development of a urethral diverticulum and the possibility of a urethroperineal or urethrorectal fistula, all of which may require later open surgical repair.

## IV. Malignancy of the Prostate

The total removal of a carcinoma localized to the prostate gland can be hoped for only by resort to open radical prostatectomy (Huggins, 1969). Unfortunately, only about 10% of patients with this disease have it detected at such an early state (Culp, 1967). The possibility of surgical extirpation is good if the carcinoma is present as a palpable nodule or is detected in a major portion of the tissue removed by transurethral resection in an apparently benign prostate gland (Goodwin, 1952).

It is to be noted that the patients with "incidental carcinoma", not palpable rectally but found microscopically in the specimen of an obstructive prostate removed by open or transurethral resection, do as well without any treatment as with endocrine therapy, achieving a 10 year survival about 50 percent (Emmett et al., 1960). It is doubtful that any further therapy is indicated on them, particularly in view of the hazards of estrogen administration (Arduino et al., 1967, Lehman et al., 1968).

If extensive carcinoma is detected after the removal of the prostate tissue through open transcapsular surgery, or if the disease is judged to extend lateral to the prostatic capsule by palpation, then the advantage of total surgical excision is no longer present and conservative medical therapy must be used. Clearly, the presence of detectable distant metastases also rules out radical surgery. Detailed consideration of the indications for radical surgery in carcinoma of the prostate is included later in this chapter.

Sarcoma of the prostate, whether the rhabdomoysarcoma of children or the adult forms of this rare condition (Stirling and Ash, 1939; Melicow et al., 1943) has demonstrated such rapid invasion and grim prognosis that an aggressive surgical attack with prostato-cystectomy (Miller et al., 1969) alone or in combination with chemotherapy may offer the only hope for cure (Goodwin, Mims, and Young, 1968).

# C. Preoperative Preparation

The increasing safety and success of open prostatic surgery is due in no small part to the fact such surgery is almost never an emergency procedure. It is the duty of the surgeon to provide the optimal preoperative diagnostic and therapeutic measures in respect to various sources of possible complication.

## I. Evaluation of Renal Function

The patient with significant obstructive uropathy is likely to have damage to his renal function. This will be routinely demonstrated by determination of the concentration of urea in the blood and a creatinine clearance. Various clinics are now limiting themselves to the accurate determination of serum creatinine and omitting the determination of blood urea nitrogen. The presence of an elevated serum creatinine in someone with obstructive symptoms is a sufficient and imperative indication for the establishment of catheter drainage to the bladder. It is a common experience to document a progressive decrease in the creatinine levels after the placement of the catheter. It is to be remembered that the creatinine level may not return to normal but establish a plateau at a lower level and that prolongation of catheter drainage at this point is of no help to the patient. It is likely in such cases that there is sufficient obstruction of the terminal ureters by the prostate so that drainage of the bladder has limited effectiveness. Prolongation of such drainage only increases the chances of urethral infection, epididymitis, or ascending infection into the partialy obstructed upper urinary tract. The same considerations make it unreasonable to resort to the old practice of two-stage prostatectomy in which placement of a suprapubic cystos stomy preceded by weeks or months an attempt at the surgical relief of the obstruction.

An intravenous urogram should be performed in all cases provided that there is no allergy to the contrast agents. The presently available contrast agents may be considered safe even in the presence of impaired renal function. If the serum creatinine is elevated above 3 mg percent, adequate visualization of the upper tracts may not be achieved in spite of the administration of large doses of contrast agents by the infusion technique. It is to be remembered, however, that the absolute value of the creatinine is not a contraindication if the serum creatinine level has been dropping as a result of the relief of obstruction by catheter drainage. The establishment of catheter drainage and the use of large doses of contrast agents combined with nephrotomography will provide enough information in many uremic patients so that retrograde pyelograms need not be done. Retrograde pyelograms carry an increased risk and greater technical difficulty in cases of prostatic obstruction. But they become necessary when there is a suspicion from the intravenous urogram of associated upper tract pathology such as calculi or tumors.

Serum electrolytes should be obtained in any patient with impaired renal function who is treated with preliminary catheter drainage. The accompanying postobstructive diuresis is occasionally marked by severe sodium depletion which can rapidly lead to hypovolemia, CNS depression, and vascular collapse (Wilson, 1951; Eiseman, 1955). Also detected occasionally is a syndrome of inappropriate secretion of antidiuretic hormone in which symptomatic hyponatremia and water intoxication can occur due to the persistent excretion of hypertonic urine in spite of the dilution of the serum to hypotonic levels (Murphy, 1968). Such patients probably have a hypothalamic disfunction rather than renal impairment.

## II. Preoperative Infection

Urinary infection and its potential for gram negative septicemia will have to be prevented or controlled in all cases before the risk of prostatic surgery is reduced to its potential minimum. Because there is such an overlap in the symptoms of obstruction and lower tract infection, a routine bacteriological culture of the urine should be obtained in all cases being prepared for prostatic surgery. Antibiotic sensitivity tests, preferably those using dilution techniques, should be carried out on all positive cultures.

Patients who are candidates for prostatic surgery and have negative urine cultures should be spared from preliminary catheter drainage, if at all possible, in order to avoid introducing an infection. Clearly, however, the presence of impaired renal function, significant clot retention or bladder decompensation are overriding considerations in favor of catheter drainage in such cases. When catheter drainage is established, effective prophylaxis against infection is now available by the use of closed sterile drainage (Finkelberg and Kunin, 1969), and the use of the proven adjuvants of hydration and urinary acidification.

When preoperative infection is present, the surgeon must make the judgment as to whether it represents an active inflammatory process of the urinary organs or simply a bacteriuria without tissue invasion. Active tissue infection requires both antibiotic therapy and a consideration of measures to improve the drainage of any obstructed and infected urine as a prelude to any consideration of open surgery. Such measures will include catheter drainage of the bladder and epididymectomy. Suprapubic cystostomy has a definite place in the situation when there is tissue infection in the prostate or urethra added to the preexisting urinary obstruction. The presence of bacteriuria without tissue invasion permits the safe performance of surgery as long as antibiotic therapy specific for that potential infection is initiated with and maintained after surgery.

## III. Coagulation Defects

Every effort is made to avoid preventable blood loss from a coagulation defect. Such a defect is particularly suspected if hematuria has been a presenting symptom. A complete blood count is required to permit the preoperative determination of anemia or blood dyscrasia. The routine determination of prothrombin time is useful and may suggest the preoperative use of vitamin K in this age group. The presence of bleeding suggests the added determination of a platelet count, bleeding and clotting times, and the storage of a blood clot at room temperature for possible fibrinolysins. The presence of hemophilia is now no longer the awesome problem which it represented in the past, due to the availability of antihemophilic factor concentrates.

Again, the presence of a clotting defect deserves ample time allotted to its correction so as to lower considerably the risk of open prostatic surgery.

## IV. Cardiopulmonary Reserve

The extent of the cardiovascular and pulmonary impairment present in the age group being considered for prostatic surgery deserves careful evaluation. Prophylactic measures can improve the chances of uncomplicated surgery. A chest X-ray and an electrocardiogram should be obtained routinely. The presence of significant emphysema or pulmonary fibrosis signals the consideration of the transurethral or perineal routes of surgery. If the nature of the prostatic disease or associated bladder pathology demands an abdominal approach, then preoperative respiratory exercises and the clearing of accumulated secretions may be extremely helpful in preparing the patient. Respiratory function studies performed preoperatively will give a quantitative estimate of the patient's reserve.

The preoperative electrocardiogram is mandatory to provide a baseline for comparison and evaluation of potential cardiovascular difficulties. It will also permit the preoperative discovery of cardiac arrhythmias and their control under optimal conditions. Digitalization can and should be accomplished in a leisurely manner in any preoperative patient with any evidence of congestive failure or with certain types of arrhythmia.

### V. Cystoscopy

It is elementary to point out that cystoscopy must be done prior to any open prostatectomy. The findings are often relied upon for determining the choice of operative technique. However, when other indications point to open prostatectomy, it is easier on the patient and more efficient to perform the examination immediately preceding the surgery and under the same anesthesia.

### VI. Miscellaneous Factors

A determination of the total acid phosphatase and of the prostatic fraction in the serum must be determined routinely in order not to overlook prostatic cancer in apparently benign prostatic conditions. The presence of a definite elevation of acid phosphatase must be checked with a repeat determination in two or three days because of the occasional instances of a false positive elevation due to prostatic infarcts in benign tissue. (Howard and Fraley, 1967). In cases with a clearly suspicious prostatic nodule or induration, preoperative evaluation for metastatic disease must include high quality bone X-rays. Radioisotope bone scans with strontium-85 or fluoride-18. (Williams and Blahd, 1967; Williams et al., 1968) have increased the diagnostic clues available in the search for metastatic cancer of the prostate; but they do not yet have the specificity or definition to require their routine use or to permit the replacing of undue weight on their evidence if it seems to be contrary to the other tests mentioned.

A routine preparation of the lower bowel in the form of an enema the night before surgery is usually indicated. In cases of radical retropubic surgery or perineal prostatectomy, it is considered wise to add to such preparation by giving a retention enema of 0.5% Neomycin to decrease the morbidity of a rectal injury and to increase the chances of a successful intraoperative repair.

## D. Techniques of Open Prostatic Surgery

### I. Transvesical Suprapubic Prostatectomy

The first complete intracapsular enucleation of the prostate for relief of prostatic obstruction was credited to Fuller (1895) and the technique was popularized by Freyer (1896). The procedure was a blind suprapubic transvesical enucleation of the gland with the fingertip after cutting through the mucosa at the vesical neck with the fingernail. Although in popularizing the procedure Freyer pointed out that hemorrhage was not an overwhelming problem and that the prostatic fossa contracted in a manner compared to that of the uterus after childbirth, there were many departures from such an ideal postoperative course so that mortality rates as high as 50% were observed in the early years of its acceptance. It is no credit to the urological profession that such a blind prostatectomy is still practiced to this day. Although variations in the technique were introduced and heralded as great contributions, such as the use of hemostatic bags, hotpacks, and the use of a finger in the rectum, such techniques are best relegated to a historical shelf and should be mentioned only to be discarded in present day practice. It was Thompson-Walker in 1909 who originated the performance of suprapubic prostatectomy under direct vision and the control of bleeding by suture ligature of the vesical neck. Various modifications and additions to this technique have been added and variably adopted by different groups.

## 1. Indications and Contraindications

This approach is limited to the treatment of benign hyperplasia of the prostate. It is relatively indicated when the adenoma is both (a) estimated larger than 40 gm and (b) largely intravesical. These findings weigh against transurethral or retropubic approaches as first choice. The added presence of a large bladder diverticulum, large vesical calculi, or a previous cystostomy usually make suprapubic prostatectomy the procedure of choice. The procedure is relatively contraindicated when the obstruction is due mainly to a small or fibrous, intracapsular prostate; in such cases the combined, retropubic, or transurethral approaches are preferable.

## 2. Technique

Under spinal or general anesthesia the patient is surgically prepared over the lower abdomen and the genitalia. A catheter is introduced into the bladder and the bladder gently distended with sterile saline. Either a vertical or transverse incision may be used to approach the anterior face of the bladder. In a thin muscular patient, the transverse incision is more comfortable and permits a wide exposure. In an obese patient, the vertical incision is favored to permit extension of the incision for greater exposure and to avoid maceration of the wound by abdominal folds. The transverse incision is made just above the transverse skin crease above the pubis. The double leaf of fascia anterior to the rectus muscles is cut with heavy scissors for the full extent of the skin incision and then fascia is the dissected off the recti with blunt dissection so as to permit lateral retraction of the muscles in the vertical incision. The fibrous septum between the muscles is cut down to the symphysis pubis, and the muscles and their overlying fascia retracted laterally. At this point, with the bladder exposed and still slightly distended with fluid, it is advisable to dissect down its anterior face toward the bladder neck with gentle blunt dissection so as to define and control the friable veins which bridge the space of Retzius. Dissection and control of these potential bleeders at this point facilitates the closure at the end of the procedure and permits, if necessary, the extension of the cystotomy through the bladder neck and into the prostatic capsule as described under the combined prostatectomy.

A self retaining retractor is used to maintain the exposure. An incision is made into the anterior wall of the bladder and its contents aspirated. This incision is to be made adequate for a proper exposure of the intravesical operative field. The usual incision is a vertical one of at least 10 cm in length. A transverse incision has been advocated but is not generally used. After inspection of the bladder wall a gauze pack is placed in the dome of the bladder and used to support a retractor, preferably a heavy blunt spade retractor which will draw the bladder cephalad and place on tension the posterior wall. It is very useful here to introduce two curved deep retractors, such as narrow Deaver retractors, on each side of the cystomy inferiorly to provide wide exposure on the bladder outlet. For this purpose, it is most convenient to have a second assistant. Also helpful is the suture of the sides of the bladder to the edge of the muscles spread laterally by the self-retaining retractor.

The ureteral orifices ought to be identified. It is poor practice to routinely probe them, unless there is a question of their identification. The mucosa and submucosa tented up by the prostate gland is now incised with scalpel or cutting cautery in a tight circle being careful to leave a generous flange of mucosa posteriorly for the subsequent plastic repair of the bladder neck. This incision is to be made deep into the substance of the prostatic adenoma so that there is no question as to the plane between the adenoma and bladder neck posteriorly. If the incision is too shallow, or too close to the bladder neck, there is the danger of establishing a dissection plane which carries the inexperienced surgeon posterior to and outside of the prostatic capsule. With a tonsil tip suction and delicate long dissecting scissors the plane between the adenoma and the capsule is demonstrated to the surgeon's satisfaction and the enucleation of the prostate begun posteriorly by spreading of the scissors. This dissection may be continued with scissors if it is easy and under continued direct vision. Certainly, if the gland is fibrotic and fused to the capsule, sharp dissection with scissors is often the only alternative. More usually, however, it is best to use fingertip dissection in the plane started by the scissors. The finger can then quickly and safely separate the adenoma from the capsule posteriorly and laterally, down to the apex of the gland if possible. Anteriorly, the capsule may be quite thin and firmly attached to the substance of the prostate. To separate the adenoma from the midline anteriorly it is wise to return to sharp dissection under direct vision, with good exposure retracting the anterior bladder neck from the gland. The adenoma is grasped with a double tenaculum and gently lifted with a rocking motion so as to deliver it from the prostatic capsule posteriorly, still attached to the prostatic capsule anteriorly. The fibers attaching the gland to the capsule are divided progressively down towards the apex of the gland, advancing the double-hooked forceps towards the apex as needed. It is most important to avoid undue traction which might tear the membranous urethra and lead to incontinence. If the gland is not too large, it is usually possible to retract the anterior capsule caudad and depress the gland posteriorly so as to visualize the stretched urethra at the apex and to divide it transversely with scissors under direct vision. In a large gland it is often wiser to guide the long Metzenbaum scissors beyond the apex by a touch alone and with the tips sever the last attachment of the prostate to the urethra. Unless it is of extraordinary size, the adenoma should be removed in one piece and examined for obvious defects that might suggest that a significant nodule of hyperplasia has been left behind attached to the capsule.

Two or three gauze sponges should now be packed into the prostatic fossa to control the venous bleeding from the capsular wall. It is imperative that arterial bleeding be directly visualized and controlled by the surgeon. Fortunately, the arterial inflow penetrates the prostate just below the rim of the bladder neck and such opened arteries can be directly visualized.

A long Allis forceps is used to grasp the center of the posterior bladder neck and with traction careful examination of the adjacent quadrant of the bladder neck and with traction careful examination of the adjacent quadrant of the bladder neck is possible. If there is a prominent lip of fibrous tissue in this area it is advisable to place additional Allis forceps into its substance and to excise it with sharp dissection. The penetrating arterial supply is visualized accurately when the fibrous tissue is cut back in this manner, so that there is no question as to where hemostatic sutures must be placed. Having visualized the main arterial inflow in each posterior quadrant the bleeding is controlled by a Fig. 8 hemostatic suture with 00 or 000 chromic catgut (Fig. 1). Using these sutures and

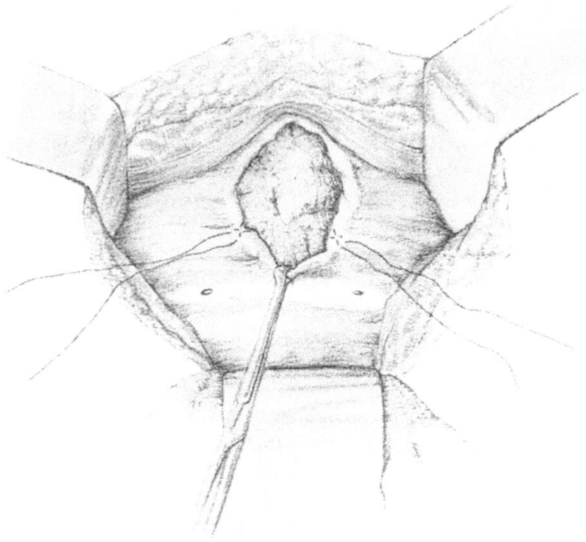

Fig. 1. Suprapubic prostatectomy. Control of arterial bleeding at the bladder neck is illustrated for emphasis on the positioning of figure of 8 suture ligatures in the posterior quadrants of the denuded bladder neck where the arterial bleeders can be visualized. Gauze packing is kept in the depth of the fossa as shown and an Allis clamp applied to the posterior bladder neck to aid in the arterial visualization. With very large adenomata, arterial bleeders may be visualized in the anterior quadrants

the Allis forceps for traction, the anterior quadrants of the bladder neck are examined for possible additional arterial bleeders. These are frequently seen only when the adenoma removed was of a very large size. The smaller anterior bleeding points may also be controlled with suture ligatures or with cautery.

At this point, with the hemostatic sutures in place and the gauze pack controlling the venous bleeding from the depths of the capsule it should be possible to carry out a plastic repair of the bladder neck without troublesome bleeding. The purpose of the repair is to cover over some of the denuded surface of the capsule with an apron of mucosa and at the same time to smooth out the lip of the bladder wall and prevent the complication of an obstructive veil forming at the bladder outlet. To perform the plastic repair, the gauze sponges are removed from the prostatic capsule to expose the posterior surface of the capsule. It is sufficient for the repair to take 4 or 5 interrupted sutures of 000 chromic catgut catching the edge of the mucosa and the movable submucosa with the first bite and then reaching down to take a good bite of the fibrous capsule directly below the lip of the opening. It is usually not necessary to carry the repair to the anterior quadrants of the bladder neck because of the scarcity of redundant tissue in this area. The repair may also be conveniently performed by running a 00 chromic catgut continuous suture along the entire posterior semicircle of the bladder neck, securing the mucosa and the mucosa down to the capsule to provide good hemostasis, at the same time avoiding constriction of the bladder outlet. A more extensive repair is routinely attempted by some surgeons and involves the approximation of the bladder neck to the very apex of the prostatic capsule, in an effort to completely exclude the raw surface of the posterior capsule. Such suturing of the vesical neck to the area of the urethral stump was advocated as long ago as 1906 by DUVALL and LEGUEU, revived by HARRIS (1930) with the use of a boomerang needle, and still practiced today by various surgeons with the use of a boomerang or a Reverdin needle to place the anchoring suture into the capsule just proximal to the verumontanum. There is no question that this procedure when successful eliminates some of the postoperative venous ooze and that it may yield postoperative cystourethrograms with smooth funneling in the wall of the prostatic fossa. However, the suture is always placed under definite tension and it is frequently found to have pulled out after the catheter is removed. In addition, the anchoring suture is placed deeply in the area where it can affect the ejaculatory ducts, and risk either a periprostatic abscess or a rectourethral fistula.

A Foley catheter is now introduced into the bladder through the surgically prepared penis and the balloon is inflated to a sufficient size so as to prevent its retraction into the prostatic fossa. Usually, a 30 $cm^3$ balloon inflated to 45 $cm^3$ will do nicely. The balloon is an effective aid in postoperative hemostasis if properly used. Its most effective function is to separate the prostatic fossa space from the bladder cavity and the ureteral orifices. This permits venous oozing from the capsular wall to form a secure clot in the capsule and avoid brushing off such hemostatic clots with urine or irrigating fluid. Some surgeons routinely place the balloon within the prostatic fossa and inflate it there to apply tension against the capsular wall. This maneuver negates the beneficial effect of the postoperative contraction of the smooth muscle elements in the prostatic capsule. It also tends to drive potentially infected fluid into the extracapsular space if there has been a tear in the capsule. Further, it increases the chance of damage to the elastic fibers of the membranous urethra and therefore the possibility of postoperative incontinence. A number of specially designed hemostatic bags were used in an effort to compensate for the inadequate surgical hemostasis so frequently seen in the performance of the "blind" suprapubic prostatectomy. They should now be considered historical curiosities.

Another technique tried by surgeons intent on improving hemostasis by separation of the prostatic fossa from the bladder cavity is the suture technique of HRYNTSCHAK (HRYNTSCHAK, 1955), especially as modified by MALAMENT (MALAMENT, 1965). A sturdy nylon suture is passed in purse-string fashion around the circumference of the bladder neck, with both long ends brought out suprapubically and tied over a plastic bridge on the skin. The suture purse-strings the bladder neck around the tube of the Foley catheter, very definitely separating the bladder cavity from the raw prostatic fossa and to some degree controlling the oozing of the opened bladder neck vessels by the purse-string constriction of the tissue. The nylon suture is removed in 24—48 hours by cutting one end and pulling out the purse string. Demonstrated difficulties with the technique of HRYNTSCHAK include secondary fibrosis of the bladder neck (BECK, 1969). Whether these will be frequent enough after the temporary

Malament suture to discourage the proponents of the technique remains to be see (Cohen et al., 1969). The nylon suture is available commercially with an appropriate curved needle and sufficient length of the suture for this specialized use.

Closure of the bladder cavity is carried out only after a careful final inspection of the ureteral orifices to assure that urine is flowing. Some surgeons routinely ask the anesthesiologist to inject indigo carmine or a similar dye at this point to visualize the orifices again. The bladder cavity is emptied of gauze sponges and inspected for significant lacerations from surgical retraction. The cystotomy is closed in water-tight fashion. We prefer to close in two layers, using a 000 plain catgut running suture for the mucosa and submucosa, followed by continuous or interrupted sutures of 00 or 000 chromic catgut to the bladder muscle. This double layer does provide mucosal hemostasis and a very secure closure which will withstand the challenge of subsequent bladder irrigations if necessary. The bladder is filled at this point and additional sutures placed if necessary to make the incision watertight.

The use of a suprapubic tube is still widely practiced because of occasional advantages, although its disadvantages should make its use unnecessary in most cases. Poor control of hemostasis or the presence of unexpected amounts of venous oozing can be more serenely accepted by the surgeon who leaves a large caliber suprapubic tube for through and through irrigation and drainage. Another advantage is found in the cases in which the bladder wall has been noted to be fibrous and leathery suggesting poor postoperative bladder tone and contraction and the need for very prolonged postoperative drainage. In such a case, the suprapubic tube may be left in long after the urethral catheter is removed and provide more comfortable drainage with less risk of urethral stricture.

Drainage of the prevesical space is of great importance. The recognition of this imperative has greatly reduced the morbidity attendant to greater mobilization of the bladder and dissection in the space of Retzius. A soft rubber tube drain is folded into both sides of the bladder and brought out suprapubically, preferably through a separate stab incision.

The wound is closed in routine fashion with special attention paid to avoiding potential undrained spaces were infected urine may lead to difficulty. Running sutures to the fascia or skin should be avoided because of the possible need for opening one portion of the wound in the event of a localized wound infection.

During the closure and frequently for a few hours thereafter in the recovery period it is of some advantage to maintain very gentle traction on the Foley balloon to hold it against the bladder neck and insure the separation of the prostatic fossa from the bladder cavity. This is readily accomplished by using rubber band traction of the catheter to the patient's leg. Heavier traction, with nonelastic lines and weights, or any prolonged traction, are to be avoided because of their danger of serious injury to the sphincter mechanism and urethra.

## II. Retropubic Prostatectomy

Retropubic prostatectomy is the term applied to the technique in which the prostate is approached anteriorly through its capsule without transecting the bladder wall. As in the case of the perineal approach, the term "simple" is used to refer to the enucleation for benign disease, while the terms "total" and "radical" retropubic prostatectomy refer to the more extensive removal of the capsule and seminal vesicles, respectively, along with the entire prostate gland. Various surgeons described an extravesical transcapsular approach to the prostate in the past before MILLIN established and popularized the procedure 25 years ago (MILLIN, 1945). The previous reports failed to establish the procedure, perhaps because of the fact that surgeons were then less prepared to control the potential complications of that approach, particularly those of bleeding, postoperative infection, and damage to the membranous urethra. While the credit for developing the technique into the most widely used open approach to the prostate certainly belongs to MILLIN, the contributions of VAN STOCKUM in 1909, MAIER in 1924, and JACOBS and COOPER in 1933, deserve recognition.

## 1. Indications

The retropubic transcapsular approach is indicated in cases of bladder outlet obstruction by lateral lobe hypertrophy of the prostate which leads to a largely extravesical enlargement of the gland to a degree which makes it unsuitable for complete transurethral resection usually above 40 g. A favorable situation for such an approach can be determined by the cystoscopic and radiographic findings of a large prostatic capsule and gland with relatively little intravesical or middle lobe enlargement. In such a situation, the approach has the decided advantage of better exposure of the prostatic fossa, bladder neck, and apical tissue, permitting more definitive hemostasis, avoiding tearing of the membranous urethra, and allowing a careful repair of the posterior bladder neck.

Obesity or the presence of a narrow deep pelvis may make the exposure unduly difficult. The presence of a small fibrous prostate, prostatic calculi, or the fibrous bladder neck obstruction seen with small fibrotic glands and after transurethral resection all suggest improving the approach by the use of the combined (transvesical and transcapsular) operation described later in this chapter.

## 2. Technique

The patient is positioned with a sand bag or a blanket roll under his lumbosacral region so as to tilt the pelvis for better exposure. The bladder is not filled, in distinction to the transvesical approach. There is again a choice of either a vertical or transverse incision but in either case the rectus and pyramidalis muscles are separated in the midline and the incision carried well down to the attachment of the muscles into the pubis. The incision is kept open with a self-retaining retractor such as the MILLIN or JACOBSON retractors. The prevesical fascia is a filmy areolar layer which is dissected off the anterior aspect of the bladder neck with gentle, blunt dissection. Lateral dissection in the space of Retzius is accomplished by a sweep of the finger against the pubic ramus. The anterior face of the prostatic capsule is exposed with gentle blunt dissection and any penetrating veins crossing into the space of Retzius are ligated or coagulated. The loose areolar tissue can be kept lateral and posterior to the vesicoprostatic angle by pushing it into that corner with one or two gauze packs small enough to be completely tucked into the space and maintain the retraction of the fatty tissue and the stabilization of the prostate. The anterior wall of the bladder is retracted under a gauze pack by the third blade of the self-retaining retractor or by the spade retractor held by the assistant.

A transverse incision is to be made in the anterior face of the prostatic capsule. The use of a transverse incision was a modification introduced by MILLIN which is considered to be important in avoiding extension by tearing into the membranous urethra during enucleation. Lateral extension of the transverse incision may occur but can be easily repaired. Large caliber veins are encountered running along the anterior face of the prostatic capsule and within the outer layers of this capsule. Many surgeons prefer to suture-ligate these veins on either side of the proposed incision and before incising the capsule. It can be done with deep figure 8 sutures of 000 chromic catgut. Another technique involves the division of the capsule with a blend of coagulating and cutting currents from the electro-surgical unit. The caliber of some of the veins makes this difficult at times and it is then useful to apply a Millin capsule clamp to the bleeding cut edge of the capsule and apply a suture ligature behind it. Blood loss can be considerable if there is too much hesitation or inactivity on the part of the surgeon at this point. Suctioning alone will not control the bleeding.

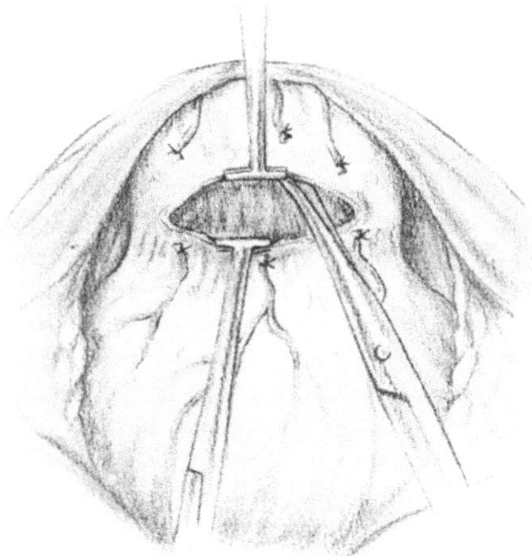

Fig. 2. Retropubic prostatectomy. After ligation of superficial capsular vessels, the capsule has been incised transversely and the edges controlled with Millin clamps. Dissection is started with the scissors to establish the plane of enucleation. Such sharp dissection is continued under direct vision of much fibrosis is present

Having made the capsular incision to the extent of about three fourths of the width of the anterior face of the capsule, and achieved reasonable hemostasis, scissors are used to begin the dissection of the plane of enucleation of the adenoma (Fig. 2). If much fibrosis or calculi are present, the greater part of the dissection has to be sharp. Usually, however, the plane of dissection from the adenoma is established and then digital enucleation is carried out with care to avoid an avulsion of the apex from the membranous urethra. When such digital dissection has freed up the apex except for the attachment of the urethra, small Deaver retractors or capsule clamps are used to retract the inferior margin of the capsular incision and the urethra is cut under direct vision with long scissors. The apical portion of the adenoma is now delivered from the capsule, grasped with a double hook tenaculum and the plane of dissection is followed upward to the bladder neck. The limiting roof of bladder mucosa is cut or ruptured anteriorly and then can be cut under direct vision circumferentially. It is possible to leave a generous cuff of mucosa and submucosa in this procedure so as to stay well away from the ureteral orifices and to permit a plastic repair of the bladder neck. The adenoma is usually delivered in one piece or, if very large, one lateral lobe at a time. It is important to inspect the prostatic fossa for any residual nodules of adenoma and to carefully palpate the bladder neck for residual middle lobe tissue or subtrigonal adenoma. Immediately after the enucleation and inspection, the prostatic fossa may be packed with gauze for a few minutes to decrease the amount of venous oozing obscuring the field. Then the packs are removed from the upper fossa and the midpoint of the posterior bladder neck secured by a Allis forceps or traction suture. The bladder neck must now be evaluated for excess fibrous tissue and the presence of a median bar. This can

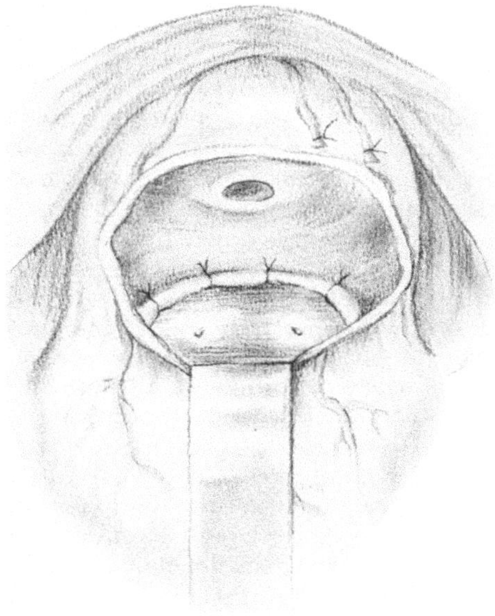

Fig. 3. Retropubic prostatectomy. Diagrammatic illustration of the plastic repair of the bladder neck after transection of the apical urethra and enucleation of the adenoma. The mucosa and submucosa of the bladder neck are sutured down to the posterior capsule with interrupted absorbable sutures. This maneuver provides a mucosal apron to cover the denuded bladder neck and the previously placed hemostatic sutures

easily be resected sharply under direct vision through this exposure and the hemostasis accomplished immediately thereafter. Both posterior quadrants of the bladder neck are carefully inspected and any obscuring fibrous tissue further resected if necessary so as to locate and suture-ligate the principal arterial bleeders, as described earlier for the suprapubic prostatectomy. Further plastic repair of the bladder neck is now carried out, bringing the apron of the mucosa and submucosa down into the prostatic fossa and securing it with interrupted or running sutures of 000 chromic catgut, taking care to avoid undue tension or damage to the terminal ureters (Fig. 3). Intravenous indigo carmine will aid in the inspection for adequate outflow from each orifice.

All gauze packing is removed from the exposed prostatic fossa and its cavity carefully examined. Some venous oozing is inevitable, but the advantage of this approach is in part that it permits careful visualization of any major open channels which can be coagulated or suture ligated. As described in the case of suprapubic prostatectomy, some surgeons elect to eliminate the raw surface of the posterior fossa more completely by heavy traction sutures drawing the bladder neck down to the area of the verumontanum.

A 22 French Foley catheter with a 30 $cm^3$ balloon is introduced through the urethra across the open fossa and into the bladder and the balloon inflated to a size sufficient to avoid its slipping back into the fossa, usually up to 45 $cm^3$. Again, gentle traction of the balloon against the bladder neck will separate the bladder cavity from the prostatic cavity and permit undisturbed clotting of the venous oozing in the prostatic fossa. The capsular incision is now closed with either interrupted or running sutures of heavy chromic catgut. The thick capsular tissue, unless shredded by excessive retraction or weakened by coagulation, will permit a firm and water tight closure. Care must be taken during the placement of these capsular sutures not to injure the large veins still present posterior to the lower arch of the symphysis. A stout, small needle on 00 or 000 chromic catgut is recommended. Some surgeons use a boomerang needle effectively at this point; but with good exposure and care that instrument is not essential and may in some cases of inexpert use lead to further tearing and bleeding. The capsular closure should be tested by instillation of saline into the bladder without tension on the balloon. If leaking occurs at the corner, further sutures should be taken because the torn capsular corner may have opened up vascular channels which will bleed secondarily and lead to hematoma formation and periprostatic infection.

It is imperative to drain the periprostatic space generously with a loose, soft rubber penrose drain, brought out through the lower corner of the wound in a vertical incision or through a separate stab incision below the transverse incision.

Before closure of the abdominal wound, the inlying catheter should be irrigated and adequately clear return obtained. If, in spite of gentle traction against the bladder neck, bloody returns are obtained, then it is wise to reopen the capsular incision and identify and secure the arterial bleeder which has probably been missed at the bladder neck. It is certainly an advantage of this approach to have such direct access to such potential sources of bleeding and the option to control them directly during the operation. The wound is closed avoiding the use of nonabsorbable material and the use of running sutures to the fascia or skin which might prevent the release of localized infection in the postoperative period.

## III. Combined or Transvesico-Capsular Prostatectomy

The combination of the extra-vesical, retropubic approach with the transvesical route is credited to HYBBINETTE in 1935. Further reports of this combined technique and a careful definition of its indications were published by WARD in 1948, HAND and SULLIVAN in 1951, BOURQUE in 1954 and the LEADBETTERS in 1959. The combined technique simply adopts the advantages of both the previously described techniques in order to add exposure and also to make it possible to modify the closure so as to perform a Y—V plasty on the bladder neck with no additional dissection.

### 1. Indications

Advocates of the combined technique suggest that it should be considered whenever some difficulty in dissecting the prostate from its capsule is anticipated, because of previous scarring from surgery, chronic prostatitis, or calculous disease. The presence of a large bladder diverticulum with such a gland would also indicate the availability of adequate transvesical exposure. A bladder neck obstruction of the type which may develop after transurethral resection, with residual periurethral adenoma, is best approached with this technique.

Because the procedure involves more extensive dissection and longer closure, it would seem to be unnecessary in a straight-forward case of prostatic enlargement. It is to be considered in any transvesical procedure which runs into unexpected difficulty with exposure of the prostatic capsule; and, conversely, a retropubic transcapsular approach may be converted to a combined approach without hesitation by adding a midline vesico-capsular incision.

## 2. Technique

A vertical midline incision or a low transverse abdominal incision may be used. In the transverse incision, it should be made no more than two finger widths above the symphysis and the rectus fascia should be well dissected off the substance of the muscles to permit wide retraction of the muscles right down to their insertion in the symphysis. It is well to have some fluid in the bladder in the early stages of dissection so as to be accurate in positioning the cystotomy slightly off the midline and slanting like the arm of a Y. The arm of the Y is carried down to just above the junction of the bladder muscle and prostatic capsule. The incision is then continued as a vertical capsulotomy. It is to be noted that because of the copious branching of the capsular veins, bleeding from them is just as much of a problem in this incision as in the transverse one. Suture ligatures should be adequately and promptly placed as the capsulotomy is carried down to the midportion of the anterior face of the

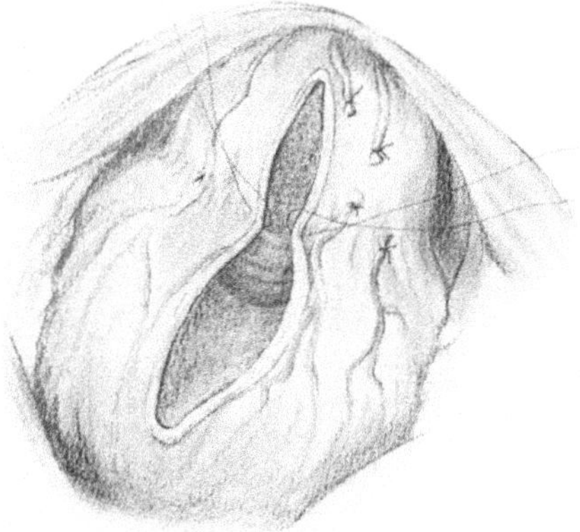

Fig. 4. Combined transvesico-capsular prostatectomy. A slightly diagonal incision of the lower anterior wall of the bladder has been extended longitudinally into the proximal half of the prostatic capsule. Traction sutures identify the area of the bladder neck. The incision provides direct exposure of the prostatic dissection and of the posterior bladder neck arterial bleeders. A Y—V plasty can be easily added as described in the text

capsule. The more distal capsule should be protected from tearing by application of a heavy chromic catgut suture at the end of the vertical capsulotomy. It is also useful to place a traction suture at each side of the divided bladder neck anteriorly, both for hemostasis and for guidance in subsequent repair (Fig. 4). The direct overhead approach to both the bladder neck and the apical area of the prostate permits the careful, sharp dissection of the abnormal prostatic tissue from the surgical capsule and the direct division of the junction of the prostatic apex and the membranous urethra without tension.

The prostatic fossa can be handled just as in the retropubic prostatectomy, with direct suture ligature of the arterial bleeders of the bladder neck, trimming of the fibrotic or band-like tissue from the posterior bladder neck and laying down of the apron of vesical mucosa over the posterior bladder neck under optimal exposure.

After the removal of the diseased contents of the prostatic fossa and plastic repair of the posterior bladder neck, approximation to each other of the angles of the anterior bladder neck previously divided will reveal whether further widening of the bladder neck is indicated. Certainly, in cases of a tight fibrotic bladder neck, it is best further to insure the patency of this area by converting the closure into a Y-V plasty. To do this, it is only necessary to incise the anterior bladder wall to complete the Y incision. It is technically important to avoid making too narrow a Y which may compromise the circulation at the tip of the V. The tip of the V is then sewn to the apex of the capsular incision with three interrupted sutures of 00 chromic catgut. These sutures are not tied until after all three are carefully placed. The sides of the V can then be closed with two running sutures of 000 plain catgut to the mucosa and interrupted 00 or 000 chromic catgut sutures to the bladder muscle. The space of Retzius is carefully drained with a soft rubber tube and the wound is closed in layers using interrupted heavy chromic catgut sutures to the muscle and fascia.

A suprapubic tube should not be required routinely in this procedure for the control of postoperative bleeding. However, in cases in which a Y-V plasty is done we usually do leave such a tube because there may be established fibrosis and loss of pliability of the bladder wall, and it is advisable to avoid balloon pressure on the V-flap.

## IV. Radical Retropubic Prostatectomy

The use of the retropubic approach for en bloc removal of the prostate and seminal vesicles was a natural extension of the demonstration of the adequacy of exposure and hemostasis in the simple retropubic prostatectomy. The radical approach was pioneered by Memmelaar and Lich in 1949. Development of this approach provided the first real alternative for the radical removal of the early carcinoma of the prostate by the perineal route. Many among the present generation of surgeons find themselves much more at ease with this exposure, particularly those accustomed to dissecting out the prostate from above in radical bladder surgery.

### 1. Indications

The usual indication for radical retropubic prostatectomy is the presence of a biopsy-proven early carcinoma of the prostate without fixation of the gland or extension of the tumor. The procedure is uniquely indicated in those patients in whom the exaggerated perineal position is not feasible because of orthopedic problems or in whom there is an unusually narrow space between the ischial tuberosities.

Although the retropubic approach makes it theoretically possible to perform a pelvic node dissection to attempt to encompass the spread of prostatic carcinoma to the regional lymph nodes, such additional surgery has not found many proponents. The known lymphatic outflow of the prostate includes drainage to the pararectal and hypogastric lymph nodes as well as pathways to nodes in the presacral region, making a complete segmental resection a formidable if not impossible task unless a radical cystectomy or pelvic exenteration is being carried out. Such radical surgery is not indicated in early carcinoma of the prostate, and more advanced cases are best treated with hormonal therapy or radiation.

## 2. Technique

The patient is positioned as for a simple retropubic prostatectomy and a generous midline vertical incision or a wide transverse incision is carried out. In the vertical incision, which more readily allows extension for additional exposure, it is useful to increase the exposure of the retropubic area by incising the tendinous portion of the recti as they insert into the pubis. In this maneuver it is best to leave a generous cuff of the tendinous insertion attached to the pubis and to mark the corner of the transverse tendinous incision for subsequent repair during the closure.

The dissection of the periprostatic space described for simple retropubic prostatectomy must be greatly expanded laterally and inferiorly so as to free up the gland laterally and leave it attached anteriorly by the puboprostatic ligaments. The bridging puboprostatic veins and the lateral venous plexus on each side must be identified, clamped, and ligated. The reflection of the endopelvic fascia lateral to the prostate must be perforated with the index finger and the lateral wall of the prostate followed down and posteriorly to the point at which the rectal wall is felt to be close to the prostate, leaving the dissection of the posterior aspect of Denonvillier's fascia for later dissection after separation of the urethra.

The puboprostatic ligament must be divided with great care to maintain hemostasis. It usually contains a large branch from the deep dorsal vein of the penis which will be carrying an additional flow after the large veins of the lateral venous plexis have been ligated on either side. Several maneuvers are recommended for the division of the puboprostatic ligament. A very effective one is to first place it on a stretch, slowly but steadily pulling it away from the symphysis so as to stretch the ligament, without tearing it, and leaving space for the application of a curved Kocher clamp across the full width of the ligament. The ligament is then cut on the prostate side of the clamp with scissors or scalpel and the slight back bleeding from the prostatic capsular surface is coagulated. Suture ligation of the puboprostatic ligament held by the curved clamp is then carried out with 00 chromic catgut. Occasional or smaller venous bleeders noted after the suture ligature is placed can be controlled by light coagulation or temporary packing with gauze. Other surgeons prefer simply to apply smaller clamps to the right and left portions of the puboprostatic ligaments and to electrocoagulate them and divide them until the entire ligament is cut and the apex of the prostate falls away from the symphysis. Still others prefer to cut across the ligament rapidly and then to apply a pad of gauze under a retractor to maintain hemostasis while the urethra is divided and then to replace the retractor with an inflated Foley catheter balloon placed on traction through the urethra to maintain hemostasis.

With blunt fingertip dissection the apex of the prostate is carefully defined and the left index fingertip can be passed between the urethra and the rectal ampulla without difficulty. It is well to have a catheter in the urethra at this point to aid in its definition and dissection. A pair of traction sutures of 00 chromic catgut placed into the substance of the membranous urethra help to identify it after it is divided and to maintain traction during the subsequent anastomosis. With curved scissors and under direct vision the membranous urethra is now cut across very close to the apex of the prostate (Fig. 5). The urethral catheter is withdrawn out of the way during the transection of the urethra and then it is advanced into the field and pulled up and over the symphysis, and clamped to itself in a circle, maintaining gentle traction thereby against the subsymphysial veins. A doublehooked tenaculum is applied to the apex of the prostate and the prostate is carefully dissected with blunt dissection away from the anterior rectal wall. Most surgeons are content in this situation to follow the plane between the two layers of Denonvillier's fascia, leaving the

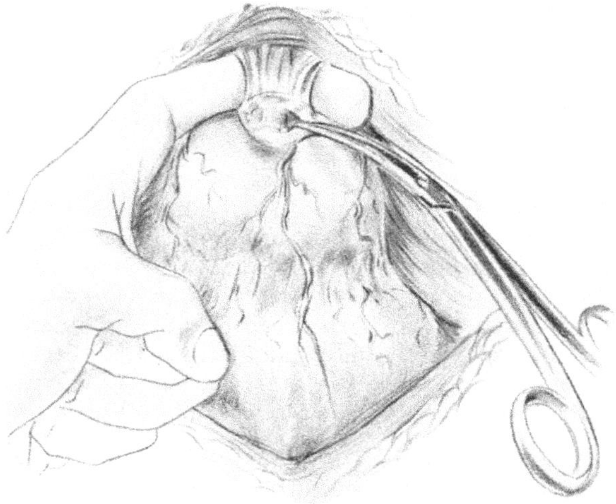

Fig. 5. Radical retropubic prostatectomy. Diagrammatic illustration of the separation of the apex of the prostate from the membranous urethra after the pubo-prostatic ligament has been divided and the left finger has been insinuated between the membranous urethra and the rectum. The inlying Foley catheter is seen but not cut and can be used for hemostasis of distal veins when its balloon is inflated

posterior layer of the fascia as a shining layer protecting the rectum from injury. The posterior blunt dissection is carried out as long as it is easy and comfortable to the base of the seminal vesicles which are covered with the anterior layer of Denonvillier's fascia. This blunt dissection is carried back behind the bladder neck without attempting to free up the seminal vesicles from this approach. It is now best to open the bladder just above the bladder neck anteriorly in a transverse fashion, with care not to enter the prostatic substance. Hemostasis presents no problem to this point. A penrose tube is now passed through the prostatic urethra and brought out again through the anterior bladder opening and clamped to itself (Fig. 6) to provide a handle for gentle retraction on the prostate and vesicles. With traction on the prostate and bladder neck a clamp is applied just lateral to the bladder neck to encompass the arterial supply from the inferial vesical artery and remaining branches from the lateral venous plexus. Suture ligation of the lateral pedicles is performed with care to stay well away from the terminal ureters which can be observed directly, and probed with ureteral catheters if there is any question. The posterior bladder neck is now transected exposing the anterior surface of the seminal vesicles and the ampullae of the ejaculatory ducts. With blunt dissection the base of the bladder can now be pushed away from the prostate and the tips of both seminal vesicles freed up sufficiently to permit the accurate application of a right angle clamp to their vascular supply up to that point. If the dissection of the bladder base encounters any difficulty, it is helpful to isolate, clamp, and divide the ejaculatory ducts first, leaving the specimen attached only by the seminal vesicles which can then be drawn out of the wound most successfully and the right angle clamp applied across the vascular pedicle entering just medial to their tip. The enbloc resection of the prostate and seminal vesicles is thus complete.

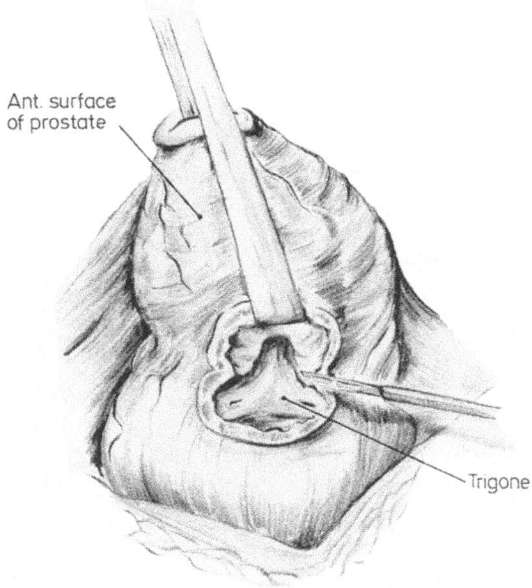


Fig. 6. Radical retropubic prostatectomy. The body of the prostate has been freed from the rectum posteriorly and the prostate is separated from the bladder neck by a circumferential incision beginning anteriorly as shown

The first step in the reconstruction of the bladder outlet is to tailor the resultant opening after the removal of the bladder neck to such a size as can be accurately connected to the stump of the urethra. A varying amount of plastic alteration will be necessary depending on how close to the bladder neck the specimen was excised. Certainly if the tumor is thought to be diffusely spread through the lobes of the prostate and if there is the possibility of extension into a seminal vesicle, it is unwise to cut across the posterior bladder neck too close to the prostate; and it is advisable to cut across close to the ureteral orifices, leaving a margin of 1 cm to permit repair without obstruction of the orifices. If that margin is not obtainable, the surgeon should be prepared for exicision of the terminal ureter and reimplantations of the ureters further back in the bladder.

The new bladder opening is made from the anterior bladder wall and the excess opening closed to itself in the form of an inverted Y so as to prevent undue tension and constriction of the terminal ureters. The new bladder opening can now be anastomosed to the membranous urethral stump with 4 to 6 interrupted 000 chromic catgut sutures, placing all of them before any are tied

(Fig. 7). If this proves difficult, the bladder can be successfully apposed to the urethral stump over the inlying Foley catheter. Gentle traction can hold the new junction together while healing takes place, but it is advisable and desirable to stabilize this apposition, whether or not a direct anastomosis has been carried out, by the addition of 2 perineal traction sutures of heavy nylon. These are made to pass through the substance of the lateral wall of the bladder and then passed out on a large straight needle through the perineum behind the scrotum and there tied over a gauze pledget. The angle of traction of these sutures

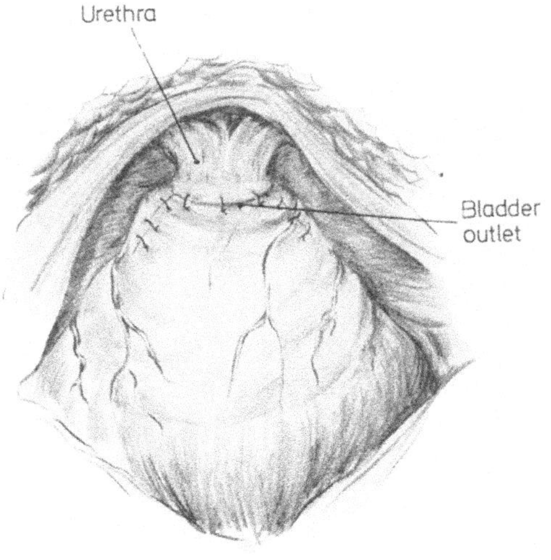


Fig. 7. Radial retropubic prostatectomy. Reconstructed bladder outlet with the opening tailored to fit the caliber of the urethra

is preferable to that achieved by Foley balloon traction. Postoperatively the traction sutures and the Foley catheter will be left in place 10 to 12 days. The wound is closed with careful drainage of the space of Retzius.

If the repair required sutures to be placed close to the ureteral orifices, it is wise to close with inlying ureteral catheters in place and brought out through a small stab incision of the anterior bladder wall and abdominal wall. These can be removed after 3 to 5 days and prevent even transient ureteral obstruction during the early postoperative course.

## V. Perineal Prostatectomy

The performance of perineal prostatectomy has many elements of a colorful ritual drawn from the contribution of many giants of urological surgery. The perineal approach to removal of stones from the bladder base was developed in ancient times. A curved perineal incision similar to that reintroduced by HUGH YOUNG was used by the physician CELSUS in 25 A.D. A blind enucleation analogous to the blind suprapubic prostatectomy was described by GOODFELLOW in 1891. He used a median perineal urethrotomy and reported a series of 72 cases. At the turn of the century, both PROUST in France and HUGH YOUNG in the U.S. improved the procedure by the design of better instruments which made direct visualization of the operation possible. Young adopted the curved perineal incision and standardized the procedure to provide the necessary exposure for reliably successful surgery. In 1908 he described 128 consecutive cases of perineal prostatectomy without a death. It was YOUNG (1903) also who described the radical perineal prostatectomy for use in cases of early carcinoma, a technique so simple and carefully conceived that it has remained in use to this day without significant modifications. Another outstanding contribution came from HANS WILDBOLZ who in 1906 brought about a great improvement in the results of conservative perineal prostatectomy with respect to postoperative incontinence by avoiding damage to the membranous urethra. He also advocated suture of the vesical neck to the stump of the urethra within the prostatic fossa, a clear concept of the importance of direct hemostasis and plastic closure of the bladder neck.

The last great recognized contribution to this operation was made by BELT (BELT, 1939) who demonstrated the anatomical and practical advantage of moving YOUNG's incision further back in the perineum so as to approach the prostate by developing a cleavage plane between the external anal phincter and the longitudinal fibers of the rectum. This approach is thought to have greatly reduced the incidence of inadvertent injury to the rectum and at the same time to have avoided inadvertent intrusion into the area of the voluntary urethral sphincter by the more anterior incision. The exposure to be described here does incorporate the modification introduced by BELT.

## 1. Simple Perineal Prostatectomy

### a) Indications

There is no absolute or overwhelming indication for simple perineal prostatectomy. Although it remains the procedure of choice in some European and American clinics, in most areas it has lost favor either to the open retropubic approach or to transurethral prostatectomy. Some relative indications for adoption of the technique exist, however, and these should be heeded by surgeons in order to develop and maintain their familiarity with the perineal approach because of its value in radical prostatectomy for cancer. Appropriate candidates for the procedure include older men no longer sexually active who have a large extravesical gland, considered to be larger than safely resectable by transurethral surgery. Since postoperative incisional discomfort is minimal and does not interfere with pulmonary ventilation after this procedure, the approach is relatively indicated in any patient with chronic lung disease whose ventilation and oxygenation can be assured during the surgery itself. Most appropriate also is the patient with a large gland who has had a colostomy performed since the colostomy may contaminate an abdominal wound and such a patient carries no risk of rectal complications.

There are some relative contraindications to the perineal approach. One is the desire by the patient to continue sexual activity since there is good evidence that this approach is the most likely to lead to impotence (FINKLE and MOYERS, 1960; DAHLEN and GOODWIN, 1957), with an incidence estimated at 30% for the simple prostatectomy. The exaggerated lithotomy position provides a contraindication in a patient with ankylosis of the hip or spine. The position also provides a relative contraindication for a patient with congestive heart failure or significant cardiac disorder. The nearly upside down position can compromise cardiac function in a way which is not easily controlled during anesthesia. A careful preoperative perineal and rectal examination will also rule out those patients who have extensive perineal scarring from previous abscesses or patients whose pelvic configuration is such that there is a very narrow space between the ischial tuberosities.

### b) Technique

The preoperative preparation of the patient must include careful cleansing of the rectum and it is advisable to add a short bowel preparation—we use enemas-to-clear the day before surgery followed by a small retention enema of 0,5% neomycin the night and early morning before surgery. Careful shaving of the perineal area is necessary; frequently it has to be completed by the surgical team with the patient in perineal position.

The position for the operation is ideally an exaggerated lithotomy position in which the lumbar-sacral area is brought out to the end of the table and elevated with sandbags so that the weight of the patient is largely on his upper back and shoulders. The knees are bent back over the patient to the point where the perineum is almost parallel to the floor. Positioning is greatly facilitated by the use of a perineal board, particularly the type designed by PALMER which allows for easy shifting of the degree of the position during the operation. The anterior flexing of the pelvis onto the abdomen is maintained by the use of the perineal posts around which the patient's legs are hooked and to which they are secured in such a way as to prevent pressure damage, using foam rubber and elastic bandages. Shoulder braces are very useful to prevent backsliding of the patient and should be heavily padded and applied to the acromio-calvicular part of the shoulders rather than to the supralavicular area. This placement of the shoulder braces and extreme care to avoid abduction of the arms by the anesthetist is required to prevent nerve damage to the brachial plexus.

Some clinics still perform simple prostatectomies through a much less exaggerated lithotomy position in which the plane of the perineum is little different from that in female surgery in the lithotomy position and where the surgeon sits for the operation. The major advantage of this less exaggerated position is that it permits surgery with relative comfort to the patient under spinal anesthesia. Such clinics will choose this approach as the procedure of choice for simple perineal prostatectomy in extremely poor risk patients. The exaggerated lithotomy position provides a most welcome increase in the exposure obtained and is particularly necessary for the safe performance of the radical perineal prostatectomy so that its routine use in the simple perineal is desirable. At the same time, the position makes it advisable to use general anesthesia with intubation, and if necessary, muscle relaxants and complete control over the respiration of the patient to insure adequate ventilation.

Many specialized instruments have been designed and used for perineal prostatectomy. As a practical requirement, the only absolutely necessary special instruments are prostatic tractors. These are usually some modification of the Young tractor, such as the curved and the straight tractors of Lowsley.

The placement of the inverted U perineal incision is important in determining the type of perineal approach to be used. In the approach of BELT, considered preferable here, the incision is made about 1.5 cm anterior to the anal margin. The incision for the classic approach of YOUNG is made about 3 cm anterior to the anal margin. The anal opening is to be draped out of the way by a tightly clipped towel or by use of the self-adherent plastic drapes now available. One such drape is available with a finger cuff extension for examination of the rectum during the procedure. While such examination is seldom necessary, the less experienced surgeon should not hesitate to carry it out to reestablish his landmarks and the position of the rectum when necessary. Once the perineal incision is carried through the superficial and deep fascia of the perineum, the lower flap is turned back and sewed to the taut towel drape with a running subcutaneous suture of silk so as to minimize possible contamination of the wound from the anus.

The incision is deepened with a knife to each side of the central tendon into the usually abundant fatty tissue. Once the deep fascia is cut, it is then possible to dissect bluntly with the index finger to loosen the loose fatty stroma anterior to the rectal wall and to pass one finger across to the other side underneath the central tendon (Fig. 8). The central tendon is then divided transversely where it is tented over the finger. As the lower flap of tissue falls back one sees the longitudinal fibers of the rectum in the depth of the wound where they have been cleaned off by the finger dissection. A 22 French urethral sound or

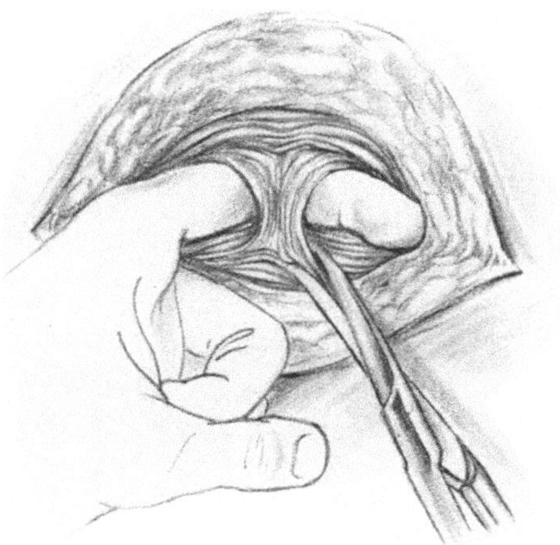

Fig. 8. Perineal prostatectomy. A finger has been passed under the central tendon and in front of the rectum. In dividing the central tendon, this approaches the prostate through a cleavage plane between the circular fibers of the external anal sphincter, as introduced by BELT

a curved Lowsley tractor with the blades closed is introduced into the bladder and slipped back so that the tip is in the prostatic urethra and can be used to apply leverage to the prostate and stabilize it in the subsequent dissection. The sound or urethral tractor is entrusted to the second assistant who stands to the surgeon's left. Narrow right angle retractors are placed laterally at the ten and two o'clock positions, one held by each of the assistants. They are to be instructed to avoid retractor pressure in the anterior midline where damage can result to the sphincter. The posterior flap and rectum which are continuously visualized can now be gently retracted by the left hand of the operator with a gauze pad over the wide blade retractor. This retractor is usually best controlled by the left hand of the surgeon to avoid injury to the rectum. With careful symmetrical retraction, the reflection of the rectal wall onto the mass of the prostate can usually be seen and felt. The midline rectourethralis fibers can be gingerly transected with the knife as the reflection of the rectum is kept under tension. Then with sweeping motions of a scalpel handle the decussating fibers of the levator ani are carefully and progressively swept sideways, exposing the dull white surface of the posterior layer of Dennonvillier's fascia.

The simple and radical procedures are the same up to this point. In the simple procedure, once the posterior layer is exposed, it is perfectly simple to open it with a transverse incision entering the space between the two layers and exposing the glistening white surface of the anterior layer of Denonvillier's fascia. The plane between these two layers allows for rapid and safe blunt dissection with the fingertip to separate the rectal wall posteriorly and to expose the entire posterior face of the prostatic capsule. By this point, the dissection has been deep enough to use small curved Deaver retractors pulling symmetrically to each side of the midline and a deeper posterior retractor, flat to protect the rectum, is introduced with careful padding. The mass of the prostate is stabilized with the urethral sound or curved tractor and the capsular incision is made, preferable in the shape of a inverted wide V with the apex of the V well

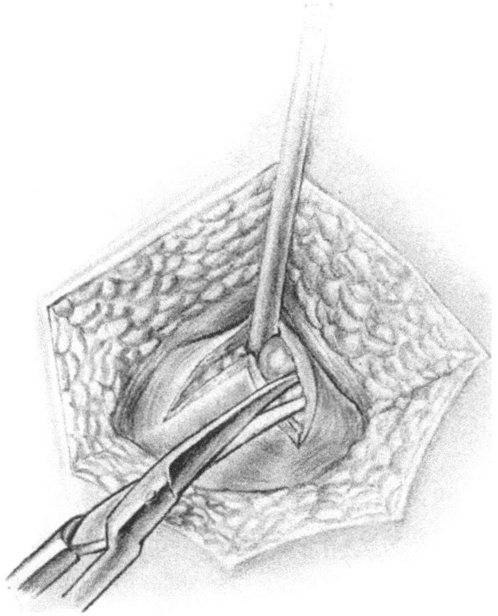

Fig. 9. Simple perineal prostatectomy. A straight tractor has been introduced into the prostatic urethra through the capsular incision and used to stabilize the gland. A plane of dissection for enucleation is started with the scissors as shown. In this plane the apical urethra will be found and cut under direct vision without risk of avulsion

below the prostatic apex so as to avoid damage to the membranous urethra (Fig. 9). The incision is carried through the capsule and substance of the prostate until the metal of the sound is reached. Light cautery on the edge of the capsule is sufficient for hemostasis. Under direct vision, the curved Lowsley tractor or urethral sound is withdrawn and through the wound a straight prostatic tractor is introduced into the prostatic urethra and its blades opened in the bladder.

With the straight tractor in place, it is a simple matter to establish a plane between the capsule and the adenoma first anteriorly towards the membranous urethra, carefully dividing the junction of the adenoma and the urethra under direct vision with scissor and then proceeding posteriorly and towards the bladder neck by a combination of blunt dissection and spreading of the scissors. When the bladder neck mucosa is reached, it is cut anteriorly by levering the freed up adenoma downward and the mucosal incision thus started is continued laterally to each side to the posterior bladder neck where an effort is made again to leave a cuff of mucosa for plastic repair. The adenoma is thus removed, usually in one piece and carefully examined for evidence of tissue left behind. Through the capsular opening the bladder neck is visualized and grasped with a long Allis clamp at the posterior midline position to avoid trauma to the ureters. With this traction on the Allis clamp, the bladder neck can be brought out to be examined under direct vision without difficulty. Hemostatic suture ligatures of 00 chromic are placed at the points where the arterial bleeders are visualized in each posterior quadrant (Fig. 10). Consideration is then given to whether a wedge of the posterior bladder neck is to be resected if there is a suggestion of bladder neck obstruction.

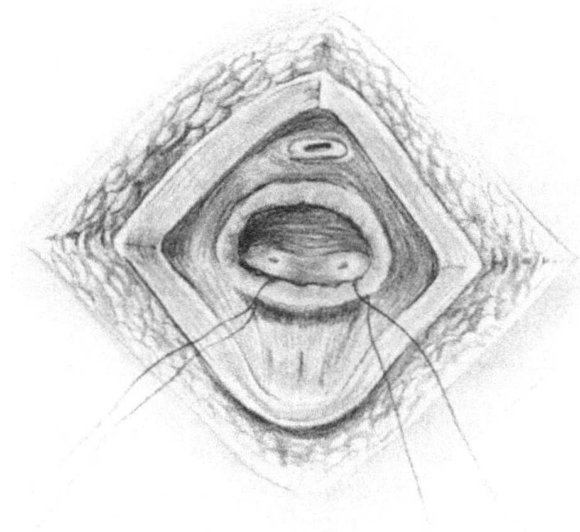

Fig. 10. Simple perineal prostatectomy. Diagrammatic representation of the placement of hemostatic sutures at the bladder neck after removal of the adenoma. Good hemostasis is readily afforded by this approach if the bladder neck is brought into view through the opening in the prostatic capsule, as shown

Repair of the bladder neck can be performed in a variety of ways but it is quite simple from this exposure to apply sutures which attach its overlying mucosa and submucosa to the substance of the exposed posterior capsule. Three or four mattress sutures are thus placed using 00 chromic catgut and accurately imbricating the posterior bladder neck to the capsule across some of the raw fossa. As explained earlier, some surgeons have practiced the complete imbrication of the posterior raw space by attaching these bladder neck sutures to the apical capsule by the stump of the urethra. Again, we feel these are tied under undue tension and may compromise the function of the external sphincter.

Before closure of the capsule, the patency of the ureteral orifices is ascertained with dye excretion or passing of ureteral catheters. The cavity of the bladder is irrigated clean of any clots or any other debris. Then a 22 Foley catheter with a 30 $cm^3$ balloon is passed through the urethra and under direct vision into the bladder and the balloon inflated so that it will not be drawn back beyond the bladder neck. The inverted V capsular incision is closed with interrupted 00 or 000 chromic mattress sutures carefully applied to take the full thickness of the capsule and to provide a hemostatic and watertight closure. If a tear has occurred laterally, it is carefully exposed so that the capsular closure will be complete and avoid later hemorrhage and extravasation.

In closing the wound, a small rubber penrose drain is laid against the capsular space and brought out through one corner of the incision. The fibers of the levator ani muscle are sutured in the midline with wide bites to provide a good sling support and to provide accurate separation of the capsule from the rectum. The rest of the wound is closed with two or three layers of interrupted 000 chromic sutures to reconstitute the fatty dead space and the approximation of the slit fibers of the anal sphincter. Some surgeons place an imbricating suture to the fibers of the sphincter so as to reinforce the structure but this is usually not necessary. We prefer to close the skin with a running subcuticular suture of 000 plain catgut and to seal the incision with a spray of plastic dressing. A gentle rectal examination at this point should be carried out to be sure that there is no free blood in the rectum. If blood is noted, an inadvertent tear in the rectal wall may have occurred and it is wise to reopen it and carefully examine the rectal wall until the damage is found. Because of the previous bowel preparation, a careful two layer closure with catgut sutures to both the mucosa and the rectal muscle will usually heal without fistula formation. If such rectal injury has occurred and been repaired in such fashion, copious washing of the wound with neomycin-bacitracin solution and a gentle dilatation of the anal sphincter are advisable precautions against fistula formation.

## 2. Radical Perineal Prostatectomy

### a) Indications

A well performed radical perineal prostatectomy is undoubtedly the most satisfying treatment for a localized and early carcinoma of the prostate (Huggins, 1969). Because alternative conservative therapy does often provide an acceptable measure of temporary and even prolonged control, we do not advise radical prostatectomy in a patient whose life expectancy may well be expected to be less than the expected control from conservative therapy. This usually means that a patient over 70 years of age is not offered the radical perineal procedure unless he happens to be an unusually vigorous and physiologically young specimen. Younger men may expect a survival after radical perineal prostatectomy which is very similar to the general population of the same age (Berlin et al., 1968).

Radical perineal prostatectomy is occasionally resorted to as a definitive measure for the treatment of intractable chronic prostatitis where pain and recurrent infection have become intolerable. Some surgeons accept a lesser procedure which involves leaving behind the seminal vesicles and is labelled a "total" perineal prostatectomy in contrast to the usual "radical" procedure taking the vesicles. The frequency with which the vesicles are similarly involved in such a chronic and inflammatory process and leave a focus for continued pain and inflammation makes it advisable to carry out the "radical" procedure even in the presence of this benign disease.

Ankylosis of the hip or spine are again contraindications to this approach because of the demands of the position. Interference with sexual potency is not a valid consideration in the face of a cancer, particularly because the conservative hormonal therapy can also be expected to bring such activity to an end. It is true that when sexual potency is a strong consideration, some surgeons are willing to consider the alternative of radiation therapy in an attempt to clear a localized and primary carcinoma (del Regato, 1967). We feel strongly that this modality of therapy is not to be recommended as a reasonable alternative in aiming for a cure of the carcinoma. Such radiation certainly affects the local tissue planes to such a degree that later radical perineal surgery is no longer readily feasible if the radiation has failed to control the tumor; in addition, impotence does occur after radiotherapy.

### b) Technique

The preoperative preparation, operative position and incision for the radical procedure is the same as that described under the simple perineal prostatectomy. The procedure is modified after the posterior layer of the Dennonvillier's fascia is exposed by lateral dissection of the decussating fibers of the levator ani muscle.

In operating for cancer, we think it is advisable to expose the posterior bulk of the prostate gland by following the posterior layer of Dennonvillier's fascia instead of opening into the space between the two layers. Although the dissection is a little more tedious because there is no ready made plane, this modification has the dual advantage of providing one extra fascial layer to protect against the inadvertent dissection into carcinoma and at the same time carry the surgeon further laterally and posteriorly in a plane which reaches further around the prostate gland and gives ready access to the troublesome vascular pedicles. It must be pointed out, however, that many surgeons do proceed to enter the space between Dennonvillier's fascia and to carry their dissection in that plane in order to rapidly eliminate the possibility of rectal injury.

Open perineal biopsy is carried out and submitted for a frozen section diagnosis. It is to be noted that this biopsy does in fact violate the fascial planes overlying the tumor and therefore the point of biopsy must be well exposed, and kept completely dry to avoid the washing of tumor cells into the wound. A useful maneuver is to apply a ring of dry gauze to be held by the tension of the soft tissue surrounding the face of the prostate. The most suspicious area is biopsied by taking a rectangular wedge through the capsule and into the substance of the prostate. With continuous suction to prevent spilling of blood, the resulting defect is extensively cauterized and then closed tightly with interrupted heavy chromic catgut sutures. The modern technique of frozen section which permits the application of standard and familiar histological stains has greatly improved the reliability of the all-important decision needed at this time. The experienced urological surgeon may indeed be quite capable of making the diagnosis himself and should consider leaving the operating theater to look at the section himself if the pathologist is equivocal or gives a diagnosis which is inconsistent with the gross clinical findings.

After the positive diagnosis, the surgeon proceeds to break through the endopelvic fascia lateral to the apex of the prostate with his fingertip or forceps and to dissect bluntly around the prostate retropubically. With the apex of the prostate thus well defined, gentle blunt dissection is used further to define the proximal membranous urethra with the curved Lowsley tractor in place. This done, the urethra is transected at the junction with the apex and the curved tractor replaced by the straight tractor introduced through the wound (Fig. 11). Before completing the transection of the anterior wall of the urethra, a pair of 000 chromic catgut sutures are placed on each side of the cut urethral stump so as to provide easy access to the urethra which tends to retract into the urogenital diaphragm. The puboprostatic ligament with its accompanying veins is defined by tact, clamped with a curved Kocher clamp and divided on the surface of the anterior prostatic capsule. The back bleeding on the capsule is controlled by fulguration. The ligament is suture ligated with a heavy chromic catgut suture before the clamp is released. Dissection is continued in retrograde fashion at the surface of the prostatic capsule. Tilting the prostate to one side and then to the other, the vascular pedicles are defined with blunt dissection and clamped up through the level of the lateral bladder neck. This step is of great help in controlling subsequent bleeding, and if properly accomplished effectively stops the inflow of blood to the prostate (Fig. 12).

The bladder neck is incised anteriorly by tilting down on the straight prostatic tractor, the blades of which define the junction of the prostate and bladder. This incision is carried around to each side and narrow Deaver retractors are placed through the open bladder neck into the bladder to permit visualization of the posterior bladder neck and the ureteral orifices. With the orifices well in sight, the circular transection is completed with sharp dissection, being sure to cut

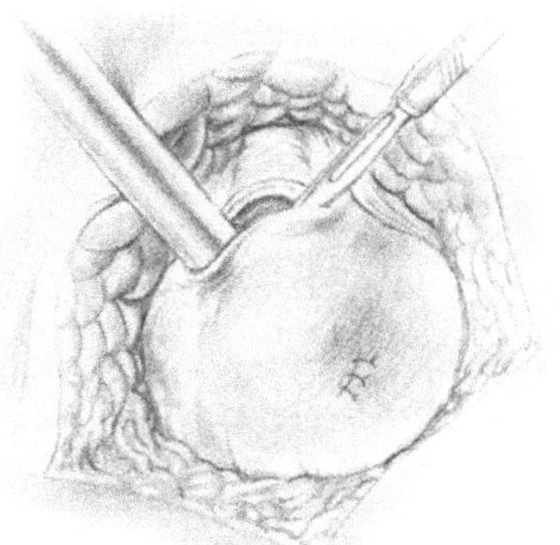

Fig. 11

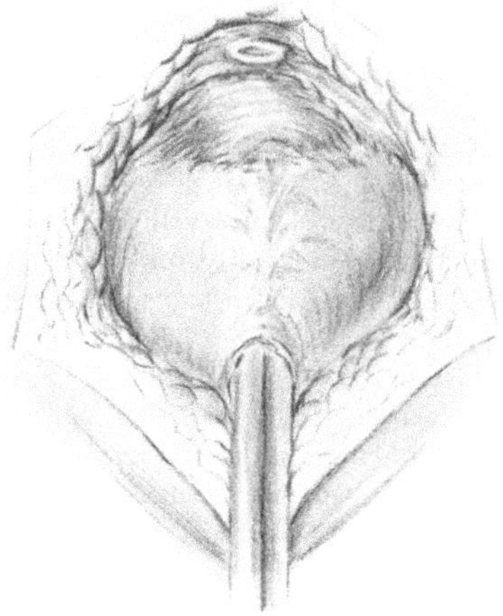

Fig. 12

Fig. 11. Radical perineal prostatectomy. After biopsy proof of the malignancy, a straight tractor is introduced into the urethra and down into the bladder by an incision at the apex and the separation of the prostate from the urethra is made by sharp incision as shown

Fig. 12. Radical perineal prostatectomy. The anterior aspect of the prostatic capsule has been freed from the pubo-prostatic ligament. This permits the lower portion of the anterior bladder wall to be brought into the field as shown, tented up by the open tractor blade

through the full thickness of the posterior bladder neck and controlling the penetrating arterial bleeders with suture ligatures. The straight tractor is replaced with a Penrose rubber drain to permit more delicate traction on the prostate which is still attached by the seminal vesicles and the ejaculatory ducts.

The ampullae of the vas deferens on each side of the midline are dissected with a right angle clamp and then the bladder base is pushed back with blunt dissection so that the terminal vas can be clamped and divided well away from the prostate (Fig. 13). If the rectum has been properly dissected completely off the posterior layer of Denonvillier's fascia, a finger can now be introduced in he space between the seminal vesicles and poked through into the space dissected behind the bladder base. At this point, depending on the degree of fusion of the peritoneum, the peritoneal cavity may be entered but this is of no consequence. A second Penrose rubber drain can be introduced through this opening to provide further traction of the prostate which now is attached only by the seminal vesicles. Careful blunt dissection, avoiding rupture of the fragile vesicles, allows the surgeon to follow each seminal vesicle to its apex where there is a vascular pedicle. This vascular pedicle is clamped beyond the tip of the vesicle on each side, and the vesicles are thus taken *en bloc* with the specimen. The specimen is removed and closure can begin. If the peritoneum was entered it can now be closed accurately. The transected bladder outlet is carefully defined and prepared for the vesicourethral anastomosis.

If the surgeon has transected the bladder outlet right at the junction with the prostatic capsule, then the bladder opening may be small enough to permit an end to end anastomosis with the urethral stump without the need for remodeling

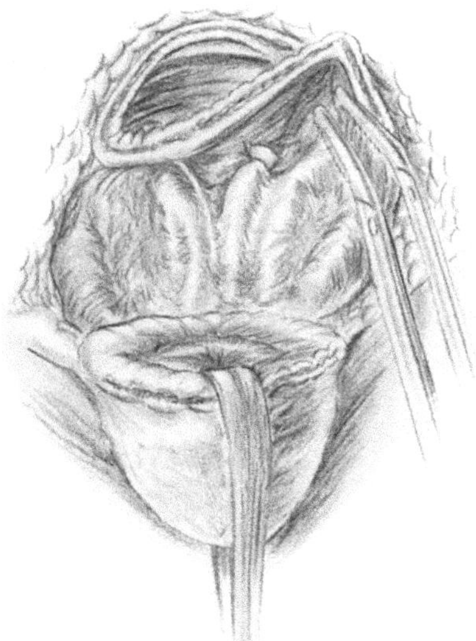

Fig. 13

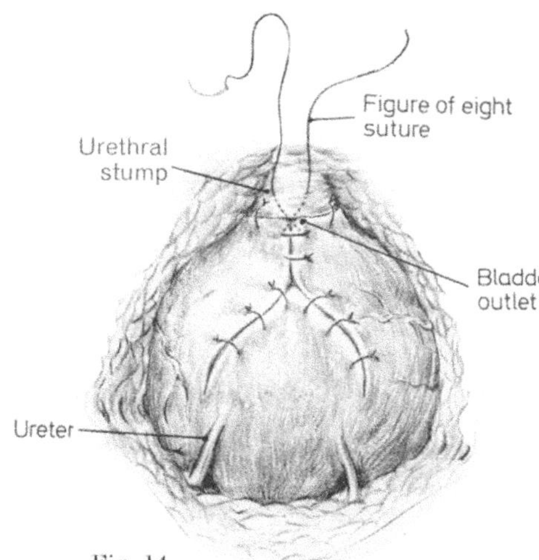


Fig. 14

**Fig. 13.** Radical perineal prostatectomy. After circumferential incision of the bladder neck to separate the prostate from the bladder, the bladder is pushed up bluntly and the vas deferens and seminal vesicles are taken with the specimen as shown

**Fig. 14.** Radical perineal prostatectomy. Illustration of reconstruction of bladder outlet and anastomosis to urethral stump. Plication of a large bladder outlet defect in this fashion prevents undue tension and distortion of the ureteral orifices

of the outlet. More usually, especially if a cuff of bladder has been taken to insure a good margin, the bladder outlet will be much too large and only a portion of it is to be used for anastomosis to the urethra. With good lighting and in a dry field, two or three interrupted sutures are placed to join the anterior edge of the bladder outlet to the anterior half of the stump of the membranous urethra. These are placed so that the knots will be outside of the new lumen. A Foley catheter is now brought through the urethra and into the bladder and the row of interrupted sutures is continued posteriorly to close the bladder outlet to the urethral stump. The last suture is placed in the manner described by JEWETT as a figure-of-eight (JEWETT, 1963) which pinches together the bladder outlet to conform to the urethral diameter. The redundant excess of the bladder outlet is closed to itself in a single layer of interrupted 000 chromic sutures. To prevent excessive traction and deformity on the ureteral orifices, this may be done in the form of a inverted Y (Fig. 14). It is wise to clean out the cavity of the bladder of any blood clots before completing this closure. The balloon is inflated and the bladder irrigated to demonstrate a water tight closure. The wound is closed and drained as described above for the simple perineal prostatectomy.

The special sutures for this vesico-urethral anastomosis described by VEST have as their purpose the avoidance of suture-constriction of the external sphincter mechanism. By the careful definition of the membranous urethra and the accurate placement of the interrupted sutures as here described, many surgeons have been able to omit the use of VEST's sutures.

### VI. Other Techniques

The posterior or transcoccygeal approach has become obsolete in most centers though occasional reports of present-day usage do appear (MARSHALL, 1965; CAMPBELL and MACGREGOR, 1969). No superiority of results is claimed by its proponents.

Cryosurgical prostatectomy introduced by GONDER et al. (1966) is to be considered as a transurethral instrumentation procedure and in fact is often complimented by transurethral resection in recent reports in the literature. It has not been described further in this chapter although some of the early reports described the application of transvesical freezing of the prostate.

## E. Postoperative Management

### I. Antibiotics

The routine use of systemic antibiotic therapy after open prostatectomy has come into general use and we personally endorse it. Rather than a prophylactic medication, such practice can best be considered in the light of the almost certain contamination of an open wound from the necessary passage of urethral catheters and the proximity of the rectum even in cases with apparently sterile urine. It is our practice to give a broad spectrum antibiotic such as a tetracycline or ampicillin for three to five days and then change the patient over to a milder drug such as one of the sulfa drugs or nitrofurantoin which is maintained three to four weeks, as long as there are inflammatory cells in the urine attesting to the presence of as yet unepithelialized areas of the prostatic fossa or the bladder wall incision. In practice this has led to a drastic reduction in the number of significant clinical infections, particularly in the perivesical space or ascending into the kidneys.

### II. Fluids and Diet

From the time of surgery, the generous administration of fluids maintains a good urine flow to minimize clot formation and at the same time may aid in the avoidance of ascending infection. It is quite safe to administer three to four liters of fluid intravenously during the first 24 hours, taking care to use balanced electrolyte solutions to avoid electrolyte derangements, particularly hyponatremia. The use of an indwelling venous catheter for the determinations of central venous pressure has made it easier to avoid the occasional problem with fluid overloading in the aged patient.

As a rule the patient can be allowed a liquid diet on the day following surgery and a rapid progression to his usual diet with the addition of a large intake of oral fluids to maintain a urine output of 2 to 3 liters per 25 hours.

Blood hematocrit determinations are performed repeatedly as long as there is loss of blood into the urethral catheter, starting with a determination the evening after surgery and at least daily thereafter. We feel that it is important to maintain a hematocrit above 30% in this age group to avoid anoxia and hypotension.

### III. Catheters and Drains

The Foley catheter is removed 5 or 6 days after the suprapubic or retropubic simple prostatectomy, as long as the urinary drainage is clear. The catheter is left in place 7 or 8 days after a simple perineal prostatectomy. In the case of radical retropubic or radical perineal prostatectomy the catheter is left in for a longer period which depends in part on the amount of difficulty which was encountered in anastomosing the bladder to the urethra. Ten to twelve days is a prudent interval in the optimal cases and the period may be extended to two weeks if there is doubt about the anastomosis.

A suprapubic tube which is left in place in addition to the Foley catheter for the control of bleeding can usually be removed one or two days after surgery. In those cases in which the bladder wall was found at surgery to be fibrotic and leathery, it is often wise to leave the suprapubic tube in place until after the Foley catheter is removed and after the patient has demonstrated that he can void adequately. In some cases this means leaving the suprapubic tube in place for several weeks while the bladder regains effective contractility.

The Penrose drains left in the space of Retzius are advanced and then removed as soon as there is no significant further drainage, usually the second or third days after surgery. In the perineal operations, we make it a practice to remove the Penrose drain even sooner, one to two days after surgery, striving to avoid the contamination of the perineal wound.

When the Foley catheter is removed in any of these cases it is wise to monitor the voiding pattern of the patient in order to determine whether he requires reinsertion of the catheter and more time for the bladder to regain effective emptying. We often fill the bladder with sterile saline at the time of catheter removal and have the patient void immediately after the removal so as to estimate the contractility of the bladder and the amount of postvoid residual urine. We ask the nursing staff to collect each voiding, record its volume, and keep the last three voidings in separate plastic containers for the doctor's inspection. If the urine is grossly bloody, or the volumes are consistently less than 100 $cm^3$, or there is a suggestion of bladder retention on physical examination, then the catheter is reintroduced. If there is gross bleeding, or a residual urine of over 100 $cm^3$, the catheter will be left in place for another 48 hours or longer. In those cases in whom there has been a significant amount of chronic bladder distension and failure to pass this voiding test, we will not hesitate to send them home on catheter drainage, to return for a followup visit in one or two weeks at which another attempt will be made for the successful removal of the Foley catheter.

## F. Postoperative Complications

### I. Bladder Spasms

As in any procedure in which the bladder wall is sutured, bladder spasms can occur with every form of prostatectomy but are particularly common after the transvesical procedures of the suprapubic or the combined prostatectomy.

In addition to their severe discomfort, the patients with the bladder spasms are likely to precipitate fresh bleeding from their bladder wall and bladder neck.

To decrease the incidence of spasms, we reduce the amount of fluid in the Foley catheter balloon on the first postoperative day down to about 15 $cm^3$. If traction has been applied on the Foley catheter in the early postoperative period, this is also an acknowledged cause of spasms and its discontinuation will be of help.

Anticholinergic drugs are effective in the treatment and prevention of bladder spasms. We prefer Banthine or Probanthine, first intramuscularly and then by mouth, every 4 hours. On occasion we have felt justified in giving Banthine intravenously to a good risk patient having prolonged and severe spasms, usually with welcome relief. Analgesics are given at the same time. The most worrisome side effect of the anticholinergic drugs is the tachycardia which they can produce. It is to be remembered that the severe discomfort and the potential imitiation of postoperative bleeding from severe spasms may be more taxing to the patient's myocardium than the tachycardia alone.

## II. Bleeding

Unexpected blood loss can occur rather frequently after open prostatectomy, but particularly in the cases of simple prostatectomy where the prostatic fossa is left as a large denuded surface with multiple potential sources of delayed bleeding. The ability to deal with such bleeding has been greatly increased by the advances in the understanding of coagulation defects. In the rare instances of severe bleeding, however, the source is arterial and requires surgical acumen and courageous reintervention, not the imprecise diagnosis of an unknown clotting problem and the continuation of self-defeating conservative measures.

The direct visualization of the principal arterial branches just below the bladder neck at the time of surgery is the most important measure in preventing serious postoperative bleeding. *This cannot be stressed enough.* In large glands, significant arterial bleeders may be present in the anterior quadrants of the bladder neck and will be missed unless the area is carefully inspected at the time of surgery. Severe bleeding arising from the capsule below the bladder neck is unusual but must not be ignored. A slight venous ooze will be controlled, as described earlier, by separating the bladder from the prostatic fossa with the Foley catheter balloon, allowing the blood to clot in the fossa. But if arterial bleeding is suspected in that area, before the wound is closed, with blood forcing its way into the bladder or around the Foley catheter down the urethra, then it will be unwise to depend on traction alone and it is indicated to open the capsule anteriorly so as to permit direct suction and inspection of the bleeding area, looking for an unsuspected tear in the capsule or an unusual arterial bleeder. Direct fulguration and suture ligation can then be carried out before closing.

If the patient has a known coagulation defect, preoperative preparation with the appropriate plasma factors and transfusion, as needed, with fresh blood permit the performance of elective prostatectomy. It is to be noted that this prostatectomy should probably be a total prostatectomy, either perineal or retropubic, removing the capsule and permitting a direct and hemostatic anastomosis of the bladder to the apical remnant of the capsule. All too often, in spite of the apparently optimal preparation, the denuded capsular surface refuses to stop bleeding and requires reexplorations and secondary capsulectomy.

The more usual bleeding problem is the bleeding in the patient in the first 12 hours after surgery. Clots form in the catheter and set up a vicious cycle of obstruction, distention, spasms, and further bleeding. Some surgeons believe that the secondary bleeding is initiated by straining and spasms occurring as the anesthesia wears off and the patient is overactive. The use of generous analgesia and anticholinergics can do much to avoid such problems.

If the early postoperative bleeding is not arterial, it will respond to conservative measures. These should include the thorough irrigation of all bladder clots, with deflation and deeper insertion of the Foley catheter and, if necessary, the change to a larger lumen such as that available in a 24 or 26 French whistle-tip nephrostomy tube. Once the bladder is clear, the balloon catheter is placed on slight but continuous traction achieved by attaching several common rubber bands to the catheter and then anchoring the rubber bands under slight tension to the lateral aspect of the lower leg, using a long wide strip of adhesive tape. The traction is designed not to occlude arterial bleeders, but to separate the prostatic fossa and the bladder cavity. If bleeding is thus controlled, it can be assumed to be venous in origin. It is to be noted that such traction is uncomfortable, increases the severity of spasms, and if prolonged will certainly traumatize the urethra, particularly at the peno-scrotal angle. It should be discontinued the first postoperative morning.

If venous postoperative bleeding has been sufficient to require the institution of traction, or alternatively if the Foley catheter drainage on the first post-operative day has enough blood in it to lose its transparency or to threaten the formation of clots in the tubing, we believe that systemic therapy with epsilo amino caproic acid (EACA) should be initiated and maintained for several days. This is readily accomplished by administration of 8 gm added to the intravenous fluid bottle followed by 3 to 4 g by mouth every 6 hours. It is important to recognize that the rationale of this therapy is not the presumed existence of circulating fibrinolysins, which might be demonstrated by secondary lysis of clotted peripheral blood, but rather the local effect of urokinase, which by its local conversion of plasminogen to plasmin is enhancing a local lysis of freshly formed blood clot in the opened veins. Extensive double blind prospective studies have been published which leave no doubt as to the value of EACA in reducing the average blood loss in all open prostatectomies with no significant side effects or any evidence for pathological thrombosis or thromboembolic phenomena (Vinnicomb and Shuttleworth, 1966; Kirkman, 1967; Hedlund, 1969). The effect of this medication can be dramatic as demonstrated by the rapid clearing of the drainage followed by the reappearance of bleeding if the medication is stopped too soon. We usually maintain the medication for 3 or 4 days and do not hesitate to reinstitute it for 48 hours if bleeding reappears when it is stopped. While the published evidence might suggest that this therapy should be used in every case, we prefer to continue to use it selectively under the conditions described.

When arterial bleeding is present in the first 21 to 24 hours, as suggested by the rate of bleeding, its color, and its lack of response to the gentle traction, we feel that the patient should be taken to endoscopy; then under spinal anesthesia the bladder is carefully evacuated of all clots through a resectoscope; the adhering clots are lifted off from the bladder neck and capsule until the offending arterial bleeder is visualized; and this is then fulgurated. A previous water tight closure of the surgical incision in the bladder wall or capsule makes this secondary intervention quite safe and usually effective.

The onset *de novo* of signs of a diffuse bleeding tendency, with easy bleeding from other mucous membranes and formation of petechiae of the skin, is an infrequent but real complication, particularly in patients with carcinoma of the prostate or gram negative septicemia. Here the surgeon must consider the possibility of either a diffuse and severe effect of circulating fibrinolysins or, alternately, the presence of a consumption coagulopathy. The latter involves the spontaneous formation of platelet-fibrin aggregates in the blood, with trapping in vital capillary beds, and a secondary rapid depletion or circulating fibrinogen and platelets as well as an increased formation of fibrinolysins. It is in these cases that expert hematological consultation is very valuable. If a decreased circulating level of fibrinogen and platelets is found, along with a moderate increase in the prothrombin time, the life saving medication is intravenous heparin, while EACA alone can only make things worse (BROOKS, 1969).

## III. Infection

The routine use of antibiotics and the recognition of the importance of adequate drainage has virtually eliminated wound infection as a significant problem after prostatic surgery. Certain problems do remain, however.

Retropubic and suprapubic prostatectomy patients may show signs of wound infection 4 to 6 days after surgery, particularly in obese individuals and in those in whom postoperative hematoma has accumulated in the extravesical space. This should be treated by the removal of several of the interrupted sutures, evacuation of any purulent material or old blood, and loose packing with iodoform strip gauze, with subsequent daily changes of the gauze and repeated irrigation with antiseptic solutions.

Osteitis pubis is also an infrequent but dramatic complication. Acute inflammation, of uncertain origin, is localized to the symphysis pubis and brings about the typical combination of local tenderness, pain on walking, and X-ray changes in the appearance of the symphysis. The treatment of bed rest, antibiotics and corticosteroid therapy is usually sufficient to eliminate the problem. Occasionally, curetting the symphysis and even symphysiectomy has been resorted to for persistent cases.

Epididymitis is also relatively rare as a postoperative complication particularly when both vasectomy and antibiotics are used routinely. Although carefully controlled studies long ago showed the value of vasectomy in the prevention of epididymitis, many surgeons have abandoned its routine use because of the efficacy of antibiotics (CASTEEL et al., 1965). We still use it because we are impressed by the fact that infected fluid is frequently present in the posterior urethra with an inlying catheter and have seen epidydimitis occur in cases treated with antibiotics but without vasectomy. Although usually a self-contained infection, it can pose a serious threat to the aged and debilitated patient. When it occurs, it is best treated by a specific change of antibiotics according to reported sensitivities and the use of bed rest and scrotal support. If prompt response is not obtained, we do not hesitate to advise an epididymectomy or epididymoorchiectomy under local anesthesia as the least taxing course for such a patient.

A significant urethritis often develops several days after open prostatic surgery as an irritation around the Foley catheter with discomfort and drainage. Most effective in such cases would be prompt removal of the catheter. If the patient cannot void then a much smaller catheter is reintroduced with great care and with an effort to use one of a different materials in case the urethritis is a reflection of a tissue hypersensitivity to the catheter wall or to chemicals left adsorbed to it in the manufacturing process.

## IV. Incontinence

After simple prostatectomy, whether suprapubic, retropubic, or perineal, incontinence is a very rare complication but can occur. If *urgency incontinence* occurs for more than a day or two after the removal of the catheter, one must consider the possibility of a preexisting spastic bladder whose ill effects have been enhanced by the removal of the prostate. A clear-cut pattern of *stress incontinence* can be seen occasionally after these operations, particularly when the large gland was removed. The stress incontinence is marked by the loss of some urine when the patient is upright or increases his intraabdominal pressure. Not infrequently, the patient finds that he has no difficulty with the control during the night and during the first few hours of the day but loses control toward the end of the day as if he had developed fatigue of the external sphincter. The stress incontinence which is frequently noted for some time in up to 50% of cases after radical prostatectomy depends in part on the damage carried out on the urogenital diaphragm and in part on the amount of the bladder neck which has been left by the surgeon. It is wise to warn all patients of the possibility of transient incontinence and at the same time, if incontinence does occur, to support the patient through several months of waiting in the expectation that a large percentage of these cases will regain complete control within six months. The patient should be encouraged to exercise his perineal muscles and instructed in the effort desired by asking him to contrict the sphincter ani over the examining finger in the rectum. The patient is instructed to shut off his urinary stream several times every time that he voids and also to practice such sphincter exercises between voidings.

## V. Operations for Male Incontinence

Postoperative urinary incontinence in males has been a known problem ever since the days of cutting for stones in the bladder through the perineum. The variety of procedures attempted and recommended for such incontinence in this century alone are well beyond the scope of this chapter. It is fair to say that their variety and short-lived popularity attests to their lack of efficacy (Martin et al., 1963).

Before describing some procedures more recently proposed for the surgical treatment of such incontinence, it is valuable to consider two kinds of appliances which may be offered to the patient to control his problem prior to surgery or, in fact, in lieu of surgery if the patient is satisfied with their use. Widely used in America is a penile clamp made of two bands of soft metal hinged at one end, padded with sponge rubber, and latched at the other end with several notches which permit adjustment of the closing tension to just what is needed to prevent an accident during stress. This clamp has been called the Cunningham clamp. It is curious to note that its design and use has not changed in over 200 years since it was illustrated in Heister's Textbook of Surgery in 1739, as shown in Fig. 15a. The surgeon is advised to patiently instruct the afflicted patient in the proper molding of the clamp and the use of the minimal closing pressure which is necessary to control his problem in order to avoid pressure necrosis of the skin or undue edema of the penile skin beyond the clamp.

Another type of appliance which is widely used, and may be necessary in more severe cases where the clamp is not tolerated or must be applied with undue pressure, is a sheath applied like a condom to the penis and emptying into a bag attached to the leg. The newer and softer synthetic plastic sheaths now available have greatly decreased the annoying skin irritation and odor produced by the older forms of such sheath appliances. Nevertheless, the acceptance of the sheath remains poor.

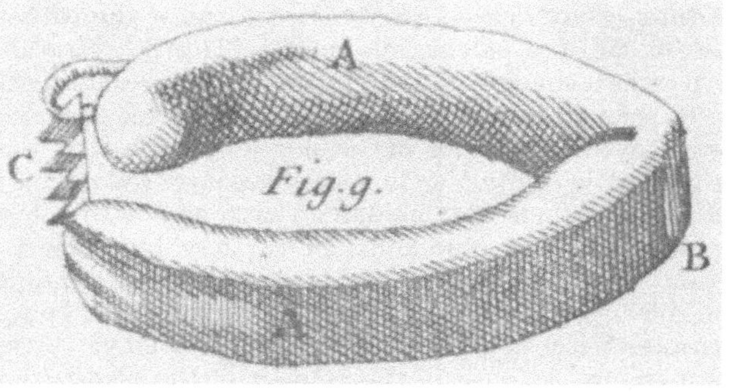


a

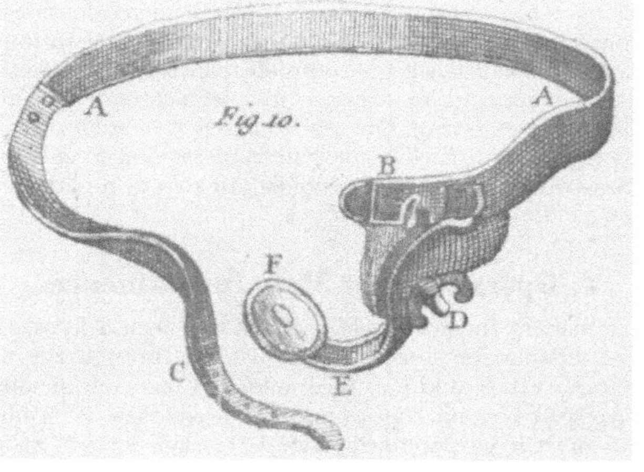


b

Fig. 15a and b. Illustrations reproduced from the Textbook of Surgery by Heister, of the early XVIII. Century. a Adjustable penile clamp for incontinence. b Incontinence truss described as lifting up on the soft tissue of the perineum behind the scrotum with the rigid arm EF adjusted into position by the wing-nut at D

Various surgical procedures have made use of a very old observation that elevation of the perineal floor in the area of the urethral bulb could provide the added support to achieve continence in many of the patients with post-operative stress incontinence. Again in HEISTER's Textbook of Surgery 250 years ago we find illustrated an external truss which reached in behind the scrotum and lifted the perineum, as shown in Fig. 15b. In 1927, KEYES described a plication across the midline of the body of the levator ani muscles, through a perineal incision, to provide such support. More recent efforts using the locally available tissue have added the resection of a wedge of the urogenital diaphragm with a tight suture of the resultant edges to reinforce the sphincter action (PETERSON, 1967), and the transposition of the ischial attachment of the ischio-cavernosous muscles to provide a muscle sling under the urethral bulb (KAUFMAN, 1969). Although the most recent modifications await the test of time, the Keyes operation has usually provided relief measured in only weeks or months because of stretching of the supporting sling or breakdown of the imbricating sutures.

Various surgeons have attempted to achieve the perineal elevation by the insertion of a more rigid support into the perineal tissue. BERRY described the use of an acrylic plaque pressing up against the bulb and attached laterally to the ischial rami with wire or other nonabsorbable sutures (BERRY, 1961). In spite of several modifications in the mode of attachment (BERRY, 1965), the initial enthusiasm for this procedure has been dampened by the late failures due to mechanical breakdown of the supporting sutures of the Berry prosthesis with relapse of incontinence (RANEY, 1969; ENGEL and WADE, 1969). The use of a plastic or collagen mesh sling around the urethral bulb has been similarly used in recent years, with long-term results not yet reported but presumably susceptible to the same problem of a lack of a firm and permanent attachment to the rigid structures of the perineal outlet (GIRGIS and VEENEMA, 1965).

A promising solution to the problem of a permanent attachment for a perineal support has been provided by the ingenious use of an autogenous transplant of a segment of rib bone attached to the ischial rami so as to permit a bony union as described by SCHMAELZLE et al. (1968). We favor a slight modification of this technique which makes use of a groove on the inner face of each ischial ramus to allow the segment of rib to be slid into place like a shelf in a bookcase and avoid even temporary reliance on sutures or bone screws to achieve bone to bone contact and bony union. More time will have to elapse before final evaluation of this technique.

## VI. Recto-urethral Fistula

The dreaded complication of recto-urethral fistula may still be seen after either simple or radical prostatectomy. It can be avoided in radical retropubic or perineal surgery by careful inspection and continuous attention to the directly visualized rectal wall. The complication is also seen occasionally after simple retropubic or suprapubic surgery if deep sutures have been taken through the posterior capsule and into the rectal lumen, in which case the complication may not be apparent until after the catheter is removed postoperatively. For many years the STONE-YOUNG (STONE-YOUNG, 1912) operation was widely practiced for the radical cure of this complication. This procedure involved the resection of the distal rectum affected by the fistula and the advancement of the rectum which was then reanastomosed to the anal verge. Unfortunately, some of these cases were cured of their fistula only to be left with rectal incontinence. With the advent of antibiotics and careful bowel preparation, it is now possible to resect the fistula's tract through a perineal exposure, and to close the urethral and rectal wall defects separately with carefully placed inverted catgut sutures. This approach, (GOODWIN, 1958) as well as the transrectal one (TALARICO and FERNANDES, 1969), do not risk the further complication of rectal incontinence because the anorectal junction is left intact. As in the case of surgery for diverticulitis of the colon, the decision as to whether to use a preliminary diverting colostomy is to be individualized depending on the amount of local active inflammation and the extent of the fistulous defect. Certainly, a very edematous and stiff inflammatory reaction in the area will be more easily controlled and the fistula closure more likely to succeed if preliminary colostomy is carried out, followed by delayed closure after the fistula has been repaired and tested by voiding.

## References

Andersson, L., Nilsson, I. M.: Effect of EACA on fibrinolysis and bleeding conditions in prostatic disease. Acta chir. scand. **121**, 291 (1961).

Arduino, L. J. et al. (Veterans Administration Cooperative Urological Research Group): Carcinoma of the prostate: Treatment comparisons. J. Urol. (Baltimore) **98**, 516 (1967).

Atherton, L. D., Atherton, L.: Aggressive surgery for carcinoma of the prostate. J. Urol. (Baltimore) **91**, 294 (1964).

Barnes, R. W., Bergman, R. T., Hadley, H. L., Dick, A. L.: Early prostatic cander: long term results with conservative treatment. J. Urol. (Baltimore) **102**, 88 (1969).

Bauer, W. C., McGavran, M. H., Carlin, M. R.: Unsuspected carcinoma of the prostate in suprapubic prostatectomy specimens: a clinics pathological study of 55 consecutive cases. Cancer (Philad.) **13**, 370 (1960).

Beck, A. D.: A critical review of the Hryntschak prostatectomy. Brit. J. Urol. **41**, 600 (1969).

Becker, L. E., Harrin, W. R.: Prostatic abscess: a diagnostic and theurapeutic approach. J. Urol. (Baltimore) **91**, 582 (1964).

Belt, E., Ebert, C. E., Surber, A. C., Jr.: A new anatomic approach in perineal prostatectomy. J. Urol. (Baltimore) **41**, 482 (1939).

Beneventi, F. A.: Two year experience with the urethral rotation operation for correction of postoperative urinary incontinence. J. Urol. (Baltimore) **100**, 488 (1968).

Berlin, B. B., Cornwell, P. M., Connelly, R. R., Eisenberg, H.: Radical perineal prostatectomy for carcinoma of the prostate: survival in 143 cases treated from 1935 to 1958. J. Urol. (Baltimore) **99**, 97 (1968).

Berry, J. L.: A new procedure for correction of urinary incontinence: preliminary report. J. Urol. (Baltimore) **85**, 771 (1961).

— Postprostatectomy urinary incontinence and some experiences with the Berry procedure. Surg. Clin. N. Amer. **45**, 1481 (1965).

Bourque, J. P.: Transvesicocapsular prostatic adenomectomy (transcommissural): Preliminary report on 80 cases. J. Urol. (Baltimore) **72**, 918 (1954).

Bricker, N. S., Schwayri, E. D., Reardan, L. B., Kellogg, D., Merrill, J. P., Holmes, L. H.: An abnormality in renal function resulting from urinary tract obstruction. Amer. J. Med. **23**, 554 (1957).

Brooks, M. B.: Heparin in treatment of hemorrhagic diathesis associated with prostatic carcinoma. J. Urol. (Baltimore) **102**, 240 (1969).

Campbell, W. G., MacGregor, A. M. C.: Posterior prostatectomy. J. int. Coll. Surg. **51**, 1 (1969).

Casteel, C. K., Thompson, E. M., Wipfler, E. J.: Vas crush for prevention of post-prostatectomy epididymitis: an experimental and clinical study. J. Urol. (Baltimore) **93**, 476 (1965).

Chute, R.: Radical retropubic prostatectomy for cancer. J. Urol. (Baltimore) **71**, 347 (1954).

— Fox, B. M.: Nonresectable carcinoma of the prostate rendered resectable by endocrine therapy. J. Urol. (Baltimore) **95**, 577 (1966).

Cohen, S. P., Kopilnick, M. D., Robbins, M. A.: Removable purse-string suture of the vesical neck during suprapubic prostatectomy. J. Urol. (Baltimore) **102**, 720 (1969).

Cook, G. B., Watson, F. R.: Twenty single nodules of prostatic cancer not treated by total prostatectomy. J. Urol. (Baltimore) **100**, 672 (1968).

Culp, O. S.: Radical perineal prostatectomy: its past, present, and possible future. J. Urol. (Baltimore) **98**, 418 (1967).

Dahlen, C. P., Goodwin, W. E.: Sexual potency after perineal biopsy. J. Urol. (Baltimore) **77**, 660 (1957).

del Regato, J. A.: Radiotherapy in the conservative management of operable and locally inoperable carcinoma of the prostate. Radiology **88**, 761 (1967).

Duval, P.: Prostatectomie transvesicale avec suture de la vessie a l'uretre et reunion par premiere intention (Rap. de F. Legueu) Bull. Soc. Chir. Paris **32**, 651 (1906).

Eiseman, B., Vivion, C., Vivian, J.: Fluid and electrolyte change following the relief of urinary obstruction. J. Urol. (Baltimore) **74**, 222 (1955).

Emmett, J. L., Greene, L. F., Papantoniou, A.: Endocrine therapy in carcinoma of the prostate gland: 10 year survival studies. J. Urol. (Baltimore) **83**, 471 (1960).

ENGEL, R. M., WADE, J. C.: Experience with Berry Prosthesis. J. Urol. (Baltimore) **102**, 78 (1969).

FINKELBERG, Z., KUNIN, C. M.: Clinical evaluation of closed urinary drainage systems. J. Amer. med. Ass. **207**, 1657 (1969).

FINKLE, A. L., MOYERS, T. G.: Sexual potency in aging males: IV. Status of private patients before and after prostatectomy. J. Urol. (Baltimore) **84**, 152 (1960).

FLOCKS, R. H.: Carcinoma of prostate. J. Urol. (Baltimore) **101**, 741 (1969).

FREYER, P. G.: One hundred ten cases of total enucleation of the prostate for radical cure of enlargement of that organ. Lancet **1904 II**, 197.

FULLER, E.: Six successful and successive cases of prostatectomy. J. cutan. Dis. **13**, 229 (1895).

GIRGIS, A. S., VEENEMA, R. J.: Perineal urethroplasty: a new operation for correction of urinary incontinence in the male patients. J. Urol. (Baltimore) **93**, 703 (1965).

GONDER, M. J., SOANES, W. A., SHULMAN, S.: Cryosurgical treatment of the prostate. Invest. Urol. **3**, 372 (1966).

GOODWIN, W. E.: radical prostatectomy after previous prostatic surgery. Technical problems encountered in treatment of occult carcinoma. J. Amer. med. Ass. **148**, 799 (1952).

— MIMS, M. M., YOUNG, H. H.II.: Rhabdomyosarcoma of the prostate in a child. First 5-year survival. J. Urol. (Baltimore) **99**, 651 (1968).

— TURNER, R. D., WINTER, C. C.: Rectourinary fistula principles of management and technique of surgical closure. J. Urol. (Baltimore) **80**, 246 (1958).

GUTE, D. B., CHUTE, R., BARON, J. A., Jr.: Bladder neck revision for obstruction in neck. A clinical study reporting normal e-aculation postoperatively. J. Urol. (Baltimore) **99**, 744 (1968).

HAND, J. R., SULLIVAN, A. W.: Retropubic prostatectomy: An analysis of 100 cases. J. Amer. med. Ass. **145**, 1313 (1951).

HARRIS, S. H.: Suprapubic prostatectomy with closure. Surg. Gynec. Obstet. **50**, 251 (1930).

HEDLUND, P. O.: Antifibrinolytic therapy with cyclokapron in connection with prostatectomy—a double blind study. Scand. J. Urol. Nephrol. **3**, 177 (1969).

HINMAN, F., JR.: Flowmeter for automatically timed voiding. J. Urol. (Baltimore) **94**, 89 (1965).

HOWARD, P. J., FRALEY, E. E.: Elevation of the phosphate in benign prostatic disease. J. Urol. (Baltimore) **94**, 687 (1965).

HRYNTSCHAK, T.: Suprapubic prostatectomy with primary closure of the bladder by an original method: preparation, technique, and postoperative treatment. Springfield: C. C. Thomas Co. 1955.

HUDSON, P. B.: Prostatic Cancer. XIV. Its incidence, extent and behavior in 686 men studied by prostatic biopsy. J. Amer. Geriat. Soc. **5**, 338 (1957).

HUGGINS, C.: Commentary on treatment of prostate cancer (Editorial). J. Urol. (Baltimore) **102**, 119 (1969).

— HODGES, C. V.: Studies on prostatic cancer. I. Effect of castration, of estrogen and of androgen injection on serum phosphatases in metastatic carcinoma of the prostate. Cancer Res. **1**, 293 (1941).

HYBBINETTE, S.: Suprapubische Transurethral Prostatiktomie. Langenbecks Arch. klin. Chir. **183**, 145 (1935).

IVANOVICI, F., BOCANCEA, D.: The management of urinary incontinence following prostatectomy by the procedure of tubular cutaneous flap: a preliminary note of operative technique. J. Urol. (Baltimore) **103**, 202 (1970).

JACOBS, L. C., COOPER, E. J.: Prevesical prostatectomy. Urol. cutan. Rev. **37**, 729 (1933).

JEWETT, H. J.: Treatment of early cancer of the prostate. J. Amer. med. Ass. **183**, 161 (1963).

— The case for radical perineal prostatectomy. J. Urol. (Baltimore) **103**, 195 (1970).

KAUFMAN, J. J.: Personal communication, 1969.

KELLY, G. G., SILBERGLEIT, A., BERKAS, E. M., CAPUTO, J. M., BROMME, W.: Suprapubic prostatectomy: A report of 337 cases. J. Urol. (Baltimore) **92**, 215 (1964).

KEYES, E. L.: An operation for incontinence of urine following perineal prostatectomy. Surg. Gynec. Obstet. **42**, 423 (1926).

KIRKMAN, N. F.: Postprostatectomy haematuria: treatment with aminocaproic acid. Brit. J. Surg. **54**, 1026 (1967).

KRAHN, H., MORALES, P., HOTCHKISS, R.: A comparison of suprapubic prostatectomy with and without vesical neck closure. J. Urol. (Baltimore) **96**, 83 (1966).

LEADBETTER, G. W., JR., DUXBURY, J. H., LEADBETTER, W. F.: Can prostatectomy be improved? J. Urol. (Baltimore) **82**, 600 (1959).

LEHMAN, T. H., KIRCHHEIM, D., BRAUN, E., MOORE, R.: An evaluation of radical prostatectomy for incidentally diagnosed carcinoma of the prostate. J. Urol. (Baltimore) **99**, 646 (1968).

Lich, R., Jr., Grant, O., Maurer, J. E.: Extravesical prostatectomy: A comparison of retropubic and perineal prostatectomy. J. Urol. (Baltimore) **61**, 930 (1949).
Lilien, O. M., Schaefer, J. A., Kileijan, V., Andaloro, V.: The case for perineal prostatectomy. J. Urol. **99**, 79 (1968).
Limbert, D. J.: Transcoccygeal repair of prostatorectal fistula. J. Urol. **100**, 666 (1968).
Lytton, B., Eemery, J. M., Harvard, B. M.: The incidence of benign prostatic obstruction. J. Urol. **99**, 639 (1968).
MacAllister, C. L. O.: Retropubic prostatectomy without catheter drainage. J. Urol. (Baltimore) **92**, 517 (1964).
Maier, O.: Inguinal extravesical prostatectomy. Langenbecks Arch. klin. Chir. **132**, 296 (1924).
Malament, M.: Maximal hemostasis in suprapubic prostatectomy. Surg. Gynec. Obstet. **120**, 1307 (1965).
Maresca, G. M., Vallett, B. S.: Parasacral prostatectomy. Delaware St. med. J. **29**, 31 (1957).
Marshall, D. F.: Trans-coccygeal prostatectomy. J. Maine med. Ass. **56**, 193 (1965).
Martin, D. C., Turner, R. D., Goodwin, W. E.: The surgical treatment of urinary incontinence: a review of some of the pertinent literature. Urol. Surv. **13**, 111 (1963).
Melicow, M. M., Pelton, T. H., Fish, G. W.: Sarcoma of the prostate: review of literature table of classification; report of four cases. J. Urol. (Baltimore) **49**, 675 (1943).
Memmelaar, J.: Total prostatovesiculectomy. Retropubic approach. J. Urol. (Baltimore) **62**, 340 (1949).
Michener, F. R., Thompson, I. M., Ross, G., Jr.: Urethrovesical tubulerization for urinary incontinence. J. Urol. (Baltimore) **92**, 203 (1964).
Miller, A. L., Jr., Scott, F. B., Scott, R., Jr.: An evaluation of antibiotics prior to prostatectomy. J. Urol. (Baltimore) **92**, 711 (1964).
Miller, H. C., Benjamin, J. A., McEvoy, R. K.: Sarcoma Botryoides: 7-year survival. J. Urol. (Baltimore) **101**, 567 (1969).
Millin, T.: Retropubic prostatectomy. In: Campbell, M. F., Urology. Philadelphia: W. B. Saunders 1963.
— Retropubic prostatectomy: a new extravesical technique. Report of 20 cases. Lancet **1945 II**, 693.
Murphy, J. J.: Inappropriate secretion of antidiuretic hormones in urologic patients. J. Urol. (Baltimore) **97**, 755 (1967).
Parry, W. L., Dawson, C. B.: Surgery for malignant disease of the prostate. In: Urologic Surgery (J. F. Glenn, and W. H. Boyce, eds.). New York: Harper & Row 1969.
Pennington, J. W., Prentiss, R. J., Howe, G.: Radical perineal prostatectomy for cancer: significance of perineal lymphatic invasion. J. Urol. (Baltimore) **97**, 1075 (1967).
Peterson, R. A.: Plastic repair of the external urethral sphincter. A new technique for correction of postoperative incontinence in men. J. Urol. (Baltimore) **97**, 1050 (1967).
Raney, A. M.: Reevaluation of postprostatectomy urinary incontinence with Berry procedure. J. Urol. (Baltimore) **102**, 81 (1969).
Reeves, J. F., Scott, R., Scott, F. B.: Prevention of epididymitis after prostatectomy by prophylactic antibiotics and partial vasectomy. J. Urol. (Baltimore) **92**, 528 (1964).
Robards, V. L., Jr., Ross, G., Jr.: The pathogenesis of postobstructive diuresis. J. Urol. (Baltimore) **97**, 105 (1967).
Roberts, S. B., Lattimer, J. K.: Reversibility of renal functional impairment after prostatic obstruction. J. Urol. (Baltimore) **93**, 545 (1965).
Rowan, R. L., Howley, T. F.: Postoperative impotence. J. Urol. (Baltimore) **95**, 68 (1966).
Samellas, W.: Urinary control following radical perineal prostatectomy. J. Urol. (Baltimore) **95**, 580 (1966).
— Measurement of urethral pressures following radical perineal prostatectomy. J. Urol. (Baltimore) **96**, 499 (1966).
Schmaelzle, J. F., Cass, A. S., Hinman, F., Jr.: Autogenous bone graft for post-prostatectomy incontinence. I. Animal experiments. J. Urol. (Baltimore) **99**, 656 (1968).
Scott, W. W.: An evaluation of endocrine therapy plus radical perineal prostatectomy in the treatment of advanced carcinoma of the prostate. J. Urol. (Baltimore) **91**, 97 (1964).
— Boyd, H. L.: Combined hormone control therapy and radical prostatectomy in treatment of selected cases of advanced carcinoma of prostate. J. Urol. (Baltimore) **101**, 86 (1969).
Stirling, W. C., Ash, J. F.: Sarcoma of the prostate. J. Urol. (Baltimore) **41**, 515 (1939).
Talarico, R. D., Fernandes, M.: Transrectal closure of urethrorectal fistula. J. Urol. (Baltimore) **101**, 332 (1969).
Thompson-Walker, J.: Transactions Second. Congress International Association of Urology, London, 1911.

TIERNEY, T. M.: Control of bleeding after prostatectomy with special reference to the use of oxydized regenerated cellulose. J. Urol. (Baltimore) **91**, 400 (1964).
VEST, S. A.: Radical perineal prostatectomy — modification of closure. Surg. Gynec. Obstet. **70**, 935 (1940).
VICKERY, A. L., JR., KERR, W. S., JR.: Carcinoma of the prostate treated by radical prostatectomy. Cancer (Philad.) **16**, 1598 (1963).
VINNICOMBE, J., SHUTTLEWORTH, K. E. D.: Aminocaproic acid in the control of haemorrhage after prostatectomy. Lancet **1966 I**, 230.
WARD, R. O.: Vesicocapsular prostatectomy. Lancet **1948 I**, 472.
WEYRAUCH, H. M.: Surgery of the prostate. Philadelphia: W. B. Saunders 1959.
WHITMORE, W. F., JR.: The rationale and results of ablative surgery for prostatic cancer. Cancer (Philad.) **16**, 1119 (1963).
WILDBOLZ, H.: Die operative Behandlung der prostatahypertrophie. Korresp.-Bl. schweiz. Ärzt. **36**, 277 (1906).
WILLIAMS, D. F., BLAHD, W. H.: The diagnostic and prognostic value of strontium-85 photoscanning in carcinoma of the prostate. J. Urol. (Baltimore) **97**, 1070 (1967).
— — WETTERAN, L., JR.: Radioactive fluorine-18 photoscanning: A diagnostic evaluation in cancer of the prostate. J. Urol. (Baltimore) **100**, 675 (1968).
WILSON, B., RISEMAN, D. D., MOYER, C. A.: Fluid balance in the urological patients. Disturbances in the renal regulation of the excretion of water and sodium salts following decompression of the urinary bladder. J. Urol. (Baltimore) **66**, 805 (1951).
YOUNG, H. H.: Practice of urology. Philadelphia: W. B. Saunders Co. 1926.
— STONE, H. B.: An operation for urethorectal fistula: Report of three cases. Trans. Amer. Ass. gen.-urin. Surg. **8**, 270 (1913).

# The Neurogenic Bladder in Spinal Cord Injury

TH. BURGHELE and V. ICHIM

With 35 Figures

## A. The Architectonics of the Musculature of the Urinary Bladder, Terminal Ureters, Trigone and Urethra

The architectonics of the musculature of the urinary bladder, terminal ureters, trigone and urethra has been the subject of numerous studies for over 100 years.

Gaps in our knowledge of this musculature have led to contradictory opinions and discussions concerning the functions of these anatomic formations, the mechanism of vesical continence and especially of the vesico-urethral opening in the course of micturition.

Study of the anatomy of this musculature is still a subject of present interest, owing to:

1. The difficulty of following up, by dissection, the muscular fibers of the detrusor because of the crossing and changes in position and direction of these fibers.
2. The development of the trigone-orificial region formed from the smooth musculature dependant upon the detrusor, trigone and ureters, each of different embryologic origin.
3. The interconnection of these muscles in the region of the bladder neck and trigone, and the impossibility of delimiting the area of each in spite of the serial histologic studies carried out.
4. The presence of a rich connective-elastic tissue, especially in the region of the fundus and neck, forming together with the muscular tissue veritable myo-elastic rings.
5. The complex autonomic-somatic innervation of the detrusor, trigone, smooth and striate sphincters, forming the paravesical plexuses.
6. The lack of agreement between the anatomical and functional aspects, which are created to complete each other.

### I. Architectonics of the Urinary Bladder Musculature

#### 1. The Bladder Wall

The anatomical studies of HUNTER (1954) on the anatomy of the urinary bladder again brought to the fore an older concept on the architectonics of the detrusor musculature, sustained by HANCOCK (1852), GRIFFITHS (1891), VERSARI (1897) and KALISCHER (1900), who considered that an anastomosis existed between the longitudinal or external, the circular or middle bladder muscular coat and the deep longitudinal coat.

Fig. 1 shows the transition from the surface towards the depth of the muscular fibers of the detrusor, forming coats with a different orientation and position.

According to HUNTER (1954, 1968), the longitudinal ventral fibers of the bladder musculature are inserted upon the pubo-vesical ligaments, the lateral ligaments of the bladder, the fascial capsule between the pubo-vesical ligaments, the internal sphincter and capsule of the prostate. The dorsal longitudinal mus-

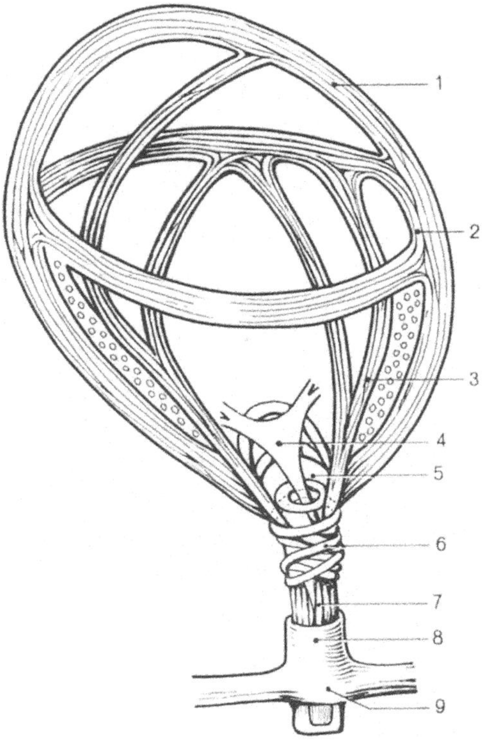


Fig. 1. Architectonics of the musculature of the bladder, trigone and urethra. *1* External longitudinal layer; *2* middle circular layer; *3* internal longitudinal layer; *4* trigone; *5* fundus ring; *6* circular muscular layer of the urethra; *7* longitudinal muscular layer of the urethra; *8* external sphincter; *9* striate perineal musculature

cular fibers of the detrusor are inserted on the middle lobe of the prostate, the tendinous ring of the uvula, the prostate capsule and parenchyma.

The muscular fibers of the longitudinal, external coat, over the bladder surface are distributed fanwise, the fibers on the right side coursing towards the left half and conversely, forming a first crossing over the ventral and respectively dorsal wall of the bladder; the fibers then run deeper, in a circular direction, the ventral fibers crossing the dorsal ones within the lateral walls of the bladder, and contributing to the formation of the deep circular coat.

At the level of the proximal urethra, TANAGHO and SMITH (1966) showed that part of the fibers of the external longitudinal fibers run obliquely over the anterior aspect of the urethra where they join the opposite fibers, forming the posterior concave loop. The fibers of the anterior longitudinal coat surround the posterior aspect of the urethra in the same way. These circular fibers of the proximal urethra gradually fuse with the striate fibers of the external circular sphincters.

The fibers of the circular layer continue on the lateral side of the bladder crossing the fibers from the ventral wall, as well as those from the dorsal wall. After this final crossing the muscular fibers run lengthwise down the urethra (Woodburne, 1967). In all there are five crossings and changes of direction and position.

It is generally admitted that the middle circular coat stops sharply at the level of the internal urethral meatus. According to Uhlenhuth, Hunter and Loechel (1953), the circular fibers in the fundus compact with the deep trigone fibers, forming the fundus ring, located below the deep trigone — the name of trigonal sphincter, given to this formation defines its role in continence during both filling and voiding of the bladder. Of interest in the fundus ring is the arrangement of the precervical muscular fibers. Tanagho and Smith (1966) showed that the anterior portion of the fundus ring is better represented than the posterior aspect. The anterior muscular fiber condensation is about 2 cm thick and can be clearly distinguished from the circular coat of the bladder that ends at the level of the urethra, as already mentioned.

Gil Vernet (1960) described the musculature in the precervical area as a muscular complex in the form of an arc, with a posterior concavity in which the muscular fibers are mixed with collagen tissue.

Most authors agree that the precervical musculature is dependant upon the circular muscular layer of the detrusor. Bro-Rasmussen et al. (1965), carrying out serial histologic studies on the anterior bladder wall slightly above the vesico-urethral orifice, noted the presence in this zone of fine bands of smooth musculature similar in structure to the musculature of the trigone. Owing to this histologic resemblance of the precervical muscular fibers with those of the trigone, the bladder orifice is surrounded by a musculature differing from that of the detrusor, which exhibits a rough fasciculation, poor in connective tissue.

The precervical muscular arc formed of fine muscular fibers is covered by the precervical musculature of the detrusor, and it is impossible to separate them from each other.

Apart from the histologic findings which demonstrate the unity of the trigono-orificial musculature, there also exists a unitary functional behaviour, as proved experimentally by Learmonth (1931) and Burghele, Ichim and Demetrescu (1959).

## 2. The Bladder Neck

Tanagho et al., (1966) in a discussion on the anatomy and function of the bladder neck state: "The precise mechanism of closure of the bladder neck and the way in which it is opened during voiding is not known; the subject remains quite controversial" (Brit. J. of Urol., 1966, XXXVIII, 1, p. 65).

Three opinions have been sustained regarding the architectonics of the bladder neck.

The first stipulates the existence of a sphincter separate from the rest of the musculature (Kohlrausch, 1854; Kalischer, 1900; Diese, 1902; Denny Brown, 1936; Uhlenhuth et al., 1953).

According to the second opinion, upheld by Wesson (1920), McCrea (1926), two muscular bands are described around the bladder neck, depending upon the detrusor fibers which form the sphincteral mechanism of the bladder neck.

The anterior band derives from the longitudinal muscular coat of the bladder and forms half a ring with a posterior concavity. The posterior band dependant upon the middle circular coat of the bladder forms a lower half ring with an anterior concavity. According to TANAGHO and SMITH (1966) the two bands are dependant upon the longitudinal muscular coat of the bladder. The third denies the existence of a sphincter at the bladder neck (LE GROS CLARK, 1883; SCHER, 1950; LAPIDES et al., 1957; LAPIDES, 1958; LAPIDES et al., 1958; and WOODBURNE, 1960).

According to these authors the function of the sphincter is ensured by the posterior urethra in men and by the whole urethra in females. Continence is

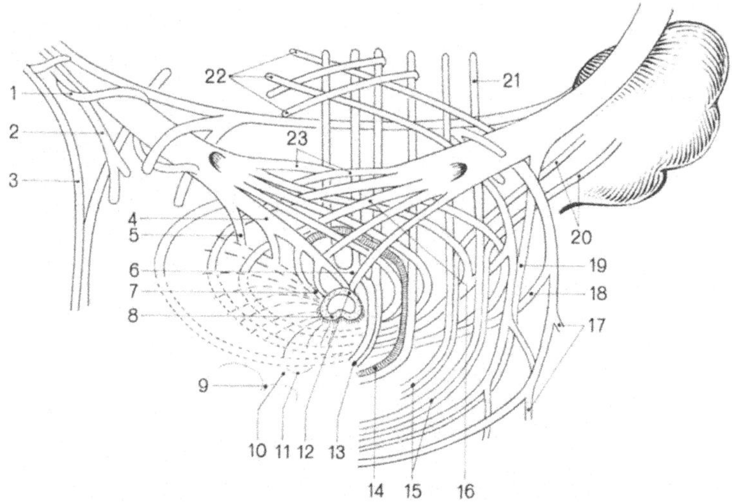


Fig. 2. Diagrammatic view of base of bladder, demonstrating distribution of ureteric and bladder musculature. *1* Circular ureteral fibres shown becoming longitudinal. *2* Longitudinal ureteric fibres entering the bladder wall. *3* Outer longitudinal ureteric fibres shown leaving the ureter and coursing with the outer longitudinal layers of the bladder. *4* Most inferiorly disposed ureteric fibres. *5* Fibres of trigonal musculature contributing to the fibromuscular plate. *6* Tendinous ring or yoke underlying the uvula which gives rise to the dorsal longitudinal musculature inserting into the trigone. *7* Fibres of the fibromuscular plate spiralling into the urethra. *8* Redundant urethral mucosa with submucosal musculature. *9* Innermost bladder musculature. *10* Fibromuscular plate. *11* Fibres of internal sphincter. *12* Bell's muscle forming portion of dorsal urethral wall. *13* Continuation of 6 into the main component of the dorsal longitudinal musculature. *14* Portion of prostatic ring coursing with dorsal longitudinal bladder musculature. *15* Dorsal longitudinal bladder musculature passing through trigonal muscle and encircling the urethral orifice anteriorly. *16* Characteristic ureteric fibres traversing trigone. *17* Origin of the deep crossed dorsal longitudinal bladder musculature from prostatic glandular capsule. *18* Elements of the deep crossed dorsal component of bladder musculature which become fused into the internal sphincter. *19* Outer longitudinal ureteric fibres shown leaving the ureter and coursing with the outer longitudinal layers of the bladder. *20* Musculature of fibromuscular capsule of the seminal vesicle which courses with the dorsal longitudinal bladder musculature. *21* Superficial uncrossed bundles of dorsal longitudinal component of bladder musculature. *22* Deep crossed bundles of dorsal longitudinal component of bladder musculature. *23* Longitudinal ureteric fibres forming Mercier's bar. (After HUNTER, 1968)

possible due to the resistance of the intraluminal urethra which depends upon the tension of the urethral wall and the radius of the lumen, according to Laplace's law, and upon the elastic connective tissue.

Fig. 2 gives the architectonics of the trigono-orificial musculature; the distribution of the muscular fibers around the urethral orifice can be noted.

The most distal muscular fibers form an almost complete ring that ends retrocervically in the apex of the deep trigone.

The arc formed by the precervical fibers situated more cranially, opens up wider and wider, the endings of these fibers terminating in the lateral and dorsal edges of the deep trigone. They do not form a complete ring. Some of the fibers course up to the urethral hiatus, below the deep trigone.

The muscular fibers of the vesico-urethral orifice which do not join on the posterior aspect to form a complete ring end in the fibro-elastic connective tissue in the trigonal area; therefore a ring is formed that is partly muscular and partly connective, the elasticity of the connective tissue fulfilling the tonicity role of the muscular tissue. The tonus and elasticity of the musculo-connective ring is sufficient to ensure continence of the bladder without contraction of the musculature.

HUTCH (1965, 1966) describes a formation surrounding the internal urethral orifice at the base plate of the bladder and demonstrates anatomically, radiologically and theoretically the role of this base plate as internal sphincter and the changes it undergoes in the course of micturition. The ventral aspect of the base plate consists of 15 to 18 stringlike bands which belong to the middle muscular layer of the bladder.

The bands situated towards the urethra form an almost complete ring whereas those towards the bladder fan out and break up into the connective-elastic tissue of the trigone.

The dorsal plate is broader than the surface of the trigone.

The investigations of KJELLBERG, ERICSSON and RUDHE (1957) demonstrated that at the radiologic examination the trigone appears more clearly because of the adherence of the bladder mucosa to the deep plane, which can also be observed anterior to the bladder orifice, so that the anterior position in the immediate neighbourhood of the urethral orifice can be considered to form part of the base plate of the bladder.

The base plate is formed of smooth muscle, collagen and elastic tissue. This structure is round and flat exept during voiding, when it is converted into a cone-shaped, funnel-like object.

Contraction of the external longitudinal musculature of the bladder, contraction of the superficial trigone, of the internal longitudinal layer and of the striate muscle of the urethra contribute to "breaking of the plate" (from flat into a funnel-shape position), of importance in the inititation of voiding.

## II. Architectonics of the Musculature of the Terminal Ureters and Trigone

According to WOODBURNE (1967) "considerable confusion exists in the literature concerning the anatomy of the uretero vesical junction" (Neurogenic Bladder, the Williams and Wilkins Company, Baltimore 1967, p. 9).

TANAGHO and PUGH (1963) describe the terminal ureter as being formed of three segments: the juxtavesical, intramural and submucous ureter. In the opinion of DEBLED (1968) the terminal ureter forms the uretero-trigonal and periuretero-trigonal musculature. The uretero-trigonal musculature includes the juxtavesical and the intramural ureter and the superficial trigone. At the level of the juxtavesical ureter there are circulatory and oblique fibers apart from the longitudinal fibers.

The anterior and posterior lip of the ureteral meatus are surrounded by oblique and spiroid fibers that cross one another giving rise to an anterior and a posterior decussation. The periureteral musculature is more developed posteriorly where the juxtavesical ureter joins the intramural one.

The longitudinal fibers of the ureter form within the bladder the superficial trigone whose fibers are distributed crosswise between the two ureteral orifices forming Mercier's bar which delimits the superficial trigone posteriorly. The lateral fibers of the superficial trigone meet along the midline and pass over the posterior lip of the urethral meatus, then continue in the posterior urethra in men, where they form the crista urethralis, which is inserted upon the veru montanum. In women the superficial trigone ends at the level of the distal collagen ring. There are no connexions between the superficial trigone and bladder neck. Worthy of note is the insertion of the muscular fibers of the superficial trigone in the bladder mucosa. This fusion of the musculature to the mucosa also extends to the marginal zones of the vesico-urethral orifice corresponding to the base plate.

Waldeyer's sheath begins 1—3 cm before the penetration of the ureter into the bladder wall. At first made up of connective tissue, Waldeyer's sheath is supplied along its course with smooth muscular fibers and, in addition, with fibers from the circular muscular coat of the bladder at its passage through the bladder wall. Within the bladder, the muscular fibers of the sheath penetrate between the superficial trigone and vesical musculature, to form the deep trigone.

Woodburne (1967) denies the existence of Waldeyer's sheath. Sections at the level of the uretero-vesical junction show a lax, free penetration of the ureters within the thickness of the bladder wall. The superficial trigone joins the anterior half of the deep trigone, and this in turn the connective and muscular tissue of the detrusor. Owing to this unity of the bladder and trigone musculature contraction of the detrusor during micturition draws up the trigone with a tendency to verticalization, so that the pressure of the bladder content is exercised upon the urethral orifice.

Although Gil Vernet (1960) admits the existence of the posterior part of the trigone, as resulting from confluence of the muscular fibers of the ureters and Waldeyer's sheath, he considers that it has nothing in common with the ureters.

The apex of the deep trigone ends at the level of the urethral meatus. The combined thickness of the two trigones is about equal to that of the detrusor (Tanagho, Smith and Meyers, 1968). According to these authors the deep trigone and condensation of smooth muscular precervical fibers of the middle circular layer of the detrusor maintain a flat surface around the bladder outlet, without playing the role of a sphincter, which is realized only by the longitudinal muscular bands of the bladder, surrounding the proximal urethra. A second function of the deep trigone, during contraction, is that of initiating tension in the anterior middle circular fibers, thus spreading the contraction to the whole musculature of the detrusor. Finally, a third function is that of transforming and maintaining the bladder neck into a funnel-like shape. Concomitant contraction of the anterior cervical fibers will help support the posterior part of the bladder neck preventing it from sagging downwards, because of the weaker posterior extravesical support.

On appraising the richness of the connective and muscular tissue at the level of the bladder neck and urethra, Woodburne shows that "In fact, muscle and elastic tissue are intermingled in the vesical neck and along the urethra, in a most intimate fashion, such as may be expressed in the little used term myo-elastic tissue" [J. Urol. (Baltimore) 84, 1, 83 (1960)].

The musculature of the superficial and of the deep trigone is of mesodermal origin. No doubts exist concerning their anatomic, histologic, embryologic, pharmacologic and neurologic origin. The only point in question is the behaviour of the trigone, especially during micturition.

According to the opinion of Wesson (1920), MacCrea (1926), and MacLeod (1942), recently sustained by Tanagho and Smith (1966), the trigonal muscle plays a part in opening the vesical neck during micturition. On contracting it draws up the posterior lip of the neck. Tanagho, Hutch, Meyers and Rambo (1965) and Tanagho, Smith and Meyers (1968) consider that the trigone contracts about 5 seconds before the detrusor. Its contraction closes the uretero-vesical orifices and draws up the posterior lip of the neck, which leads to its funnelling. Relaxation of the external sphincter and dropping of the urogenital diaphragm take place concomitantly.

Concerning the role of the contraction of the trigone in opening the vesico-urethral orifice, certain reserves must be made, since it is assumed that this contraction acts upon an elastic opening, which will be drawn entirely in the direction of the traction. It is therefore not excluded that contraction of the trigone itself should take place concomitant to contraction of the precervical muscular fibers, hence closing instead of opening the vesico-urethral orifice. Concomitant contraction of the trigone and of the smooth sphincter has, moreover, been demonstrated experimentally by electric stimulation of the hypogastric nerve (Learmonth, 1931). On the other hand, contraction of the trigono-orificial opening closes the vesico-urethral opening during ejaculation.

Gil Vernet (1960) describes the following muscles that close the vesical neck: a circular muscle, an internal sphincter forming the true smooth sphincter, a precervical loop of the detrusor fibers and urethral retro-orificial arcuate fibers, that form a complete ring with the precervical loop. All these anatomical formations are located in the highest part of the neck. Distal to these formations are other muscular elements which help to close the urethral opening, forming a deep loop dependant upon the detrusor.

Contrary to the opinion of McCrea (1926), who describes a circular vesical sphincter formed of smooth and striate fibers, Gil Vernet (1960) considers it to be a fusion of the detrusor muscle with the striate sphincter, the former gradually continuing with the latter, which becomes increasingly well represented. The bladder neck is opened by the distribution of the fibers of the plexiform layer in the region of the urethral opening, which are inserted in the periurethral fibro-elastic tissue of the verumontanum. Other dilatory fibers continuing from the detrusor belong to the external longitudinal layer of the latter and of the trigone.

Mellick et al. (1962a and b) attribute closure of the ureteral orifices to the tonus of the ureters and the power of contraction of the bladder wall. Gruber (1930), Prather (1944) and Hutch (1954, 1961) sustain the passive mechanism of ureteral continence, which depends upon the oblique position of the ureters that lie upon the bladder wall and upon which increased intravesical pressure acts, producing a flap-valve.

The pressure gradient between the ureters and bladder likewise plays an important part in the mechanism preventing vesico-ureteral reflux. At rest, endo-vesical pressure attains only 20 cm of water, whereas endo-ureteral pressure may reach 120 cm of water during contraction. Inversion of this gradient during micturition prevents vesico-ureteral flow.

Cooper (1948) and Uhlenhuth et al. (1953) attribute closure of the ureteral orifices during micturition to contraction of the detrusor muscular fibers, and, specifically to those of the internal longitudinal layer.

Tanagho and Pugh (1963) describe another mechanism in closure of the uretero-vesical orifices, which also takes into account the opinion of other authors, i.e. the action of the ureteral muscle and Waldeyer's sheath, and that of the two trigonal layers. Contraction of these two layers facilitates the outflow and prevents reflux. When the bladder is empty the tonus of the detrusor musculature is sufficient to maintain uretero-vesical continence. The accumulation of urine raises the pressure and presses upon the terminal ureter closed by the tonus of the bladder musculature. Mechanical stretching of the trigone and terminal ureter brought about by progressive distension likewise helps to maintain uretero-vesical continence.

According to TANAGHO and HUTCH (1965) active contraction of the extravesical ureter and trigone press the ureteral roof against its floor and the whole ureter against the bladder wall. This is also demonstrated by the anatomic data: the uretero-trigonal continuity, diverging of the ureteral roof fibers to the side walls to meet the floor fibers, and the ureteral-bladder angle.

BURGHELE and ICHIM (1959) showed that contraction of the trigone and internal sphincter occurs after the sensation of the need to micturate appears.

TANAGHO, HUTCH, MEYERS and RAMBO (1965) demonstrated the functional unity of the trigone, intravesical and extravesical ureter by interrupting the anatomic continuity between the ureter and trigone by incision or excisions below the ureteral orifice, by incisions and resuturing or by sympathicotomy which produces vesico-ureteral reflux. In contrast, the administration of sympathomimetics and electrical stimulation of the trigonal muscle induce contraction of the trigone and ureteral orifices by contraction of the muscular fibers that proceed from the ureteral roof to the trigone.

During micturition, these authors demonstrated by lateral cysto-urethrographies that contraction of the trigone opens the urethral outlet and closes the ureteral orifices by diminishing the distance between them. The orifices were marked by metal clips. This shortening, however, may also be produced under the action of the detrusor alone, because of its muscular continuity with the trigone.

The antireflux function of the uretero-trigonal musculature is implemented, according to DEBLED (1968) by an active muscular mechanism, stressed by slow, progressive filling of the bladder. Increase in the muscle tonus leads to a shortening of the muscular fibers and is manifested by diminution of the distance between the ureteral meatus and urethral orifice, accentuation of the ureteral angle and pressure of the ureteral roof against the floor.

DEBLED contends participation of the uretero-trigonal musculature in opening of the bladder outlet.

## III. Architectonics of the Urethral Musculature

Both the smooth and the striate muscle, and a rich fibro-elastic tissue combine to form the urethral musculature.

HUNTER (1968) defines the urethral sphincter as formed of smooth muscular fibers continuing the external longitudinal layer of the bladder and the external striate sphincter continuing the urogenital diaphragm. The levator ani muscle separates the two muscular groups: above the fibers of the internal sphincteral muscle and the distal portion of Henle's muscle, and below, the distal portion of the predominantly striate external sphincter that continues posteriorly with the transverse muscle of the perineum and anteriorly with the pubo-vesical ligament.

The fascia of the uro-genital diaphragm delimits inferiorly the distal external sphincter.

The circular muscular layer in the upper half of the urethra continues the external longitudinal layer of the detrusor, similar to the longitudinal layer of the urethra which proceeds from the internal longitudinal coat of the bladder. Interconnections exist between the two muscular layers. The junction between the smooth and striate musculature takes place along an oblique line, running antero-posteriorly.

The external sphincter is well represented both anteriorly and laterally. In men this sphincter ends in the prostate capsule. Few of the striate circular fibers can be individualized, most of them forming arcs that run in a posterior direction.

According to Woodburne (1967) Bell's muscle represents a poor contribution of the ureteral longitudinal musculature and its fibers are gradually lost within the posterior musculature of the urethra.

In women the urethra is formed of an external circular muscular layer which continues the longitudinal muscular coat of the bladder and the internal longitudinal layer that continues the internal longitudinal coat of the bladder. Hutch (1968) notes the oblique direction in which the fibers of the external urethral layer lie. In women the striate muscular fibers surround the urethra in its middle third.

The urethra has a thick collagen tissue throughout its whole length and a particular condensation of this tissue in the terminal portion.

In the opinion of Tanagho and Smith (1966), Tanagho and Smith (1968), and in agreement with Lapides (1958) and Woodburne (1960), the circular and longitudinal musculature of the urethra play the part of a sphincter.

Contraction of the longitudinal muscular fibers shortens the urethra, increases its lumen and diminishes the pressure of the urethral wall upon the latter.

Gil Vernet (1960) describes the unity of the morphofunctional vesico-prostato-sphincteral complex, provided with dilatory and constrictor muscular fibers most of them belonging to the detrusor musculature.

According to this author, closure of the membranous urethra is ensured by the external sphincter and in the second place by the fibers of the smooth musculature. The smooth sphincter of the membranous urethra is acted upon by cervico-urethral, vesico-prostato-urethral and prostato-urethral fibers.

Under the influence of these fibers the urethra becomes shorter and wider. The membranous urethra is opened by contraction of the vesico-urethral fibers proceeding from the muscular bundles of the anterior and posterior longitudinal layer of the detrusor, the precervical transverse arc and the external cervico-urethral fibers.

MacCrea (1926) showed that the external sphincter opens the bladder neck especially by its dorsal extension which joins the external longitudinal layer above the smooth vesical sphincter.

Simultaneous recording of intravesical and intraurethral pressure (Einhorning, 1961; Tanagho, Miller, Mayers and Corbett, 1966; Woodburne, 1960; Lapides, 1958; Lapides, 1960) demonstrated that during filling of the bladder the action of the sphincter extends over three thirds of the urethra in women and the prostatic and membranous urethra in men. Pressure is lower over a distance of 0.5 cm from the urethral meatus, then increases in the middle portion of the urethra and decreases again in the distal portion of the femal urethra. This is explained by the rich amount of circular and longitudinal muscle in the middle segment of the urethra.

# B. Innervation of the Urinary Bladder and Sphincters

## I. Central Innervation

The location of the nervous centers that control the activity of the bladder and sphincters is difficult to establish because of:

— The proximity of the facilitatory and inhibitory centers in the cerebral cortex, the slightest cerebral lesions affecting the function of both centers;

— The bilaterality and symmetry of these centers, the lesion of one center leaving intact the center on the opposite hemisphere;

— The reflex function of the bladder without higher control under the influence of the sacral micturition center;

— extraspinal tracts of the sympathetic innervation controlling the trigone and internal sphincter and function of the latter even when the spinal parasympathetic micturition center is a functional.

The location of the micturition facilitatory or inhibitory cortical, subcortical, mesencephalic, hypothalamic and pontine bulbar centers is determined by experimental ablation of certain areas of the central nervous system, sectioning at different levels, electric stimulation, recording of the action currents from different areas or clinical observation of the function of the urinary bladder in cerebral lesions.

### 1. Cortical Centers

The cortical centers of micturition are located in the following areas (Fig. 3 and 4):

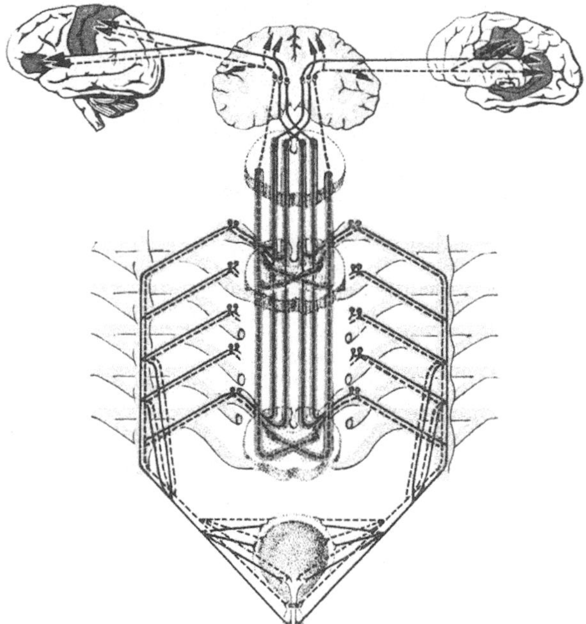

Fig. 3. Sensitive innervation of the urinary bladder. Micturition centers on the convex aspect of the cerebral hemispheres: gyrus pre- and postcentralis (top left); lobus frontalis facies inferior (bottom left). Micturition centers on the medial aspect of the cerebral hemispheres: lobulus paracentralis (top right); gyrus cinguli; gyrus hippocampi (bottom right). Centripetal spinal pathways: spinothalamic tract (dotted lines); fasciculus gracilis, fasciculus cuneatus (full lines). The sphinctero-spinal reflex center is located in the intermedio-lateral spinal grey matter in the $Th_{10}$—$L_2$ segments

— precentral gyrus (Langworthy and Kolb, 1935; Pfeifer, 1919);
— postcentral gyrus (Czyhlarz and Marburg, 1901; Friedmann, 1903);
— cingular gyrus (Kremer, 1947; Takebayashi et al., 1957; Matsumoto, 1957; Mukai, 1959; Gjone and Setekleiv, 1963);
— hippocampal gyrus;
— gyrus fornicatus (Adler, 1920; Ranson et al., 1935; Kabat et al., 1936; Henneman, 1948; Kaada, 1951);
— frontal lobe (Adler, 1920; Yamaguchi, 1960);
— paracentral lobulus (Kleist, 1918; Müller, 1919; Adler, 1920).

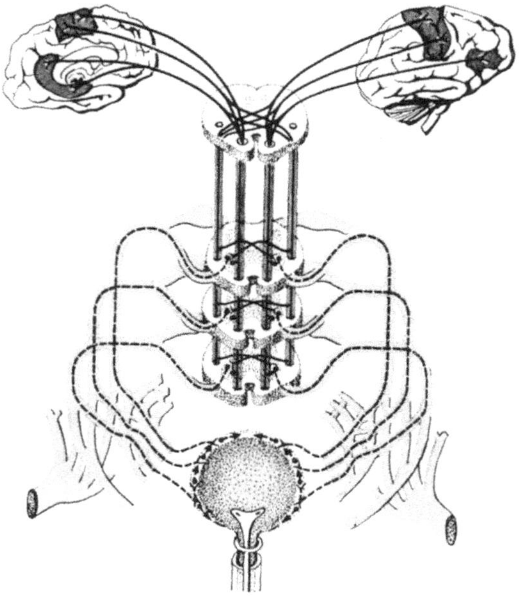

Fig. 4. Motor innervation of the urinary bladder. Micturition centers on the external aspect of the cerebral hemispheres: gyrus pre- and postcentralis (top left); lobus frontalis (facies inferior) (bottom left). Micturition centers on the medial aspect of the cerebral hemispheres: lobulus paracentralis (top right); gyrus cinguli; gyrus hippocampi (bottom right). Centripetal spinal pathways: tractus cortico-spinalis ventralis and tractus cortico-spinalis lateralis (full lines). Spinal micturition centers: sacral segments 2, 3 and 4. Peripheral motor pathways (dottes lines): anterior sacral roots and pelvic nerves. Neuronal synapse (pre- and postganglionic) in the bladder wall. The spinal parasympathetic micturition reflex center is located in the intermediolateral nucleus in the $S_2$—$S_4$ segments

## 2. Subcortical Centers

In the subcortex, electric stimulation of the anterior thalamus, internal capsule and tegmentum produces strong contractions of the urinary bladder (Bechterew and Mislawsky, 1888).

## 3. Mesencephalic Centers

The mesencephalic vesicoconstrictor area was located by Koyama et al. (1962) in the superior colliculus and intercollicular area, and the vesicorelaxer in the inferior colliculus and intercollicular area. The mesencephalic vesicoconstrictor area is connected with the vesicoconstrictor area in the medulla oblongata and has bilateral connections with the sacral vesicoconstrictor center. The mesencephalic vesicorelaxer area has connections with the pontine vesicorelaxer area.

## 4. Hypothalamic Centers and Preoptical Area

Contractions of the bladder were obtained by stimulation of the anterior hypothalamus (Beattie and Kerr, 1936), preoptical area, septum pellucidum and lateral hypothalamic area (Kabat et al., 1935), stria terminalis, anterior commissure, preoptical area, ventral aspect of the septum (Ranson et al., 1935; Kabat et al., 1936). According to Katsuki et al. (1955) accentuated vesical contractions are produced by stimulation of the preoptical area. In contrast, stimulation of the anterior hypothalamic area is accompanied by biphasic responses. In 1947, Uvnäs sustained that the anterior hypothalamus and preoptical area generated facilitatory vesical responses in terms of the frequency of the electric stimulus. Stimulation of the posterior septum pellucidum, the superior portion of the preoptical area, the supraoptical area or lateral part of the hypothalamus is followed by contractions of the bladder (Hess and Brügger, 1943). Stimulation of the posterior hypothalamus and upper midbrain (Beattie and Kerr, 1936), nucleus supraopticus diffusus (Mochida, 1957), cerebrum and midbrain (Tang, 1955), tegmentum (Tang and Ruch, 1956), middle hypothalamus and Forel's $H_1$ field (Nishiyama et al., 1959) results in relaxation of the bladder.

Stimulation of the nucleus amygdalae produces micturition in the cat, dog and monkey (Kaada, 1951). Similar observations were made by Gastaut et al. (1951), MacLean and Delgado (1953), Kaada et al. (1954), Anand and Dua (1956), Shearly and Peele (1957), Mochida (1957). According to Koikegami et al. (1957) only stimulation of the main nucleus amygdalae and of one part of the hippocampus produces micturition; in contrast, the neighbouring nuclei produce inhibition of the bladder movements.

Tang (1955) establishes a facilitatory area of micturition in the posterior hypothalamus and pons anterior. Nishiyama (1959) obtained bladder contractions by stimulation of the anterior area of the hypothalamus (ventro-caudal aspect of the septum pellucidum and ventro-lateral region of the lateral commissure). In the hypothalamus proper stimulation provokes a response only when applied in the lateral hypothalamic area, perifornix nucleus and lateral part of the mammillary body. Prompt, vigorous and sustained contractions can only be obtained, according to Yokoyama et al. (1960), by stimulation of the periventricular layer, medial mammillary nucleus, mammillotegmental tractus and lateral nucleus hypothalamicus. According to the same authors, relaxation of the bladder after stimulation or after a period of contraction is obtained by stimulation of the hypothalamic nuclei (anterior, posterior, ventromedial and dorsomedial), lateral mammillary nucleus, supraoptical nucleus, paraventricular nucleus and mammillary peduncle.

## 5. The Pons Centers

In the pons the area controlling vesical contraction is located in the pontine detrusor nucleus (Barrington, 1921) and the area controlling relaxation of the bladder corresponds to the nucleus subcoerulens ventralis (Taber, 1961). Stimulation of the pontine detrusor nucleus inhibit the discharge of the external urethral sphincter. Because of these results Kuru et al. (1963) proposed the name "pontine sphincter controlling area".

### 6. The Cerebellum Centers

Although Barrington (1921), Pressman and Shitov (1940) and Langworthy et al. (1940) concluded that the cerebellum had no direct role in the control of micturition, Chambers (1947) produced micturition on stimulation of the fastigial nucleus and nucleus interpositus, and Yokoyama et al. (1963) observed that stimulation of the pyramis and uvula resulted in contraction of the bladder. Inhibition of the bladder response was obtained by stimulation of the culmen, lobulus medius medianus and lobulus centralis of the cerebellar vermis.

### 7. Medulla Oblongata Centers

Vesicoconstrictor and vesicorelaxer centers have been described in the medulla oblongata.

Kuru (1940a, 1940b), tracing the ascending degenerations produced by antero-lateral cordotomy, found 3 nuclei in the medulla oblongata.

— nucleus paraalaris in close relation to the ala cinerea;
— nucleus juxtasolitarius, and
— nucleus lateralis externus dorsalis.

In further investigations on the existence of centers in the medulla oblongata, Kuru and Hukaya (1954), then Kuru and Ozaki (1959) obtained vesical and rectal contractions on stimulation of the dorsomedial reticular formation close to the ala cinerea and caudal end of the pyramidal decussation, and relaxation of these organs by stimulation of the ventrolateral reticular formation, between the ala cinerea and the obex.

Tokunaga and Kuru (1959) describe a vasoconstrictor center rostral to the extremity of the ala cinerea and the caudal end of the pyramidal decussation. Vesical relaxation was constantly obtained on stimulation of an area medial to the solitary fascicle at a point 1 mm rostral to the ala cinerea and obex.

## II. Peripheral Vesico-Sphincteral Innervation

### 1. The Spinal Parasympathetic Micturition Reflex Center (Cholinergic)

The spinal parasympathetic (cholinergic) micturition reflex center is located in the S2—S4 segments forming the intermediolateral nucleus close to the ependymal canal. The neurones of this center are fusiform or polygonal.

The preganglionic fibers originate from the second, third and forth anterior sacral roots, then leave them at 1—2 cm from the foramina sacralia anterior, to form the pelvic nerves, then join the hypogastric nerves to form the plexus pelvicus (ganglia pervina or plexus hypogastricus inferior).

On leaving the plexus pelvicus, the parasympathetic preganglionic fibers join the sympathetic fibers, forming the vesical nerves which are especially numerous near the entrance of the ureters into the bladder. They synapse within the wall of the detrusor with the postganglionic effector neurone.

The postganglionic neurone courses around the smooth muscular fibers of the bladder, according to Langworthy and Murphy (1939), or also to the trigone and smooth sphincter according to Kuntz and Saccomanno (1944). It appears to have an inhibitory effect upon the latter (Elliot, 1907; Learmonth, 1931).

KUNTZ (1953) showed that the urethra also receives cholinergic fibers.

The afferent pathways of the parasympathetic spinal reflex arc originate in the bladder wall receptors (Paccini type), situated in the chorion of the bladder mucosa (NICULESCU et al., 1956), and terminate in the parasympathetic sacral reflex center on the route of the posterior sacral roots.

## 2. Sympathetic or Sphinctero-Spinal Reflex Center (Adrenergic)

The sympathetic or sphinctero-spinal reflex center (adrenergic) is located in the intermedio-lateral spinal grey matter in the Th10—L2 segments (RIDDOCH, 1921), the Th11—L3 segments (PETERSEN and FRANKSSON, 1955), the Th9—L2 segments (BORS, 1952).

The sympathetic preganglionic neurones send their axons into the tenth, eleventh and twelfth anterior roots and the first, second and third anterior lumbar roots, but soon leave these to enter the paravertebral lumbar sympathetic chains via the white rami communicantes. By way of the splanchnic, lumbar and hypogastric nerves the axons reach the inferior mesenteric and inferior hypogastric plexus, where they synapse.

The postganglionic sympathetic fibers terminate in the musculature of the trigone, urethral and ureteral orifices, the seminal vesicles, ejaculation canals and prostate.

According to KUNTZ and SACCOMANNO (1944) the postganglionic fibers are also distributed to the detrusor muscle. HAMBERGER and NORBERG (1965), by means of a specific fluorescence method, observed nerve terminals of adrenergic type among the intramedial ganglia of the bladder wall.

The afferent sympathetic fibers of the sphinctero-spinal reflex center start from the receptors in the bladder mucosa, vesical peritoneum and walls of the bladder blood vessels, and by way of the vesical nerves, pelvic plexus, hypogastric nerves, pelvic splanchnic nerves, paravertebral sympathetic chains reach the sensory neurone through the posterior rami of the spinal nerves from L2 to Th10. They then synapse with the adrenergic motor neuron of the sphinctero-spinal center through a relay neurone.

## 3. Somatic Reflex Spinal Center of the Striate Sphincter

The somatic reflex spinal center of the striate sphincter is located in the anterior horn of the spinal cord, in the third and forth sacral segments. The axons of the motor neurons reach the striate sphincter by way of the third and fourth anterior sacral roots and the pudendal nerves.

The sensory fibers originating in the receptors of the posterior urethral mucosa, course along the pudendal nerves and posterior sacral roots, through the spinal ganglia and reach the somatic reflex spinal center in the anterior horn of the spinal cord.

Minute dissection of the intrapelvic innervation of the bladder (Fig. 5) reveals the abundance of the nervous fibers that form the pelvic plexus. The pelvic nerves can be exposed over approximately 2 cm, permitting the application of electrodes for electric neurostimulation of the bladder.

At the site of entry of the ureters into the bladder, a rich condensation of nervous fibers can be observed, forming the vesical nerves; this site is likewise indicated for application of the electrodes in myostimulation.

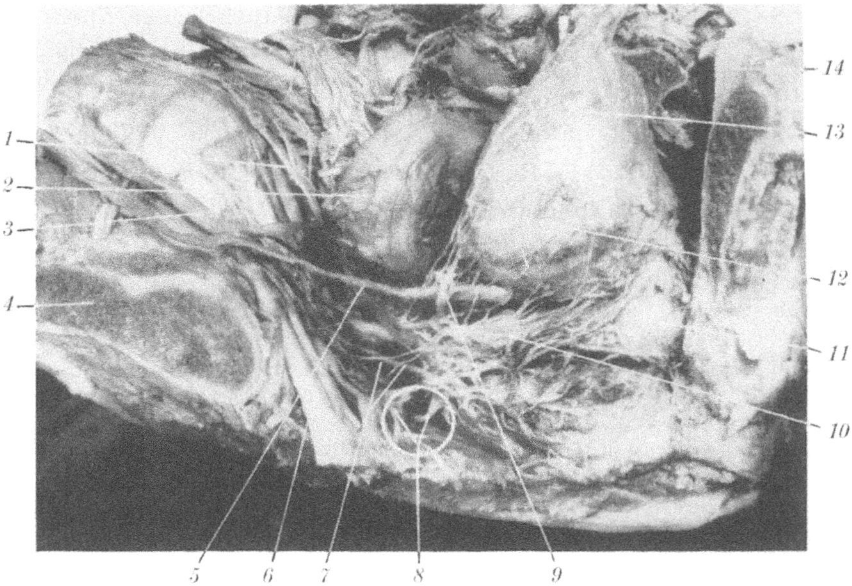


Fig. 5. Side-view of the male pelvis. Dissection of the peripheral innervation of the bladder: *1* nervus hypogastricus dexter; *2* ampulla rectalis; *3* arteria iliaca externa dexter; *4* os iliacum; *5* ureter dexter; *6* nervus ischiadicus; *7* nn. splanchnici pelvini sacralis; *8* nn. pelvici; *9* nervous loop of the ureter; *10* plexus pelvinus; *11* prostate; *12* nn. vesicalis; *13* urinary bladder; *14* os pubis

## III. Connection between the Micturition Centers in the Midbrain, Pons, Medulla oblongata and Spinal Centers

The bulbar vesicoconstrictor center receives centrifugal pathways from the vesicoconstrictor centers in the midbrain and pons, and centripetal pathways from the sacral micturition center via the sacrobulbar tractus (KURU, 1940a, 1956). The centrifugal connections of the bulbar vesicoconstrictor center with the sacral micturition center pass through the lateral reticulospinal tract (KURU and OZAKI, 1959).

The bulbar vesicorelaxer center receives centrifugal fibers from the mesencephalic vesicoconstrictor center and from it centrifugal fibers arise and descend to the sacral parasympathetic micturition center via the ventral reticulospinal tract (KURU and KAMIKAWA, 1960). Centrifugal fibers connect the pontine vesicoconstrictor center with its bulbar homologue and sacral micturition center. The connecting pathways course towards the spinal cord through the lateral reticulospinal tract. The pontine vesicorelaxer center is connected with the bulbar center and the spinal micturition center through the medial reticulospinal tract.

On the one hand, connections exist between the mesencephalic vesicoconstrictor center and the vesicorelaxer bulbar, vesicoconstrictor bulbar and vesicoconstrictor sacral centers, and on the other, between the mesencephalic and the pontine vesicorelaxer centers.

The centripetal pathways originating from the sacral micturition center participate in the sacrobulbar tract up to the paraalar, juxtasolitary and lateral nuclei. The paraalar nucleus is connected with the thalamus through the paraalarothalamic tractus and the juxtasolitary nucleus with the thalamus through the juxtasolitarothalamic fibers, that pass through the vesicorelaxer bulbar center, the pontine nucleus and the micturation facilitatory and inhibitory zones in the midbrain (KURU and YAMAMOTO, 1964).

In conclusion, the centrifugal pathways that connect the higher centers with the sacral parasympathetic micturition center and transmit facilitatory or inhibitory impulses, course within the lateral, the ventral and the medial reticulospinal tracts.

The centripetal pathway pass through the funiculus gracialis and funiculus cuneatus, lateral spinothalamic tract, dorsal spinocerebellar tract, marginal zone or Lissauer's tract.

The nervous impulses that give rise to the sensation of the desire to micturate, of imminent micturition, of fullness of the bladder, of pain and of passage of the urine through the urethra, are mediated by pathways within the spinothalamic tracts. According to BORS (1952), the nervous pathways that generate the sensation of pain course within the funiculus gracilis and cuneatus. NESBIT and LAPIDES (1948) attribute to the funiculus gracilis conduction of the proprioceptive nervous influxes.

The centripetal and the centrifugal pathways cross each other in the medulla oblongata (WANG and RANSON, 1939) and sacral spinal cord (BARRINGTON, 1933).

# C. Physiology of the Urinary Bladder and Sphincters

Study of the physiology of the urinary bladder and sphincters refers to the two phases of micturition: filling of the bladder ensured by continence and evacuation of the urinary reservoir.

Filling of the urinary bladder is done passively by propelling through the ureters of the urine secreted by the kidney. Intraureteral pressure during filling of the bladder being greater than intravesical pressure, the urine enters the urinary reservoir without difficulty.

Adaptation of the bladder to different urine volumes, without any appraisable increase in intravesical pressure, is due to the smooth musculature of the detrusor that maintains the same tension in spite of the constantly increasing volume of the bladder. Apart from the tone of the bladder its filling with variable volumes of fluid also depends upon the elastic tissue of the vesical wall.

## 1. Continence

Maintenance of the urine in the bladder in the interval between micturition is controlled by occlusion of the urethral orifice and the two ureteral orifices. The vesico-urethral orifice is closed by the smooth sphincter which physiologically functions as a smooth sphincter, although it has not the anatomic configuration of such a sphincter. Contractions of the smooth sphincter depends upon the desire to urinate. Until this sensation is perceived, the smooth sphincter maintains continence by its tone, an intrinsic property of the smooth muscular fibers. When feeling of the need to pass urine appears, but must be restrained until environmental conditions permit it, the smooth sphincter contracts reflexly under control of the sympathetic centers located in the cortex, subcortex and spinal cord.

The elastic fibers accumulated in the trigone orifice area also exert a predominant role in continence, as they complete the posterior part of the orifice ring, where the muscular fibers of the internal sphincter do not close the muscular ring completely.

When the desire to micturate is voluntarily restrained, continence may also be maintained by relaxation of the detrusor, inhibited by the parasympathetic spinal reflex center.

Continence, controlled by active contraction of the smooth sphincter after the need to urinate arises demonstrates the role of the sympathetic in the physiology of this phase of micturition denied by Nesbit and Lapides (1958), who asserted at the XI. Congress of the International Society of Urology that: "The sympathetic system has no influence on the initiation, maintenance or inhibition of urination in the human being and should be eliminated for all future discussion of the bladder physiology" (XI. Congress of the International Society of Urology, Tome I, Rapports, 1958, p. 110).

The fact that sectioning of the sympathetic innervation is not followed by incontinence does not plead for negation of the role of the sympathetic but demonstrates that occlusion of the vesico-urethral orifice is controlled under these conditions only by the tone of the smooth sphincter.

Moreover, the bladder remains continent after section of the sympathetic, parasympathetic and somatic innervation (Lapides, Sweet and Lewis, 1955), sectioning of the urethra below the bladder neck (Lapides, 1958), or paralysis of the striate sphincter and striate perineal musculature induced by curare (Fister et al., 1960). Retief (1950) showed that transection of the sympathetic may produce retrograde ejaculation due to the absence of contraction of the smooth sphincter.

The striate sphincter maintains continence either by voluntary contraction of short duration or due to the inhibitory effect exerted by the reflex center of this sphincter upon the spinal reflex center of the detrusor. The excitatory state of the external sphincter reflex center is always balanced by inhibition of the micturition spinal reflex center and conversely.

Apart from the two sphincters, continence of the bladder is also maintained by the participation of other adjuvant factors: vesico-urethral angle; resistance, length and curves of the urethra, folds or rugae of the urethral mucosa, its glands and venous plexus, the presence of the uvula and of the cavernosus bodies in the male. An adjuvant factor in the female is, the epithelium of the bladder neck of similar structure to that of the vaginal epithelium and, hence, undergoing the respective hormonal alterations.

The mechanism closing the uretero-vesical orifices is ensured by the uretero-vesical valves (Bettex, 1967), contraction of the trigone during micturition (Tanagho, Meyers and Smith, 1968), the musculature of the bladder wall at the level of the intramural portion of the ureters and the pressure gradient between the ureters and the bladder.

## 2. Voiding of the Urinary Bladder

The mechanism of evacuation of the urinary bladder still focusses to-day the attention of a number of urologists, physiologists, anatomists and neurologists.

Goetzen and Boeminghaus (1954) stated: „Letzten Endes bleibt der Miktionsvorgang insbesondere Öffnung und Abschluß der Blase in seiner Dynamik und neurologischen Steuerung weiterhin ein noch nicht restlos geklärtes Problem" [Z. Urol. **47**, 132 (1954)].

Emmet, in the same year, shows that "The solution of one great mystery concerning the mechanics of micturition would no doubt classify the subject. This is identification of the unknown factor that causes relaxation of the vesical neck when the detrusor muscle contracts so that the urine can be expelled. Anyone who discovers the explanation for this reciprocal action between the detrusor muscle and vesical neck will pave the way for final explanation of the mechanics of micturition" (Urology, vol. II, p. 1269. Philadelphia and London: W. B. Saunders Company 1954).

LAUX and MARCHAL (1953) state: "Le mécanisme qui règle le jeu si complexe des réservoirs pelviens situés aux frontières de l'inconscient et du conscient, est certainement très complexes lui-même, et ne peut plus être assimilé à un trop schématique antagonisme entre les système ortho- et parasympathiques" [LAUX and MARCHAL, Montpellier méd. **46**, 3—4, 123 (1954)].

TANAGHO and SMITH (1966) studying the architectonics and function of the bladder and sphincters asserted that "The precise mechanism of closure of the bladder neck and the way in which it is opened during voiding is not known; the subject remains quite controversial" [Brit. J. Urol. **38**, 1, 65 (1966)].

In spite of the studies on the architectonics of the detrusor musculature, bladder neck and urethra, including electrical stimulation of the autonomic or somatic nerves of the bladder or sphincters, recording of the action currents from different nervous or muscular vesico-sphincteral components, measuring of urethral resistance, urinary flow and time, static and kinetic radiologic observations and the action of drugs upon vesico-sphincteral dynamics, the mechanism of opening of the bladder neck during micturition has not yet been solved, for the following reasons:

— intricacy at the level of the bladder neck of smooth muscles of different embryonic origin, belonging to the detrusor, trigone and smooth sphincter;

— inexistence of a smooth circular sphincter at the bladder neck although, functionally, the musculo-elastic formations at this level act as a sphincter;

— intricacy of the parasympathetic, sympathetic and somatic innervation, each with its own specific action;

— concomitant contraction of the detrusor and relaxation of the smooth sphincter brought about by the nervous parasympathetic influx;

— irradiation of the electric stimulus in experimental investigations resulting in errors of interpretation in studies of electrophysiology.

The interest to which the difficult problem of the physiology of micturition gave rise is demonstrated by the great number of investigations carried out during the last ten years, using new techniques and a complex electronic equipment for measuring intravesical pressure and the rate of flow of urine during micturition, by means of an urethral catheter (VON GARRELTS, 1956, 1957; ARBUCKLE and PAQUIN, 1963), suprapubic puncture of the bladder (SANDØE et al., 1959), by an entirely intravesical measuring device (HOLM, 1961) or by radiotelemetry (GLEASON et al., 1965). With the same end in view, investigations were carried out on urethral resistance during micturition (PIERCE et al., 1963), exit pressures (GLEASON and LATTIMER, 1962). The velocity and fritional pressure loss of the effective urethral cross-sectional area, according to various laws governing the flow of fluids through tubes (RANKIN, 1967). Continuous recording by air cystometry was also resorted to in order to avoid the artefacts produced by the turbulence effect at points of changing diameter, and the viscosity of the fluid, velocity of flow, length of the fluid path were also measured (BRADLEY et al., 1968).

Opening of the bladder neck during micturition was explained by contraction of the detrusor and relaxation of the bladder neck (DENNY-BROWN and ROBERTSON, 1933), by relaxation of the cervico-trigonal region following abolition of the sympathetic nervous inflow (LEARMONTH, 1931), by traction upon the posterior lip of the neck by the superficial trigone (YOUNG and WESSON, 1921), by contraction of the dilatatory muscles of the neck and relaxation of the constrictor muscles (GIL-VERNET, 1960) or by pressure of the urine which overcomes the resistance of the bladder neck (LAPIDES, 1958; WOODBURNE, 1960).

A first factor that unquestionably interferes with opening of the bladder neck is contraction of the detrusor, which "breaks the base plate" (HUTCH, 1955, 1966). A second important factor in the initiation of micturition is pressure of the urine upon the bladder neck, a point of minima resistance.

The longitudinal distribution of the muscular fibers of the detrusor on the surface, followed by a circular and finally by a longitudinal or plexiform distribution in the depth, produces a sufficient intravesical pressure by contraction to overcome the resistence of the sphincteric system. Contraction of the longitudinal muscular fibers forces the liquid to act upon the internal bladder surface, especially in the vertex-vesical neck direction, tending to push the bladder content towards the internal urethral opening.

Contraction of the circular fibers develops a force in the intravesical fluid that acts centrifugally. Contraction of the longitudinal layer is opposed to this centrifugal force, pressing the urine in the vertex-neck direction. The plexiform fibers enhance the action of the longitudinal and circular fibers.

On the other hand, contraction of the detrusor tends to raise the trigone in a vertical position so that the urine pressure is exercised upon the vesico-urethral orifice.

Opening of the bladder neck or the initiation of micturition therefore takes place on the one hand owing to the anatomy of the bladder and in the other to the pressure of the urine, provided the latter is realized by contraction of the detrusor and not by intra-abdominal pressure.

## D. Electrophysiology of the Urinary Bladder and Sphincters

Electric stimulation is one of the best methods for studying the physiology of micturition; it replaces the nervous inflow from different segments of the central or of the antonomic nervous system, which as a rule ensures continence of the urinary bladder in the interval between micturition and its evacuation when the need to void is felt.

In a correct experiment an essential condition is the use of an electric stimulus of a given intensity, duration and frequency, closely resembling that of the nervous inflow.

Electric stimulation of the various segments of the central or of the autonomic nervous system was applied as far back as 1863 (GIANUZZI, 1863; BUDGE, 1864; ECKHARD, 1863; GRIFFITHS, 1894).

These authors determined the motor or the sensory component of the vesico-sphincteric nerves by electric stimulation.

Following the technical advance made, action currents from the vesico-sphincteric nerves were recorded with the help of a cathodic oscilloscope (ABUREL and CHAUCHARD, 1931; TALAAT, 1937; EVANS, 1941).

Applying electric stimuli to the pelvic nerves or the hypogastric nerve, closely resembling the nervous inflow, HEGRE and INGERSOLL (1949), then INGERSOLL et al. (1954, 1955, 1957) followed up the effect of stimulation upon the detrusor.

The investigations of KABAT, MAGUN and RANSON (1936), KREMER (1947), UVNÄS, B. (1947), HENNENMAN (1948), HESS (1949), GASTAUD (1952), VIGOUROX et al. (1952) dealt with the location of the excitatory or inhibitory centers of micturition within the nervous system.

During the work of these investigators, the cortical and subcortical areas controlling micturition were established.

The investigations of BURGHELE, ICHIM and DEMETRESCU (1958, 1962), carried out in view of obtaining evacuation of the urinary bladder by electric stimulation, i.e. experimental micturition, opened new prospects in the electrophysiology of the urinary bladder.

Since no data exist concerning the parameters of the electric stimulus which would produce powerful and prolonged contraction of the bladder without injury to the pelvic nerves, a series of experimental investigations were carried out by these authors to determine the optimal parameters of electric stimuli.

It is known that the electric properties of the autonomic nerves essentially differ from those of the somatic nerves. Their excitability is in general lower and repetition of the electric stimulus is necessary.

The conduction speed in these nerves is of 1 to 30 meters per second faster in the parasympathetic than the sympathetic system. Their chronaxie differs from that of the effector organ, and the ratio of the nerve chronaxie to that of the organ may attain 1/500. This likewise demonstrates the necessity of iterative electric stimulation.

Electric stimulation of the parasympathetic exercises its effect upon the organ stimulated by this nerve within a few hundreds or thousands of a second. The response of the effector organ to stimulation of the sympathetic is delayed a few second up to one minute and disappears more slowly than that obtained by stimulation of the parasympathetic, when the return to normal is almost immediate.

Finally, a net difference exists between the exitability and conductivity of the pre- and post-ganglionic fibers of the vegetative neurons.

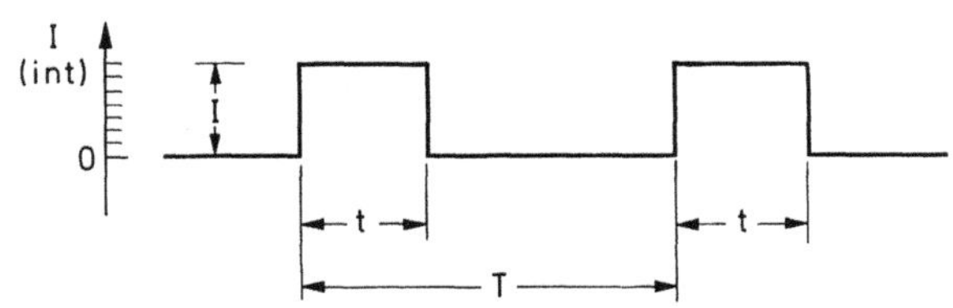


Fig. 6. Graphical representation of square wave electrical stimulus: $I$ intensity; $t$ duration; $T$ repetition rate of the electrical stimulus

In their experimental studies, BURGHELE, ICHIM and DEMETRESCU used square wave pulses with the following parameters: $t$ = duration of the stimulus; $I$ = intensity of the stimulus; $T$ = repetion rate of the electric stimulus, i.e. period of stimulation and interval up to the next stimulation. The frequency of stimulation is $f = 1/T$ (Fig. 6).

For determination of the optimal parameters of the electric stimulus, two of the parameters of the signal, which, applied to the vesical motor nerves must produce strong contractions lasting throughout the stimulation period, are assumed to be conventionally constant, and the third variable.

The effect of stimulation is appraised by the pressure obtained in the bladder, $\Delta$P.

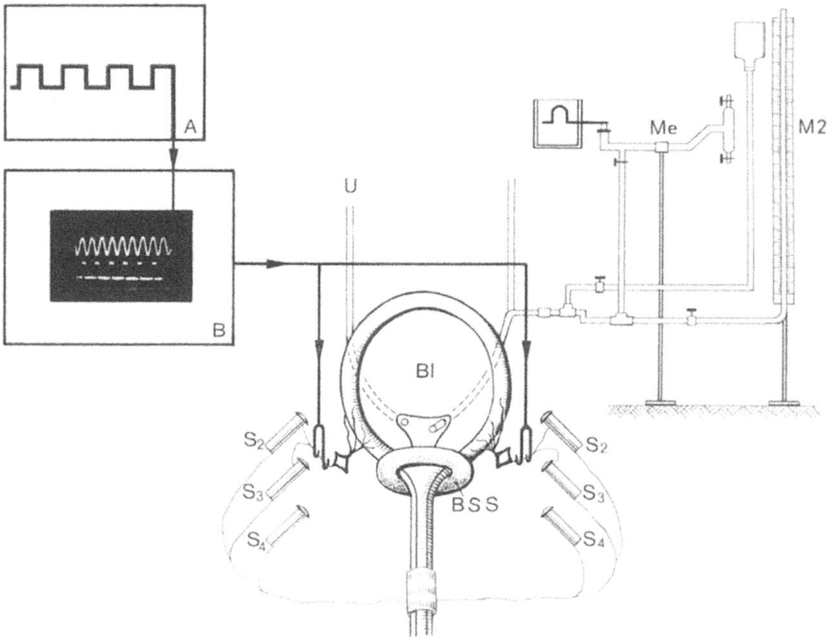


Fig. 7. Apparatus used for studying intravesical pressure during stimulation of the pelvic nerves. *A* Electrical stimuli generator; *B* oscilloscope; *Bl* bladder; *U* ureter; *BSS* smooth sphincter; *S2*, *S3*, *S4* sacral nerves; *Me* membrane manometer; *M2* water manometer

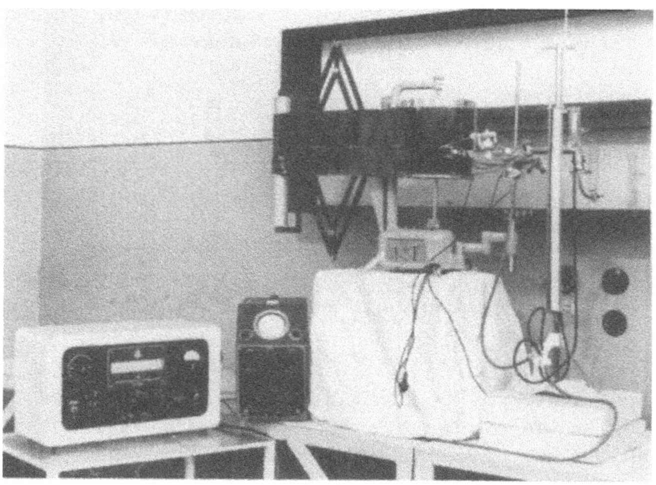

Fig. 8. Ensemble of the apparatus for experimental study of the electrophysiology of the bladder

Fig. 7 is the schematical representation of the stimulator and the apparatus for recording intravesical pressure in the experiments carried out for determining the electric parameters.

Fig. 8 shows the whole range of apparatus used in the experiments.

The electric stimulus is delivered by a neurostimulator (A). The quality and characteristics of this stimulus are monitored by a cathodic oscilloscope. The electrodes are applied uni- or bilaterally on the pelvic nerves. Intravesical pressure is recorded by means of a catheter introduced through one of the ureters, thus avoiding any foreign body in the urethra.

Endovesical pressure was recorded by a membrane manometer calibrated by a parallel connected water manometer, with direct reading. The time basis was marked by two second signs.

The horizontal lines on the diagram represent pressure values in 10 cm of water. The spaces are unequal due to the unequal displacement of the recording manometer membrane, which moves less and less with increase in the pressure of the fluid. Zero pressure corresponds to the level of the fluid in the direct-reading manometer, corresponding to the horizontal line that passes through the pubic symphysis of the experimental animal.

# I. Electric Stimulation of the Pelvic Nerve

## 1. Determination of the Parameters of the Electric Stimulus

### a) Determination of the Optimal Duration of the Electric Stimulus

Fig. 9 represents the intravesical pressure obtained by monolateral electric stimulation of the pelvic nerves with an electric signal of variable duration

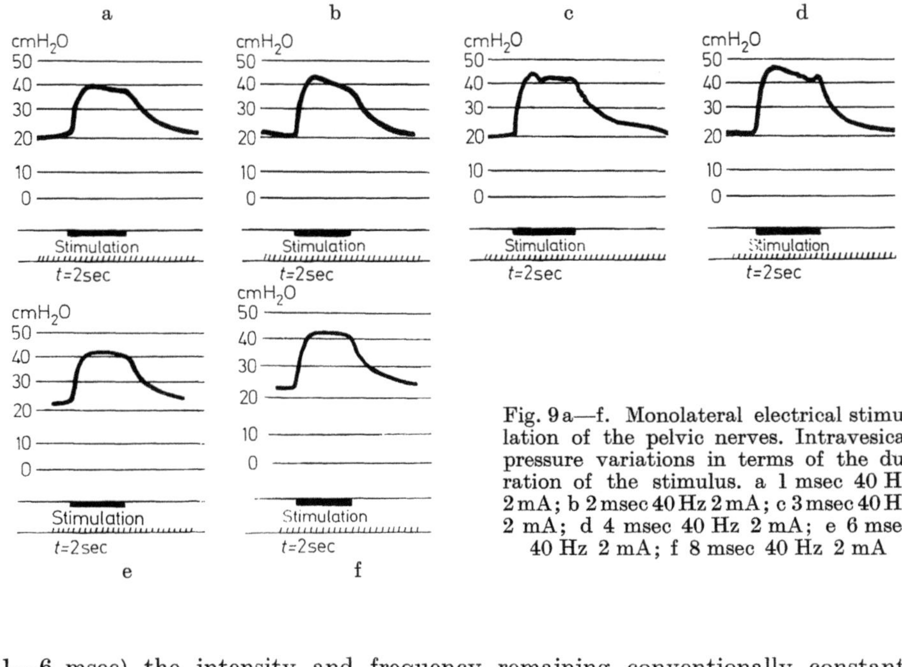


Fig. 9a—f. Monolateral electrical stimulation of the pelvic nerves. Intravesical pressure variations in terms of the duration of the stimulus. a 1 msec 40 Hz 2 mA; b 2 msec 40 Hz 2 mA; c 3 msec 40 Hz 2 mA; d 4 msec 40 Hz 2 mA; e 6 msec 40 Hz 2 mA; f 8 msec 40 Hz 2 mA

(1—6. msec) the intensity and frequency remaining conventionally constant, respectively 2 mA and 40 Hz.

The highest endovesical pressure corresponds to an electric signal of 4 msec (curve d). At a duration of 1 msec (curve a), 2 msec (curve b), 3 msec (curve c),

6 msec (curve e) or 8 msec (curve f), endovesical pressures are lower, however attaining or exceeding 20 cm of water.

This demonstrates that the optimal duration of the electric signal for monolateral stimulation of the pelvic nerve is of about 4 msec.

### b) Determination of the Optimal Frequency of the Electric Stimulus

Monolateral electric stimulation of the pelvic nerves with an electric signal having a constant duration of 1 msec and intensity of 2 mA, but a variable frequency of 10 to 40 cps (Hz) produces vesical contractions of different pressures, as may be seen from Fig. 10.

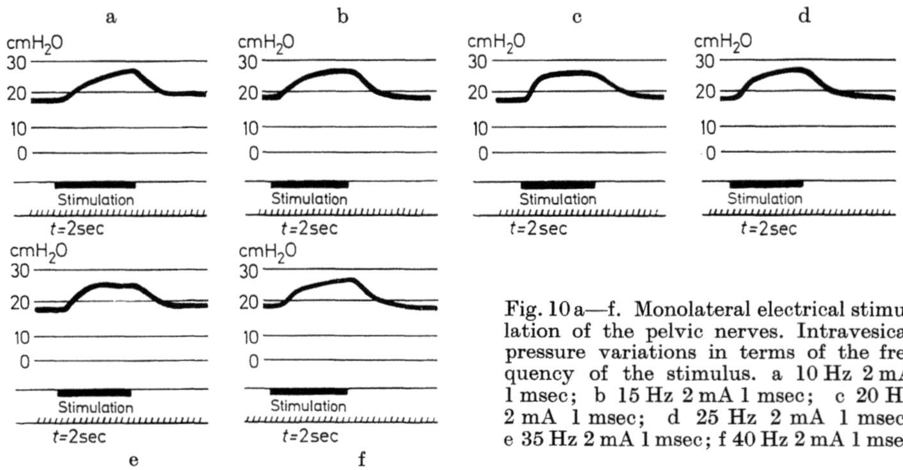


Fig. 10a—f. Monolateral electrical stimulation of the pelvic nerves. Intravesical pressure variations in terms of the frequency of the stimulus. a 10 Hz 2 mA 1 msec; b 15 Hz 2 mA 1 msec; c 20 Hz 2 mA 1 msec; d 25 Hz 2 mA 1 msec; e 35 Hz 2 mA 1 msec; f 40 Hz 2 mA 1 msec

The optimal frequency of the electric stimulus is situated approximately throughout the whole range of frequencies between 10 and 40 Hz.

Endovesical pressure remains constant throughout the duration of stimulation and returns to normal as soon as stimulation ceases.

### c) Determination of the Optimal Intensity of the Electric Stimulus

The influence of the intensity of the electric stimulus is very evident, intravesical pressures obtained with various stimulus intensities having higher values (Fig. 11).

Following stimulation of a pelvic nerve with a signal of 2 to 16 mA (pressure curves a—f) (Fig. 11) but with a conventionally constant frequency (40 Hz) and duration (2 msec), the contraction of the detrusor is minimal at 2 mA, realizing a pressure of a few cm. At intensities of 4, 6 and 8 mA, endovesical pressure gradually increases, the best response of the detrusor being obtained at 12 mA.

As may be seen from the f pressure curves, at an intensity of 12 and 16 mA, endovesical pressure exceeds 20 cm of water. It must be borne in mind that a high intensity of the stimulus, as a rule exceeding 10 mA, may damage the nerves, producing burns.

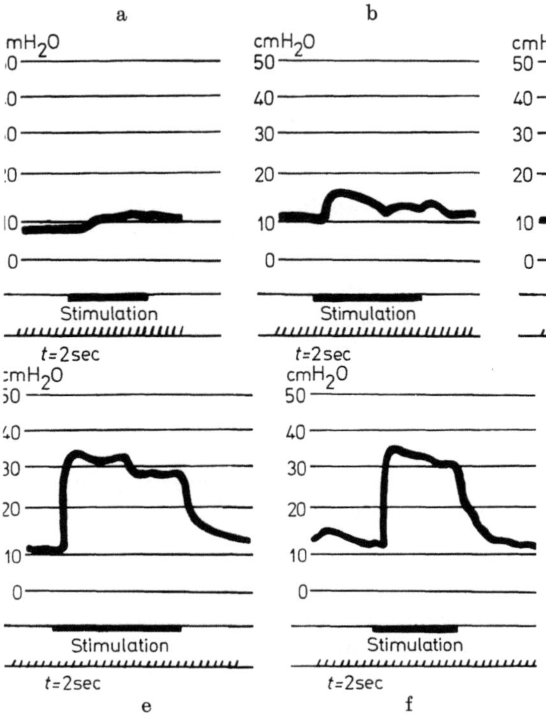


Fig. 11 a—f. Monolateral electrical stimulation of the pelvic nerves. Intravesical pressure variations in terms of the intensity of the stimulus. a 2 mA 40 Hz 2 msec; b 4 mA 40 Hz 2 msec; c 6 mA 40 Hz 2 msec; d 8 mA 40 Hz 2 msec; e 12 mA 40 Hz 2 msec; f 16 mA 40 Hz 2 msec

## d) Monolateral Electric Stimulation of Long Duration

Fig. 12 with a signal of 5 mA, 40 Hz and 2 msec, demonstrates that intravesical pressure obtained by this stimulation remains constant throughout the duration of stimulation.

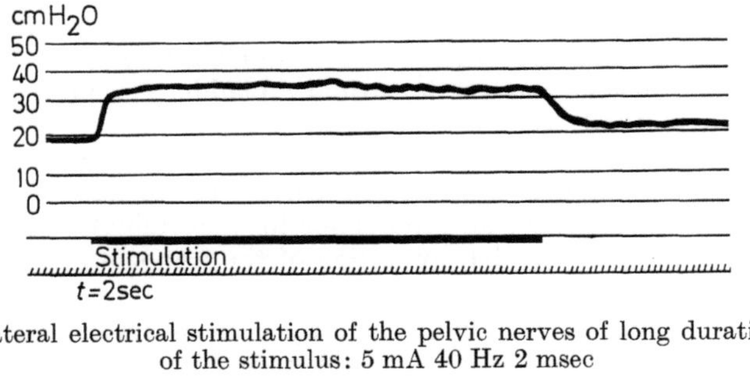


Fig. 12. Monolateral electrical stimulation of the pelvic nerves of long duration. Parameters of the stimulus: 5 mA 40 Hz 2 msec

Monolateral stimulation produces contraction of the bladder only on the stimulated side; on the opposite side the bladder wall bulges, giving the impression of relaxation.

Ingersoll, Jones and Hegre (1957) observed that stimulation of a pelvic nerve also produced weak contractions on the opposite side, after a period of relaxation. Stimulation of the peripheral end of the pelvic nerve on one side (the opposite pelvic nerve being sectioned) produces contraction of the whole bladder, the contralateral side contracting even more powerfully than when the opposite pelvic nerve remains intact.

MUELLNER (1951) and VAN DUZEN and DUNCAN (1953) explain this phenomenon by propagation of the contraction wave of the detrusor on the stimulated to the non-stimulated part. In contrast, MACDONALD and MACCREA (1930), and STEWART (1942) consider that the electric stimulus applied to the pelvic nerve on one side is transmitted retrogradely to the micturition reflex center, which induces contraction of the detrusor on the opposite side. Lending support to this assumption are the observations of INGERSOLL et al. (1957) who noted contraction of the whole bladder on stimulation of the central end of the pelvic nerve. When the pelvic nerve on the opposite side is sectioned, the phenomenon no longer occurs.

Another explanation of the contraction of the detrusor on the non-stimulated side might be the distribution of the pelvic nerve throughout the bladder and not only on one side.

Relaxation on the side opposite to stimulation is due, in the opinion of GRIFFITHS (1894) and LANGWORTHY et al. (1940), to the effect produced by the bladder fluid under pressure.

Actually, as noted by BURGHELE, ICHIM and DEMETRESCU (1958) the side opposite to stimulation becomes convex under pressure of the endovesical fluid.

However, if account is kept of the architectonics of the bladder musculature, weak contractions should also develop on the side opposite to stimulation, since the muscular fibers continue from the surface downwards and cross from one side to the other. The deep internal circular and longitudinal layers are more poorly represented than the external longitudinal layer, so that endovesical pressure readily overcomes the low resistance of these layers.

## II. Bilateral Electric Stimulation of the Pelvic Nerves

### 1. Determination of the Optimal Parameters of the Electric Stimulus

By bilateral electric stimulation of the pelvic nerves with an electric stimulus having optimal parameters BURGHELE, ICHIM and DEMETRESCU (1958) proposed to obtain artificial evacuation of the urinary bladder, in view of the clinical application of the method.

As with monolateral stimulation, the optimal value of the parameters are determined by maintaining two of these parameters constant and varying the third: for instance the intensity and frequency for determination of the duration; the intensity and duration for determination of the frequency; the duration and frequency for determination of the intensity.

As an electric stimulation of about 1 minute is necessary for evacuation of the whole content of the bladder, BURGHELE, ICHIM and DEMETRESCU (1958) studied the optimal parameters of the electric stimulus for sustained, bilateral stimulation of the pelvic nerves. Concomitant investigations were carried out in order to determine whether stimulation injures the nerve-muscle complex or whether the fatigue phenomenon develops. On testing the fatigue of the nerve-muscle complex, the intensity should not exceed the values established at mono- or bilateral stimulation. In these tests the duration and frequency were variable and the intensity constant.

## a) Determination of the Optimal Duration of the Electric Stimulus in Bilateral Stimulation of the Pelvic Nerves

In order to establish the optimal duration of the electric stimulus, the pelvic nerves were stimulated bilaterally with stimulus of constant intensity (4 mA) and frequency (40 Hz), whose duration varied from 0.5 and 16 msec.

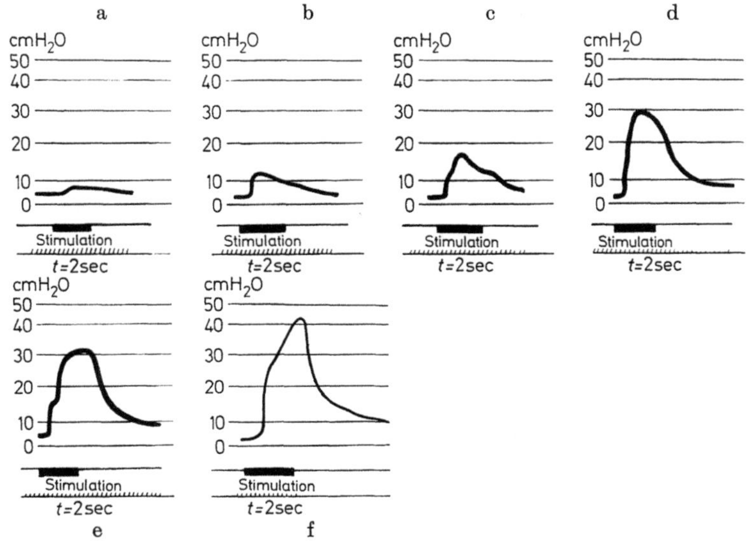


Fig. 13 a—f. Bilateral electrical stimulation of the pelvic nerves. Intravesical pressure variations in terms of the duration of the stimulus. a 0.5 msec 40 Hz 4 mA; b 1 msec 40 Hz 4 mA; c 2 msec 40 Hz 4 mA; d 4 msec 40 Hz 4 mA; e 8 msec 40 Hz 4 mA; f 16 msec 40 Hz 4 mA

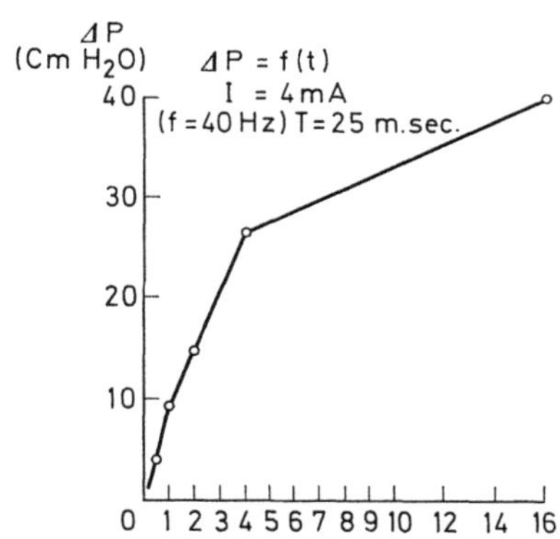


Abb. 14. Graphical representation of intravesical pressure in terms of the duration of the stimulus

There is no threshold for the duration of the electric stimulus within the range used. Contraction of the detrusor and the consequent increase in intravesical pressure begins from a duration of 0.5 msec, as in curve a, Fig. 13. At 1 msec, intravesical pressure is of 12 cm of water. It gradually increases with increase in the duration of the electric stimulus and at 4 msec it attains 30 cm of water, at 16 msec it exceeds 40 cm of water (Fig. 13).

The correlation between intravesical pressure and the duration of the stimulus is represented graphically in Fig. 14. The ordinate gives the duration of the electric stimulus and the abscissa intravesical pressures in terms of the duration of the stimuli. The inflection point of the curve appears around 4 msec; the curve then shows a tendency to run level (Fig. 14).

Hence, the best value of the duration of the electric stimulus for bilateral stimulation of the pelvic nerves is situated on the portion of the curve beyond the inflexion point (between 4—7 msec), zone in which small variations of the duration of the electric stimulus do not produce marked changes in intravesical pressure.

## b) Determination of the Optimal Frequency of the Electric Stimulus in Bilateral Stimulation of the Pelvic Nerves

Intravesical pressure was determined in terms of frequency variations of the electric stimulus maintaining the intensity and duration of the stimulus at constant values (4 mA and respectively 4 msec) (Fig. 15).

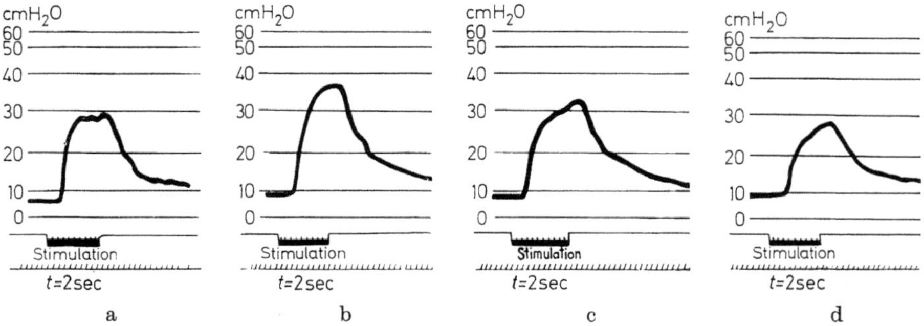


Fig. 15a—d. Bilateral electrical stimulation of the pelvic nerves. Intravesical pressure variations in terms of the frequency of the stimulus. a 15 Hz 4 mA 4 msec; b 30 Hz 4 mA 4 msec; c 40 Hz 4 mA 4 msec; d 50 Hz 4 mA 4 msec

At a frequency of less than 10 Hz, intravesical pressure increases very rapidly and is directly dependant upon the increase in frequency. For this reason, frequencies of 15—60 Hz were experimented. At the optimal frequency, strong contractions of the detrusor appear and, consequently high intravesical pressures.

The intravesical pressure curves (curve a at 15 Hz and curve b at 30 Hz) showed pressures of over 30 cm of water. When the frequency of the stimuli exceeded 30 Hz (curves c and d) the contraction of the detrusor was weaker. This is due to fatigue of the pelvic nerves, since repetition of the electric impulses at increasingly shorter intervals produces more rapid summation of the stimulus, exceeding the receptivity possibilities of the nerves.

Fig. 16 represents the ratio of the frequency to intravesical pressure. The ordinate marks the frequency of the stimulations (from 0 to 50 pulses per second). $T$ being repeated on the abscissa for each frequency $f$, i.e. duration of the stimulus + interval up to a new stimulus-repetition rate. Thus, at 15 pulses per second, $T$ is repeated 66 times, at 20 Hz 40 times, at 50 Hz 20 times, as results from $T = \frac{t}{f}$.

Intravesical pressure, represented by the above curve, indicates its gradual increase in terms of the increase in frequency, them a progressive decrease with increase in the frequency of the stimulus.

The optimal frequency of the electric stimulus that induces high intravesical pressures, of longer duration, following bilateral stimulation of the pelvic nerves, is 15 Hz.

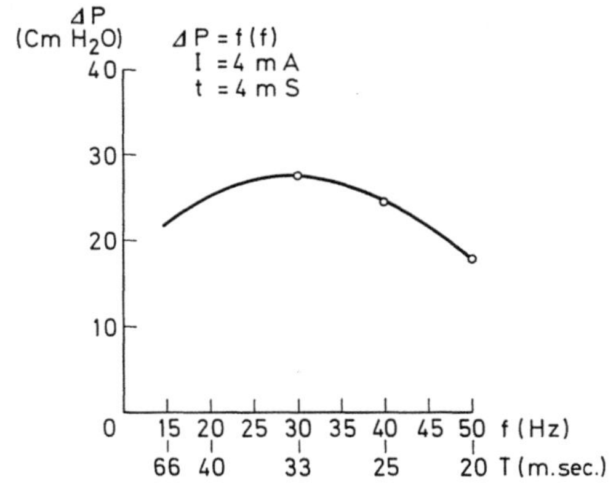


Fig. 16. Graphical representation of intravesical pressure in terms of the frequency of the stimulus

### c) Determination of the Optimal Intensity of the Electric Stimulus in Bilateral Stimulation of the Pelvic Nerves

The curves in Fig. 17 indicate intravesical pressure variations to bilateral electric stimulation of the pelvic nerves with electric stimuli of an intensity ranging between 3—10 mA. Intensities higher than 10 mA were not used in order to avoid damage to the nerves or favour irradiation of the electric stimuli to other nervous formations of the bladder or sphincters.

The curve in Fig. 17, in which the intensity of the stimulus was of 3 mA, duration 2 msec and frequency 40 Hz, shows that at this intensity, intravesical pressure is not modified and, consequently, the detrusor does not contract.

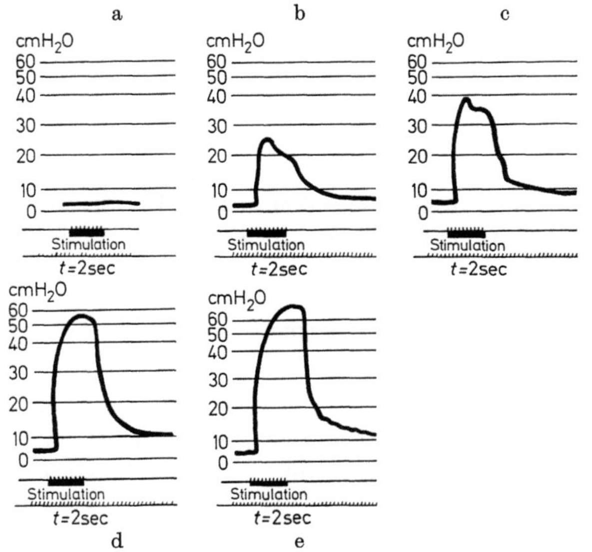


Fig. 17a—e. Bilateral electrical stimulation of the pelvic nerves. Intravesical pressure variations in terms of the intensity of the stimulus. a 3 mA 40 Hz 2 msec; b 4 mA 40 Hz 2 msec; c 5 mA 40 Hz 2 msec; d 7 mA 40 Hz 2 msec; e 10 mA 40 Hz 2 msec

With increase in the intensity of the electric stimulus to 4, 5, 7 and 10 mA (curves b, c, d and e), the contractions of the detrusor become increasingly stronger, intravesical pressure exceeding 60 cm of water at 10 mA.

Fig. 18 shows that intravesical pressure progressively increases with increase in the intensity of the stimulus up to 10 mA. The curve then tends to become stable, in plateau.

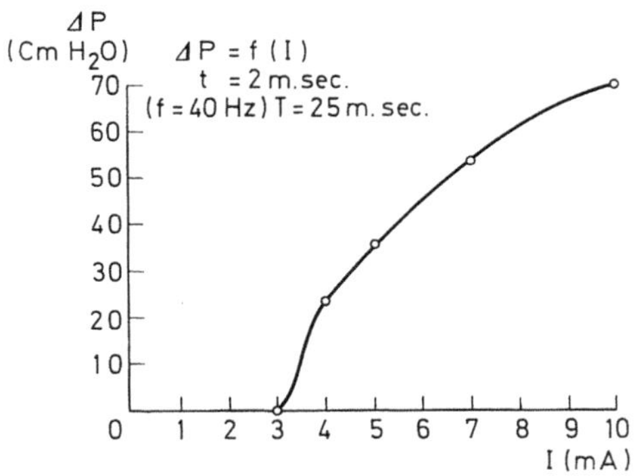


Fig. 18. Graphical representation of intravesical pressure in terms of the intensity of the stimulus

The optimal intensity of the electric stimulus for bilateral stimulation of the pelvic nerves is of 4 to 8 mA. At these intensities, the nerve is not damaged and neither does irradiation of the stimulus to the neighbouring formations occur or to the formations that interfere with the stimulated nerves.

## III. Fatigue Test of the Pelvic Nerves-Detrusor on Bilateral Electric Stimulation of the Pelvic Nerves

In order to obtain artificial micturition by stimulation of the pelvic nerves, intravesical pressures must be sifficiently high and of a long enough duration to overcome the resistance of the sphincteral system. Electric stimuli of variable frequency and duration were used (BURGHELE, ICHIM and DEMETRESCU, 1958) to assess the fatigue of the neuromuscular complex, following prolonged electric stimulation of the pelvic nerves.

### 1. Fatigue Test on Prolonged Bilateral Electric Stimulation of the Pelvic Nerves with a Stimulus of Variable Frequency

Fig. 19 gives the intravesical pressure curves at frequencies of 50, 30, 15 and 10 Hz (curves a, b, c, d), the intensity being of 5 mA and the duration of 4 msec.

The strongest and most constant contraction of the detrusor was produced at a stimulus frequency of 15 Hz.

At frequency of 10 Hz intravesical pressure remains constant throughout the duration of stimulation, but is of a relatively low value — 20 cm of water. At frequencies of 30—50 Hz, fatigue of the neuro-muscular complex takes place comparatively rapidly, whereas at less than 30 Hz this fatigue appears much more slowly. The optimal frequency of the electric stimulus for stimulation of the pelvic nerves of long duration, is of 15 Hz.

Above these frequencies fatigue of the neuromuscular complex develops; below these frequencies, fatigue appears later, but contraction, following the poorer summation, takes place more difficultly.

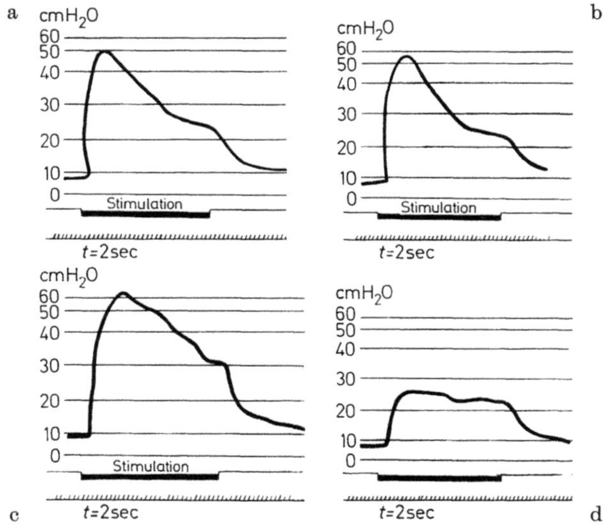


Fig. 19a—d. Fatigue test of the neuromuscular complex following longterm electrical stimulation of the pelvic nerves. Intravesical pressure variations in terms of the frequency of the stimulus: a 50 Hz; b 30 Hz; c 15 Hz; d 10 Hz. Constant intensity and duration: 5 mA, 4 msec

## 2. Fatigue Test on Prolonged Bilateral Electric Stimulation of the Pelvic Nerves with a Stimulus of Variable Duration

The optimal duration of the electric stimulus in prolonged stimulation of the pelvic nerves was determined by using a stimulus of optimal intensity (5 mA) and frequency (15 Hz), the duration varying from 2 to 16 msec (Fig. 20).

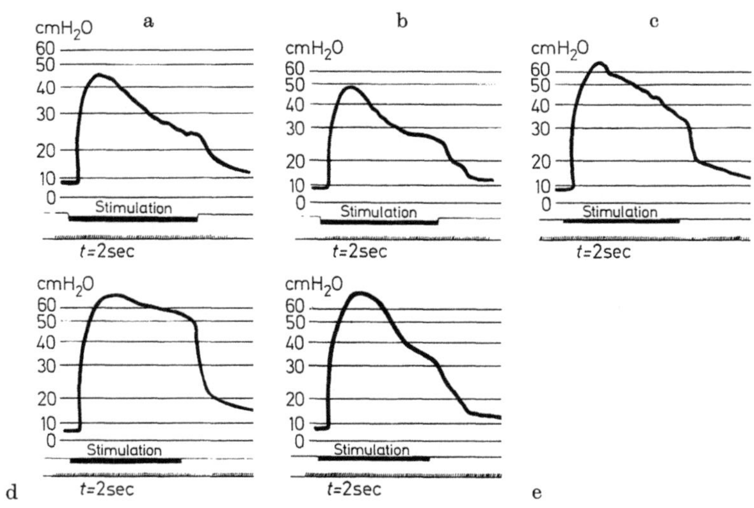


Fig. 20a—e. Fatigue test of the neuromuscular complex following longterm electrical stimulation of the pelvic nerves. Intravesical pressure variations in terms of the duration of the stimulus. a 2 msec 15 Hz 5 mA; b 4 msec 15 Hz 5 mA; c 7 msec 15 Hz 5 mA; d 10 msec 15 Hz 5 mA; e 16 msec 15 Hz 5 mA

The highest intravesical pressure that stays level throughout the duration of stimulation is obtained by a stimulus duration of 7 to 10 msec (curves c and d, Fig. 20).

Although at a duration of 2 and 4 msec (curves a and b, Fig. 20) and of 16 msec (curve e, Fig. 20) fairly high intravesical pressures are obtained, they fall rapidly.

Hence, the best duration of the electric signal for stimulation of the pelvic nerves is of 7 to 10 msec.

In conclusion, to obtain powerful, lasting contraction of the bladder with intravesical pressures of 70—80 cm of water, maintained throughout the duration of stimulation of the pelvic nerves, the electric signal must have a frequency of 15 Hz, duration of 7 to 10 msec and intensity of 5—10 mA. Below or above these values, contraction of the detrusor does not produce intravesical pressures sufficiently powerful and sustained to empty the urinary reservoir completely.

## IV. Irradiation of the Electrical Stimulus

Bilateral electrical stimulation of the pelvic nerves with a stimulus of 5—10 mA, 4—7 msec and 15 Hz produces strong contractions of the detrusor with intravesical pressures that attain up to 80 cm of water. These pressures are sufficient to overcome the resistance of the sphincteral system and to obtain artificial micturition.

Fig. 21 represents intravesical pressures obtained with a stimulus having the above parameters and recorded by an ureteral catheter; evacuation of the urine

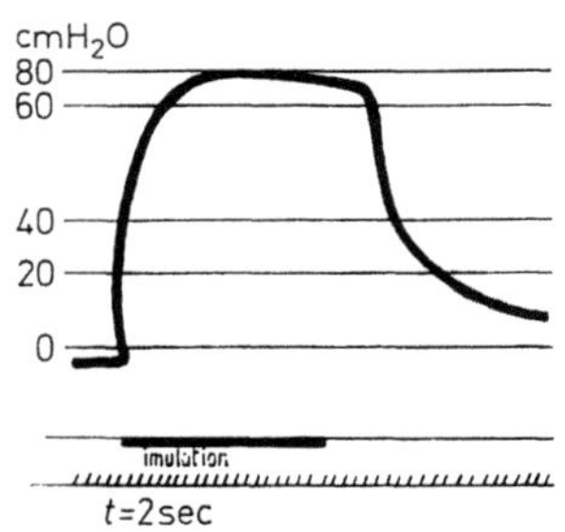


Fig. 21

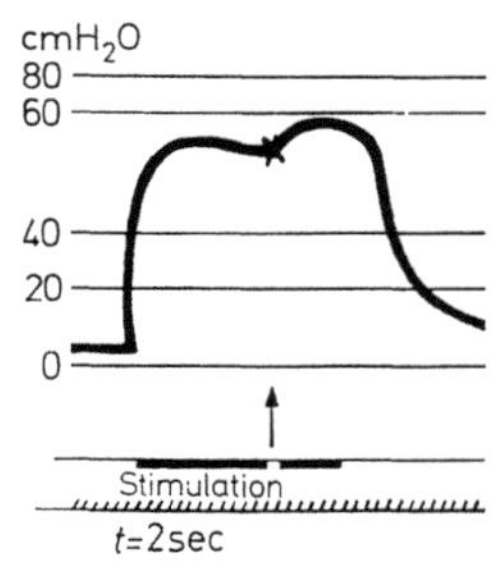


Fig. 22

Fig. 21. Intravesical pressure during bilateral electrical stimulation of the pelvic nerves with compression of the urethra. Electrical stimulus: 4,5 mA 7 msec 15 Hz; pressures recorded by intravesical catheter

Fig. 22. Intravesical pressure, with free urethra. Arrow indicates stop of micturition and concomitant increase of intravesical pressure. The same stimulus as in Fig. 21

is prevented by compression of the urethra. As soon as stimulation ceases intravesical pressure begins to fall.

Electrical stimulation of the pelvic nerves with a free urethra and the possible evacuation of the bladder content produces a lower intravesical pressure due to the variable content of the bladder. Fig. 22 gives intravesical pressures during voiding of the bladder. The pressure curve shows a sharp peak when the fluid stops flowing through the urethra.

When the bladder content exceeds its physiologic capacity a certain amount of fluid remains in the bladder. Under these conditions evacuation of the whole content is done in two or three stages with a break between, as may be seen in Fig. 23.

During bilateral electrical stimulation of the pelvic nerves the jet can be interrupted by contraction of the smooth sphincter, the striate sphincter or of both.

In order to determine the behaviour of the two sphincters, BURGHELE et al. (1958) sectioned the urethra in an acute experiment, below, at the level of and above the striate sphincter, provoking each time evacuation of the bladder by bilateral electrical stimulation of the pelvic nerves.

Interruption of the urinary jet was constantly repeated under all these conditions which demonstrates that the obstacle first occurs at the level of the vesico-urethral junction.

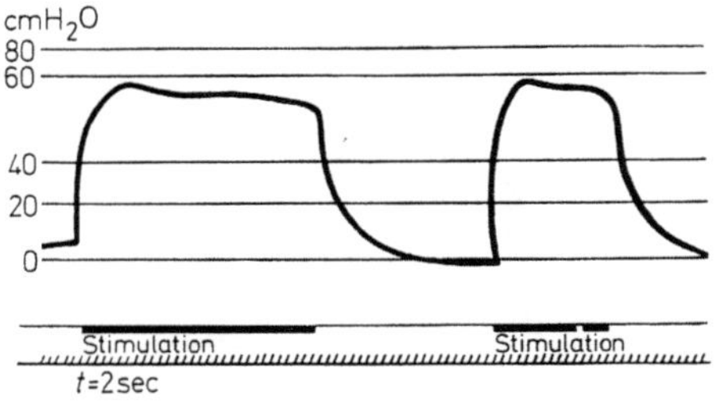


Fig. 23. Intravesical pressure during evacuation following successive, intermittent electrical stimulation

On direct observation of the urethral orifice, following section of the urethra 0.5 cm distal to the vesico-urethral junction, it was found that evacuation of the vesical fluid lasts approximately 10—15 sec, after which the orifice gradually closes. Complete closure corresponds to an increase in intravesical pressure as may be seen in Fig. 22 and is produced by contraction of the smooth sphincter.

For elucidation of the mechanism of contraction of this sphincter during stimulation of the pelvic nerves, BURGHELE, ICHIM and DEMETRESCU (1958) started from the hypothesis of an eventual irradiation of the electrical stimulus from the pelvic nerves that control the motricity of the detrusor, to the hypogastric nerves that control the contraction of the smooth sphincter, trigone and ureteral orifices. They produced concomitantly after a given interval contraction of the smooth sphincter by electrical stimulation of the hypogastric nerve, or abolished the function of the sympathetic innervation by transection, the administration of sympathocolytics or denervation of the bladder neck.

Concomitant stimulation of the hypogastric and pelvic nerves, as against stimulation of the pelvic nerves alone, produces a more rapid increase of intravesical pressure, above the evacuation level, as may be seen from the pressure curves given in Fig. 24.

The moment of concomitant application of the stimulus to the hypogastric and pelvic nerves, is indicated by (1) on the curve, (2) pointing to interruption of the urine flow and (3) the moment when both stimulations cease. The fact that a certain amount of fluid is avoided in spite of concomitant stimulation of the pelvic and hypogastric nerves is explicable by the different latency of the two autonomic nervous fibers, the sympathetic fibers having a longer latency period.

When the stimulus is applied to the hypogastric nerve 10 sec after stimulation of the pelvic nerves, the increase in intravesical pressure produced by contraction of the smooth sphincter appears later than after concomitant stimulation (Fig. 25).

In stimulation of the hypogastric nerve 10 sec after stimulation of the pelvic nerves, (1) on the intravesical pressure curve, indicates the beginning of stimulation, (2) the moment at which evacuation of the bladder starts, (3) stimulation of the hypogastric nerve, (4) contraction of the vesico-sphincteral orifice with arrested jet and concomitant increase of intravesical pressure; the pressure falls, however, as soon as both stimulations cease (5).

This demonstrates the existence of the smooth vesical sphincter and the possibility of its contraction during stimulation of the pelvic nerves by irradiation of the electrical current, at the level of the pelvic plexus, from the pelvic nerves to the hypogastric nerve.

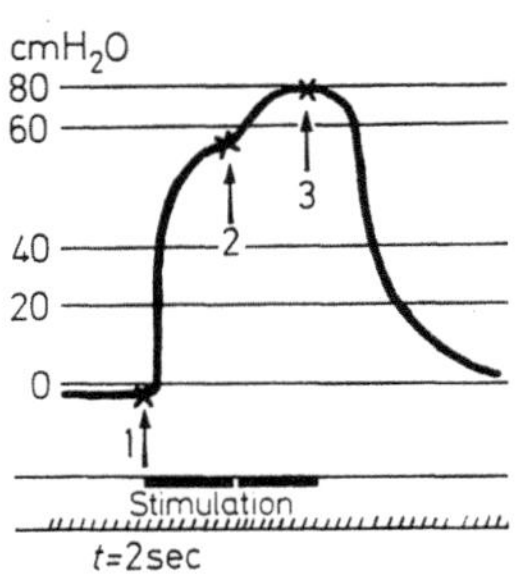


Fig. 24

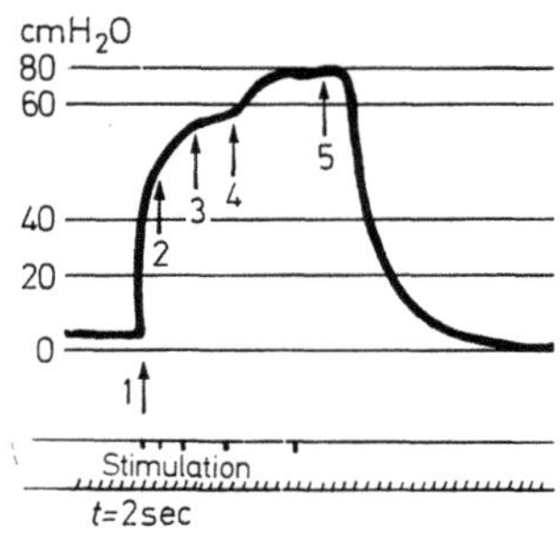


Fig. 25

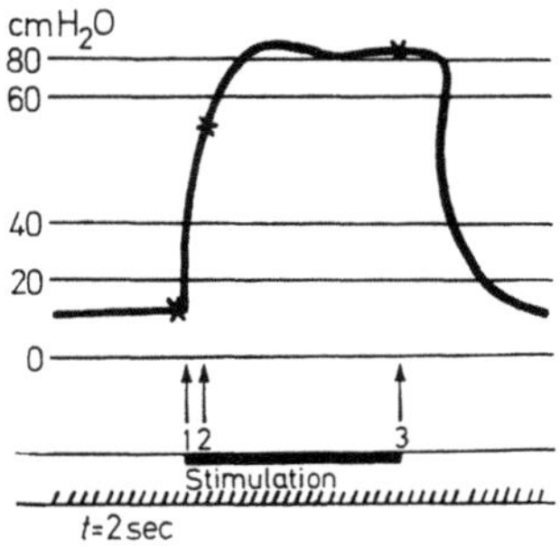


Fig. 26

Fig. 24. Intravesical pressure during concomitant stimulation of the pelvic nerves and hypogastric nerve. *1* Onset of stimulations; *2* cessation of micturition; *3* cessation of stimulation

Fig. 25. Intravesical pressure during electrical stimulation of the pelvic nerves followed by that of the hypogastric nerve at 10 second intervals. *1* stimulation of pelvic nerves; *2* start of micturition; *3* stimulation of hypogastric nerve; *4* cessation of micturition; *5* cessation of stimulations

Fig. 26. Intravesical pressure during electrical stimulation of the pelvic nerves after the administration of sympatholytics. *1* onset of stimulation; *2* onset of micturition; *3* cessation of micturition

Another proof of contraction of the smooth sphincter by irradiation of the electrical stimulus is supplied by abolition of the function of this sphincter following transection of the hypogastric nerves, the administration of sympatholytics, or denervation of the bladder neck. Section of the hypogastric does not prevent functioning of the smooth sphincter in the acute experiment, because irradiation of the electrical stimulus still remains possible, the two innervations crossing one another below the section.

On the other hand, denervation of the bladder neck annuls irradiation of the electrical stimulus during stimulation of the pelvic nerve, under these conditions, the sympathetic nervous fibers are sectioned below the pelvic plexus, and the smooth sphincter no longer contracts.

Intravenous administration of sympatholytics prevents contraction of the smooth sphincter. Intravesical pressure runs level, in a plateau (Fig. 26) and evacuation of the bladder is continuous, although taking place at much higher pressures. This implies the existence of a more distant obstacle, produced by contraction of the striate sphincter and perineal musculature, apart from the obstacle raised by contraction of the smooth sphincter. Therefore, the electrical stimulus may radiate from the pelvic nerves to the pudendal nerves, as demonstrated by

Graber and Rutishauser (1965) and Graber, Rutishauser and Wolf (1966), who showed that electrical stimulation of the pelvic nerves or the detrusor with a higher voltage is accompanied by simultaneous contraction of the striate musculature of the perineum and external sphincter. Section of the pudendal nerves improves artificial evacuation of the bladder by abolishing the function of the striate musculature.

Concomitant stimulation of the pelvic and hypogastric nerves after the administration of sympatholytics lowers the effect of stimulation of the hypogastric nerves and the bladder is better voided than when no sympatholytics are administered.

In conclusion, the experimental studies carried out have confirmed the functional existence of a smooth vesical sphincter. Contraction of this sphincter during stimulation of the pelvic nerves is brought about by irradiation of the electric stimulus at the level of the pelvic plexus.

### Behaviour of the Urinary Bladder during Bilateral Electrical Stimulation of the Pelvic Nerves

Bilateral electrical stimulation of the pelvic nerves produces contraction of the detrusor after 5—7 sec latency; this contraction includes the whole bladder, but is more evident along the dome-neck axis, increasing the angle between the anterior bladder wall and urethra.

After increase of intravesical pressure, the base of the bladder, at the insertion of the detrusor musculature, is pushed downwards be the pressure of the vesical fluid in this area.

The vesico-urethral orifice opens under the influence of this pressure which overcomes the resistance of both the smooth and striate sphincters.

## E. Electrical Stimulation of the Neurogenic Urinary Bladder

Electrical stimulation of the urinary bladder in cases of spinal cord injury has aroused great interest during the last ten years, as a method able to replace catheterism of the bladder which generally results in infection of the urinary tract.

In 1958, Burghele, Ichim and Demetrescu published the first experimental investigations in dogs regarding voiding of the bladder, in normal animals and in animals with sectioned spinal cord, induced by electrical stimulation. Starting from the notion that the nervous inflow can be replaced by electrical stimulation, they stimulated the pelvic nerves by bipolar platinum electrodes, fixed on the pelvic nerves.

In 1878, in Klinik-Chirurgie, Saxtorph reported on direct stimulation of the urinary bladder with an intravesical and a suprapubic electrode for the treatment of urine retention.

Katona (1958) introduced endovesical electrical stimulation in clinical therapy. One electrode was placed within the bladder by means of a catheter and another on the lower abdomen.

Ascoli and Federici (1964) likewise applied endovesical electrical stimulation with two electrodes: one was the cystoscope, the second was an electrocoagulation probe placed upon the internal aspect of the bladder. The electrical stimulus had a duration of 5 msec, a frequency of 20—50 Hz and an intensity of 20—30 mA.

Endovesical electric stimulation has certain drawbacks and the hazards of infection of the urinary tract due to intermittent catheterism are high.

BRADLEY, WITTMERS, CHOU and FRENCH (1962—1963) and SCHOENBERG, YOUNG and MURPHY (1962) report on their experimental results obtained by direct stimulation of the detrusor with electrodes applied on the bladder wall. SCHAMAUN and KANTROWITZ (1963) and BOYCE, LATHEM and HUND (1964) stimulated the detrusor with stainless steel wire electrodes, introduced within the thickness of the bladder muscle. HABIB (1963) resorted to stimulation of the second, third and fourth anterior sacral roots and obtained efficient contractions of the bladder on stimulation of only one root.

Starting in 1962 the number of works concerning direct electrical stimulation of the detrusor became more numerous: BRADLEY et al. (1962), BOYCE et al. (1963), KANTROWITZ and SCHAMAUN (1963), HABIB (1963), ELLIS et al. (1964). Concomitant clinical applications were attempted using electrical stimulation by means of external electrical conductors, or by induction at distance: BRADLEY et al. (1963), HABIB (1963—1964), BOYCE et al. (1964), SCOTT et al. (1965), PEDERSEN et al. (1965), POTEMPA and DITTMAR (1965), MARKLAND et al. (1966), STERNBERG et al. (1967), HALD et al. (1967), SUSSET and BOCTOR (1967), WISCHNEWSKY et al. (1967), CHOU et al. (1967), BURGHELE and ICHIM (1967).

The clinical applications evidenced a number of drawbacks and even failures. Hence, the experimental studies were taken up again in order to correct the mistakes and avoid the failures, encountered especially in electrical myostimulation of the bladder.

A sequence of studies appeared on experimental electrical stimulation: HALD and ROSSEL (1964, 1965), KANTROWITZ and SCHAMAUN (1964), POTEMPA and DITTMAR (1965), SCOTT et al. (1965), ELLIS et al. (1965), ALEXANDER and ROWAN (1965), GRABER and RUTISHAUSER (1965), HALD et al. (1966), WISCHNEWSKY et al. (1966), MARKLAND et al. (1966), JONCE et al. (1966), STAUBITZ et al. (1966), SUSSET and BOCTOR (1967), WEAR et al. (1967), HOLMQUIST and OLIN (1968).

In order to extend the clinical application of the method, different authors attempted to solve the following problems:

a) to obtain complete evacuation of the bladder;

b) to chose the most efficient stimulus for stimulation of the detrusor or pelvic nerves;

c) to prevent irradiation of the electric stimulus to the neighbouring nerves or muscles;

d) to avoid the pain produced by stimulation.

Urethral resistance induced during electric stimulation, which prevents complete evacuation of the bladder content, was studied by ALEXANDER and ROWAN (1965), HALD et al. (1966), GRABER et al. (1966), ROHNER and SCHOENBERG (1966), MALLOY et al. (1967), HOLMQUIST and STAUBITZ (1967), HOLMQUIST and OLIN (1968). BURGHELE, ICHIM and DEMETRESCU (1958) drew attention to the obstacle raised by contraction of the smooth sphincter, and SCHOENBERG et al. (1962) to contraction of the perineal musculature. It is owing to the endeavours of these different authors that at present, the indications and contraindications of electrical stimulation of the neurogenic urinary bladder have been outlined.

# I. The Difference between Neuro- and Myostimulation of the Urinary Bladder

Burghele, Ichim and Demetrescu (1958) in electrical stimulation of the pelvic nerves demonstrated that the electrical stimulus should have certain parameters in order to produce long and powerful contraction of the detrusor, with constant intravesical pressures throughout the duration of stimulation. A stimulus not possessing these parameters may produce contraction of the detrusor without however obtaining complete voiding of the bladder.

Moreover, they demonstrated that unilateral electrical stimulation, even with optimal parameters, cannot produce sufficient intravesical pressures to evacuate the whole bladder content.

There is a great difference between electrical stimulation of the pelvic nerves and of the detrusor. On stimulation of the pelvic nerves the entire electrical energy is transmitted to the area within which these nerves are distributed.

On direct stimulation of the detrusor, the electrical stimulus has a maximal effect in the stimulated area. The contraction of the muscle is stronger at the level of the electrode and decreases distal to the stimulated area.

Hald et al. (1966) measured diffusion of the electric current within the bladder wall in the course of myostimulation and found it was more accentuated around the electrodes and increased in terms of the voltage.

In order to obtain a long and powerful contraction of the detrusor by direct stimulation, it is necessary to use either a high voltage, which brings with it certain drawbacks (pain and contraction of the perineal muscles or lower limbs), or a large number of electrodes. Most authors used 4—6 electrodes (Table 1).

Table 1. *The electric stimulus and its parameters*

| Authors | Year | Parameters | | | Site of stimulation | No. of electrodes | Electric stimulus |
|---|---|---|---|---|---|---|---|
| | | Voltage or intensity | Duration | Frequency | | | |
| Burghele, Ichim, Demetrescu | 1958 | 5—10 mA | 4—7 msec | 15 cps | Pelvic nerves | 2 | Square-wave pulses |
| Bradley, Wittmers Chou, French | 1962 | 10—25 V | 1—5 msec | 20—25 cps | Detrusor | 2—6 | Square-wave pulses |
| Schoenberg, Young, Murphy | 1962<br>1963 | 60 mA<br>18—25 V | 0.5—2 msec | 600 cps<br>25 cps | Detrusor | 2 | Square-wave pulses |
| Boyce, Lathem, Hund | 1963 | 10—15 V | 0.5—1 msec | 20—30 cps | Detrusor | 4—6 | Square-wave pulses<br>Triangular<br>Sinusoidal |
| Schamaun, Kantrowitz | 1963 | 25—10 V | 3—8 msec | 15—35 cps | Detrusor | 2 | Square-wave pulses |
| Torbey, Leadbetter | 1963 | 3 V | 1.5 msec | 30 cps | Pelvic nerves<br>Sacral nerves | 2 | Square-wave pulses |
| Hald, Rossel | 1964 | 10—25 mA | 3 msec | 30—50 cps | Detrusor | 2—4 | Square-wave pulses<br>Sinusoidal |
| Ellis, Parker, Hills | 1964 | 4—6 V | 0.3—1.5 msec | 10—20 cps | Detrusor | 3 | Square-wave pulses |

Table 1 (continued)

| Authors | Year | Parameters | | | Site of stimulation | No. of electrodes | Electric stimulus |
|---|---|---|---|---|---|---|---|
| | | Voltage or intensity | Duration | Frequency | | | |
| Potempa, Dittmar | 1965 | 2—15 V<br>20—60 mA | not mentioned | 20—50 cps | Detrusor | 2—4—6 | Square-wave pulses<br>Sinusoidal |
| Scott, Quesada Cardus, Laskowski | 1965 | 5 V | 4 msec | 20 cps | Detrusor | 8—12 | Square-wave pulses |
| Graber, Rutishauser | 1965 | 4—16 V | 30 msec | 18—20 cps | Detrusor | 2—4 | Square-wave pulses<br>Sinusoidal |
| Alexander, Rowan | 1965 | 1.5—8 V | 1—2 msec | 20—25 cps | Pelvic nerves<br>Detrusor | | Square-wave pulses |
| Susset, Boctor, Rosario, Rabinovitch, Nagler, McKinnon | 1966 | 10—20 V | 1 msec | 20 cps | Detrusor | 8 | Square-wave pulses |
| Jonce, Kornelis, Berg | 1966 | 20—30 mA | 5 msec | 20 cps | Detrusor | 5 | Square-wave pulses |
| Staubitz, Cheng, Gillen, Holmquist, Zurlo, Gratbach | 1966 | 1.5—3 V | 3—4 msec | 20—25 cps | Pelvic nerves | 2 | Square-wave pulses |
| Hald, Mygind | 1966 | 1.4—3.5<br>5—13.2 V | 4 msec<br>4 msec | 20 cps<br>20 cps | Pelvic nerves<br>Detrusor | 2<br>4 | Square-wave pulses<br>Square-wave pulses |
| Wear, Kreutzmann Barquin, Bernhardt | 1967 | 2—10 V | 5—10 msec | 10—20 cps | Detrusor | 4—6 | Square-wave pulses |
| Holmquiste, Staubitz | 1967 | 3.7 V | 4 msec | 20 cps | Pelvic nerves | 2 | Square-wave pulses |
| Malloy, Komins, Rohner, Schoenberg | 1967 | 5—7.5 V | 15 msec | 15 cps | Detrusor | 2 | Square-wave pulses |
| Wischnewsky, Liwschitz, Chodorow | 1966 | 10 V | 1 msec | 20 cps | Detrusor | 6 | Square-wave pulses |
| Susset, Boctor | 1968 | 10—20 V | 1 msec | 20cps | Detrusor | 8 | Square-wave pulses |
| Holmquist, Olin | 1968 | 4—5 V | 4 msec | 20 cps | Pelvic nerves | 2 | Square-wave pulses |

When the muscles and intrinsic innervation of the bladder are intact, Boyce et al. (1964) consider that a single pair of electrodes applied to the lateral walls of the bladder is sufficient to produce a marked increase in intravesical pressure. When the bladder muscle is hypertrophic, fibrosed or decompensated by overdistension, it is absolutely necessary to have a second pair of electrodes applied upon the ventral, peritoneum-free, wall of the bladder.

## II. The Site of Implantation of the Electrodes

Some authors found that the sensitivity of the detrusor to direct electrical stimulation depends upon the site of implantation of the electrodes, and the areas, where the tension of the electric current can be lowered, have been named "trigger areas". Attention was drawn to them by SCHOENBERG et al. (1962) and HABIB (1963). They correspond to the site where the nervous filaments deriving from the pelvic plexus enter in the bladder wall.

SCOTT et al. (1965) obtained powerful contractions of the bladder wall with two electrodes placed on the posterior aspect of the bladder between the two ureters. Cineradiography showed that under these conditions electrical stimulation displaced the bladder forward. This led them to believe that implantation of two supplementary electrodes in an opposite position, on the anterior aspect, might result in complete voiding of the bladder.

JONCE, KORNELIS and BERG (1966) showed that stimulation of the bladder wall with two electrodes placed close to the ureteral-vesical junctions increases the efficiency of electrical stimulation by 60% in comparison to stimulation with a ventral and a dorsal electrode.

Application of another two electrodes on the anterior and posterior walls, under the above conditions, improves the contraction of the bladder by 10%.

Proof of the efficiency of electrical stimulation at the site of entry of the nervous fibers into the bladder wall, which is actually a neurostimulation, is supplied by drugs that block the pelvic plexus, and lower the effect of this stimulation (5 mg hexamethonium bromide/kg i.v.).

The above mentioned authors likewise observed that excitability and the response to electrical stimulation at the level of the uretero-vesical junctions, decreases after section of the sacral nerves which contain parasympathetic preganglionic fibers that synapse with the effector neurone in the bladder wall.

According to HALD, FREED and KANTROWITZ (1966) the existence of a "trigger area" is only valid for the dog in which innervation is condensed within a single nervous fiber that courses towards the bladder wall together with the blood vessels.

In man, the vesical nerves are distributed radially, in a variable number of fibers so that they cannot be covered by a disk-shaped electrode, with a diameter of 1.5 cm, even if the electrode is placed at the level of the uretero-vesical junction. For this reason, quadripolar stimulation is indicated with disk or with wire electrodes introduced within the thickness of the detrusor, towards the uretero-vesical junctions.

Investigating, in a patient with section of the spinal cord at $Th_3$—$Th_4$ level, the best place for the electrodes, SCOTT, QUESADA, CARDUS and LASCOWSKI (1965) demonstrated that stimulation with two electrodes in the "trigger area" with a 5 V signal did not produce an increase in intravesical pressure, but intense electrical discharges in the pelvic musculature, also confirmed by digital palpation of the anal sphincter. When the tension of the current exceeds 5 V, intravesical pressure increases with the voltage and number of electrodes.

These findings demonstrate that the musculature of the bladder responds difficultly to electrical stimulation and the active response is mediated by the nervous component.

On the other hand, CARPENTER (1963), reviewing the different complex and opposing opinions concerning the mechanism of direct electrical stimulation of the detrusor, considered that an electrical stimulus cannot be applied exclusively to the smooth muscular fibers since these fibers are mixed with the postganglionic nervous fibers and the intrinsic nervous plexus.

According to CARPENTER, propagation of the electric stimulus takes place along the myelin-free neural elements and not directly by depolarization of the membrane of the smooth muscular fibers.

An evident proof is the diminution or abolition of the response to direct electrical stimulation of the mouse bladder after the administration of veratrin or procaine or degeneration following transection of the postganglionic fibers.

Following electrical stimulation of the pelvic nerves, the force of contraction of the bladder musculature depends upon the chemical mediator — acetylcholine-released cut the level of the nervous endings.

The investigations of HALD, FREED and KANTROWITZ (1966) demonstrated that the electrical stimulus is distributed to the bladder wall through the nervous tissue. If the parasympathetic reflex arc is interrupted by transection of the pelvic nerves, a high voltage is necessary to obtain a response to myostimulation, similar to that prior to transection. Hence, in myostimulation, in lesions of the inferior motor neurone, the use of a larger number of electrodes is of greater importance than their site of implantation since only in this way can a good electrical covering of the bladder be ensured.

The great variability of the parameters of the electrical stimulus used by different authors in direct stimulation of the bladder muscle is due firstly to the resistance of the tissues, and secondly to a whole series of factors, such as: over-distension or prolonged drainage, thickness of the bladder wall, infection which diminishes excitability because of oedema or sclerosis, the amount of urine in the bladder, the position of the electrodes and the distance between them.

## III. Pain in Electrical Stimulation of the Bladder

Pain during electrical stimulation of the bladder wall occurs both in experimental investigations and in clinical applications.

BRADLEY, WITTMERS and CHOU (1963) showed in their experiments that during myostimulation pain is produced in lesions of the cauda equina and may be caused by the presence of electrodes in the subperitoneum. Interruption of the sensory sympathetic pathways by transection of the hypogastric nerve, diminished the pain.

BOYCE et al. (1964) report on the development of strong pains in the abdomen and penis, and contraction of the adductor muscles during electrical stimulation of the detrusor. They consider that the pain may be generated by spasm of the detrusor if evacuation of the bladder is prevented by contraction of the striate sphincter and perineal musculature. Stimulation of the adjacent somatic nerves or of the parasympathetic may likewise give rise to the sensation of an urgent need to defecate, to abdominal colics, testicular pains or painful erection.

STAUBITZ et al. (1966) noted in their experiments that pain only appears when the current has an amplitude of up to 3 V; however, they previously sectioned the presacral nerve.

Because of the pain, SUSSET and BOCTOR (1967) are against electrical myo-stimulation in incomplete spinal lesions at conus level.

In transections at the level of the cauda equina, the parasympathetic sensory pathways are interrupted, but the nervous inflow that produces the sensation of pain may continue to circulate along sympathetic pathways, the sympathetic afferences entering the spinal cord above the cauda equina. In order to remove the pain transmitted by sympathetic pathways, various experimental transections per performed.

Chou, Bradley and Markland (1967) observed that neurectomy of the hypogastric nerve in animals with section of the cauda equina attenuates the suffering produced by electric stimulation. According to Jonce, Kornelis and Berg (1966) this neurectomy has no effect upon pain which, however, no longer appears in animals with bilateral thoraco-lumbar sympathectomy.

The use of sympatholytic drugs: Nethaline HCl (10 mg/kg i.v.), Piperoxane HCl (10 mg/kg i.v.) and Pentolamine methansulphonate (1 mg/kg), used by Jonce, Kornelis and Berg (1966) to attenuate the excitability of the trigonal zone, the richest in pain receptors, did not give any significant results in experimental animals.

Neither was the discomfort produced by electrical stimulation diminished by the administration of atropin (1 mg/kg i.v.) and Hexamethonium bromide (10 mg/kg i.v.), drugs that diminish the contractility of the detrusor.

In the clinical application of electric stimulation of the detrusor pain was more frequently present in diseases of the nervous system than in spinal cord injuries. In spinal transections, pain depends upon the level of the injury and the intensity of the electrical stimulus, and also appeared in high lesions when the voltage was too great.

Pain and unpleasant sensations were noted in 9 of 26 clinical applications of electrical stimulation in spinal cord injuries and 13 diseases of the nervous system. No pain was felt during electrical stimulation in cervical or thoracic spinal injuries (Tables 3 and 4).

The pain is sometimes so strong that the patient refuses another stimulation. In the cases in which the parameters of the stimulus are specified, pain appeared at a voltage of 10 to 40 V (Habib 20—30 V on direct stimulation of the detrusor in spinal cord injury and 35—40 V in a patient with myelomeningocela).

It is worthy of note that in all the cases in which electrical stimulation produced pain, evacuation of the bladder was incomplete or did not occur, which demonstrates that apart from pain electrical stimulation increases urethral resistance by concomitant contraction of the perineal striate musculature.

Stimulation of the pelvic nerves in man, with a stimulus of 2.5 V does not provoke pain (Burghele, Ichim, 1967).

Transrectal stimulation of the urinary bladder is always accompanied by pain because of the high voltage used (Dees, 1965), which contraindicates the clinical application of this method.

Transection of the sympathetic for removing pain has not been experimented clinically, but before resorting to it the voltage of the electrical stimulus must be reduced below the threshold of pain, since this transection also has its hazards.

Montgomery and Boyce (1967) consider that pain is transmitted directly through the tissues rather than by nervous pathways since in the electrical stimulations performed by them, irradiation of the stimulus was prevented by correct implantation of perfectly insulated electrodes and individualization of the stimulus characteristics.

## IV. Erection during Electrical Stimulation

Direct stimulation of the bladder muscle is sometimes accompanied by painful erection that also persists after ceasing stimulation. Erection influences evacuation of the bladder increasing urethral resistance by angulation, by contraction of the vesico-urethral orifice, increase in the length of the urethra and decrease of its caliber and elasticity.

## V. Urethral Resistance during Electrical Stimulation of the Urinary Bladder

Obstruction of the bladder neck and urethra during electric stimulation of the urinary bladder is one of the main drawbacks in the clinical application of electric stimulation of the neurogenic bladder.

Contraction of the internal sphincter, external sphincter and perineal striate musculature was noted in experimental studies, during neurostimulation by BURGHELE et al. (1958), SCHOENBERG et al. (1962), HALD, FREED and KANTROWITZ (1966), STAUBITZ et al. (1966), HOLMQUIST and STAUBITZ (1967), HOLMQUIST and OLIN (1968), and during myostimulation by SCHAMAUN and KANTROWITZ (1963). ALEXANDER and ROWAN (1965), HALD et al. (1966), WEAR et al. (1967). Incomplete evacuation of the bladder content, consequent to increase urethral resistance, was also noted in clinical applications by BRADLEY, WITTMERS and CHOU (1963), BOYCE, LATHEM and HUND (1964), SCOTT, QUESADA, CARDUS and LASKOWSKI (1965), STERNBERG, BURNETTE and BUNTS (1967), HALD, MEIER, KHALILI, AGRAWAL, BENTON and KANTROWITZ (1967).

BURGHELE, ICHIM and DEMETRESCU (1958) demonstrated that one of the causes which prevent free flow of the urine following contraction of the detrusor stimulated via the pelvic nerves, is the coming into play of the smooth vesical sphincter. Contraction of the smooth sphincter is due to irradiation of the electric current at pelvic plexus level, where the parasympathetic fibers cross the sympathetic fibers to form this plexus. Hence, the urine jet is interrupted. GRABER et al. (1966) attribute this interruption to contraction of the bladder neck. They excluded the influence of the striate sphincter by introducing a catheter into the urethra, distal to the smooth sphincter. First, as in the experiments of BURGHELE et al. electric stimulation produced an increase in intravesical pressure with evacuation of the urine, then the urine jet suddenly ceased and intravesical pressure increased. Under these conditions the external sphincter no longer acts. The authors explain this phenomenon by constraction of the bladder neck.

ALEXANDER and ROWAN (1965), studying the intervention of the internal sphincter in direct electric stimulation of the bladder, by means of nervous transections (section of the pelvic nerves, of the cauda equina, of the cord at $Th_{12}$—$L_1$ level) practiced before stimulation, reached the conclusion that this sphincter cannot raise an obstacle. Actually, however, the nervous sections performed before stimulation of the detrusor did not affect innervation of the smooth sphincter.

The observations of LEARMONTH (1931), who demonstrated that stimulation of the hypogastric nerve was followed by contraction of the trigonal musculature and those of YOUNG and WESSON (1921), who upheld that opening of the internal urethral orifice during micturition is realized following traction of the bladder neck by the trigone, were used by MONTGOMERY and BOYCE (1967) in their hypothesis according to which the resistance of the bladder neck during electric stimulation of the detrusor may be overcome by simultaneous or sequential electric stimulation of the hypogastric nerves.

However, they did not bear in mind that on stimulation of the bladder wall at the site of penetration of the nerves into the bladder, the sympathetic nervous fibers controlling trigone and internal sphincter are concomitantly stimulated. Contraction of the smooth sphincter can only be avoided by removing the influence of the sympathetic, i.e. section below the pelvic plexus or the administration of sympathicolytic drugs and not stimulation.

Interruption of the urine jet both in stimulation of the pelvic nerves and in that of the detrusor is due not only to the obstacle raised by contraction of the internal sphincter but also to contraction of the external sphincter and perineal musculature.

HALD and ROSEL (1964), in experiments on animals, once again drew attention to the fact that stimulation of the bladder also produces contraction of the ischio and bulbo-cavernosus muscles.

Concomitant contraction of the perineal musculature and of the lower limbs was noted by KANTROWITZ and SCHAMAUN (1964). Considering this to be due to irradiation of the electric current to the surrounding tissues and bearing in mind the observations of BORS (1952), who sectioned the pudendal nerves in order to remove the spasm of the perineal muscles in paraplegic patients, they proposed sectioning of the pudendal nerves in order to ensure good evacuation of the bladder content. POTEMPA and DITTMAR (1965) likewise sustained this method.

The studies of SCOTT et al. (1965) revealed a marked increase in the electric activity of the perineal musculature during stimulation of the detrusor with two retrovesical electrodes implanted close to the vesico-ureteral junctions and another two electrodes near the bladder neck, on its anterior and posterior aspects. Contraction of the perineal muscles can also be felt by rectal touch. Stimulation of the bladder with electrodes implanted in the dome of the bladder is likewise accompanied by contraction of the striate perineal musculature.

ALEXANDER and ROWAN (1965) in their investigations on the action of the external sphincter demonstrated, by stimulation of the detrusor before and after bilateral section of the pudendal nerves, by unilateral stimulation of the pelvic and of the pudendal nerves, and by stimulation after the administration of scoline to inhibit the function of the skeletal muscles, that the external urethral sphincter only contracts when the voltage exceeds 10 volts.

In 1966, HALD et al. carried out investigations on dogs and monkeys in order to determine the effect of electric stimulation of the detrusor upon urethral resistance, in acute and chronic experiments. They demonstrated that urethral resistance increases, due to contraction of the perineal striate musculature, with increase in the voltage of the electric current. A stimulus of 0.5 V, applied directly upon the membranous urethra, interrupts the urine jet.

According to these authors contraction of the perineal striate musculature during electric stimulation of the detrusor takes place by reflex route from the detrusor to the pudendal nerves due to irradiation of the electric current, or directly via the detrusor musculature to the urethral musculature.

Section of the pudendal nerves to improve the urinary flow only had effect after a period of time; a normal flow could not be ensured because of irradiation of the electric stimulus from the detrusor to the striate sphincter. An effect similar to that of section of the pudendal nerves was also obtained by curarization, prosthesis of the membranous urethra, resection of the levator ani muscles and fatigue of the striate sphincter by electric stimulation.

The urinary jet is considerably improved by inhibition of the striate sphincter following application of a current of 150—400 Hz, 1—0.6 msec and 4—6 V on the prostatic urethra.

In another series of experiments, HALD, AGRAWAL and KANTROWITZ (1966), studying the obstructive factors of the urethra during electric stimulation, showed that direct stimulation of the detrusor and pelvic nerves is accompanied by a decrease of the urinary flow in comparison to the normal flow. The urinary flow is improved after section of the pudendal nerves. An average urinary flow of 3.1 $cm^3$/sec during stimulation of the pelvic nerves increases, under the same conditions, to 4.2 $cm^3$/sec after section of the pudendal nerves.

After section of the pudendal nerves, a substantial increase in the urinary flow was also obtained by direct stimulation of the detrusor, i.e. the average urinary flow before section of the pudendal nerves was of 1.4 $cm^3$/sec and increased to 4.6 $cm^3$/sec after section of these nerves. Moreover, the amount of residue following stimulation of the pelvic nerves fell from 36 to 14 ml, and following direct stimulation of the bladder wall from 61 to 42 ml. In agreement with Holmquist and Olin (1968), Hald et al. (1967) found no important change in the volume of the urinary flow or vesical residue after section of the hypogastric nerve. However, it is not shown whether stimulation of the pelvic nerves was done before or after section of the pudendal nerves. When the pudendal nerves are intact concomitant contraction of the smooth and of the striate sphincter occurs. Even when contraction of the smooth sphincter is eliminated by section of the hypogastric nerve, the urinary flow is not modified because the obstacle realized by contraction of the striate sphincter persists. Although the force of the two sphincters that obstruct evacuation of the urine during electrical stimulation, has not yet been evaluated comparatively, it is assumed that the striate sphincter represents a far more redoubtable obstacle than the smooth sphincter. Indeed, prolonged pressure upon the smooth sphincter forces it open, transforming the bladder neck into a funnel.

Holmquist and Staubitz (1967), then Holmquist and Olin (1968), studied the influence of different somatic or vegetative nerves, striate musculature of the perineum and of the periurethral erectile tissue, upon electromicturition.

They stimulated the pelvic nerves in animals with an intact spinal cord and with intact or sectioned hypogastric and pudendal nerves, repeated the stimulations in animals with sectioned spinal cord at $Th_{12}$—$L_1$ level, concomitantly stimulated the intact pudendal nerves with a stimulus of 3 V, 4 msec and 30 Hz and pelvic nerves, as well as the peripheral end of the pelvic nerves sectioned above the electrodes. In addition, they sectioned the bulbocavernosus muscle, producing electromicturition before and after section of the pudendal nerves and made evident the erectile tissue of the urethra by angiography of the pudendal artery, during and after section of the pelvic nerves.

The influence of the vesico-urethral nerves and striate perineal musculature upon the urinary flow was appraised by recording intravesical pressure by means of a catheter introduced through the anterior wall of the bladder, by measuring the bladder residue, by urethrocystography in lateral projection, by measuring the diameter of the urethra at the level of the external sphincter and perineum and plotting of the time-diameter curve. These experiments showed that during electric stimulation of the pelvic nerves, vigorous contraction of the detrusor occurs with evacuation of the bladder content.

Within the first three seconds after starting stimulation, the external sphincter begins to contract, without however interrupting the urine flow completely. Then, the urinary jet is interrupted due to contraction of the external sphincter, concomitant to constriction of the urethra by the periurethral erectile tissue following contraction of the bulbocavernosus muscle. The urine jet improves after section of the pudendal nerves which completely relaxes the external sphincter and after section of the bulbocavernosus muscle.

Electromicturition is not influenced by transection of the spinal cord and nor is the urethral caliber modified to any extent by section of the hypogastric nerves. Contraction of the external sphincter during stimulation of the pelvic nerves is brought about by antidromal stimulation of the reflex medullary center of the pudendal nerves, the electric current passing through the pelvic nerves in a retrograde direction to the anterior sacral roots and the medullary conus.

In female experimental animals, Holmquist and Olin (1968) noticed that electromicturition is obtained under better conditions than in the male because of a weaker striate sphincter and periurethral erectile tissue.

In order to appraise the role of the striate sphincter in spontaneous micturition and in that induced by stimulation of the pelvic nerve or the detrusor, Hald and Mygind (1967) administered d. tubocurarin and succinylcholine to dogs with intact vesico-urethral innervation and bilateral section of the pelvic and pudendal nerves or section of the spinal cord at $Th_6$ level.

After administration of 1 mg curare/kg (d.tubocurarine) the diameter of the membranous urethra increases both in the proximal and in the distal portion, thus demonstrating the action of curare upon the striate perineal musculature. The speed of the urinary flow ($cm^3$/sec) diminishes with increase in the urethral diameter. The intravesical pressure obtained by direct electric stimulation of the detrusor after the administration of succinylcholine (40—80 mg) is about 30% lower than before the administration of this product to animals with section of the pelvic nerves. On the other hand the urinary flow diminishes and the bladder residue increases.

In clinical applications Hald, Meier, Khalili, Agrawal, Benton and Kantrowitz (1967), in a patient with transverse myelitis, at $Th_9$ level, found that electrical stimulation of the bladder wall with a stimulus of 10.5 V produces a pressure of 75—133 cm of water at the external sphincter. This pressure falls to 50 cm of water after infiltration of the pudendal nerves with novocaine. In another patient with flaccid paraplegia, the powerful spasm of the sphincteral striate musculature and exaggerated reflexes of the bulbocavernosus muscles to direct stimulation of the detrusor with a stimulus of 10 V was avoided by bilateral section of the pudendal nerves.

Sternberg, Burnette and Bunts (1967) noted in one of their patients with section of the spinal cord at $C_6$ level, an increase in urethral pressure up to 20 mm Hg caused by contraction of the bladder neck or the perineal musculature

In order to remove urethral resistance brought about by propagation of the electric current during stimulation of the bladder, Rohner and Schoenberg (1966) and Malloy, Komins, Rohner and Schoenberg (1967) proposed plastic operation of the bladder neck according to the Y-V procedure. Although in the intact animals the resistance of the vesico-urethral orifice was lowered to a certain extent by Y-V plasty, in the paraplegic animals this operation did not give favourable results. In clinical applications, Burghele and Ichim (1967) reduced the resistance brought about contraction of the smooth sphincter by surgical denervation of the bladder neck, or by treatment with alcohol or phenol. This does not however inhibit the action of the perineal striate musculature.

Section of the pudendal nerves, proposed by most authors for diminishing urethral resistance, improves the urinary flow, but destroys the sexual function, The most seducing method appears to be that of electrical fatigue of the external sphincter proposed by Hald et al. (1967). Drugs can only be used for a brief interval. Particularly efficient in clinical application (Burghele and Ichim, 1967) is the method of repeated electric stimulation of the pelvic nerves with 2—5 min breaks between the stimuli, by means of which the entire content of the bladder is voided.

Perineal prostatectomy practiced by Markland, Chou, Bradley, Westgate and Wolfson (1966) does not improve evacuation of the bladder following myostimulation and cannot be accepted as a routine method.

Apart from the forementioned factors that may improve the urinary flow by lowering the resistance of the urethra, especially during myostimulation, the use of a low voltage electric current remains the best method without prejudicing the contraction force of the detrusor.

In order to obtain electromicturition by direct stimulation of the detrusor with a low voltage stimulus, care must be taken to avoid tissular lesions at the level of the electrodes and deterioration of the bladder by overdistension, infection or prolonged drainage. Of particular importance for obtaining efficient, equal contraction of the detrusor by uniform diffusion of the electric current, is the number and position of the electrodes. Irregular diffusion of the electric current deteriorates the detrusor and necessitates increase of the voltage. In the zones where the electric current spreads equally, the bladder wall becomes hypertrophic because of repeated contractions in the same area, and in the zones where it does not diffuse with the same intensity an exaggerated distension takes place due to muscular inactivity.

Hence, in myostimulation particular attention should be paid not to perforate the bladder wall and to insulation of the electrodes, which must not come in direct contact with an electrolytic solution that might produce a short circuit.

### VI. The Effect of Electric Stimulation on the Pelvic Nerves

The tolerance of the pelvic nerves to prolonged electric stimulation with optimal parameters was demonstrated by BURGHELE et al. (1958) in histologic studies.

Apart from granulation tissue around the nerve, a common tissular reaction to the presence of a foreign body, no degeneration of the nervous fibers was observed.

HALD, AGRAVAL and KANTROWITZ (1966) likewise noted the perineural granulation tissue after stimulation of the pelvic nerves, but also in the presence of the electrodes without stimulation. They asserted that deterioration of the nerves by stimulation increases their resistance and imposes an increase in the tension of the electric current. However, no data are given concerning the parameters of the electric stimulus used by HALD et al., and it is not excluded that an intensity of over 10 mA, which produces lesions of the axons, was used.

At the Symposium on the Neurogenic Bladder, held in U.S.A. in 1965, GLENN reported that intermittent experimental stimulation of the pelvic nerves for 9 months, followed by histologic study of these nerves, only revealed a minimal fibrous reaction around them (BOYARSKY, 1967).

## F. Clinical Application of Electrical Stimulation of the Neurogenic Bladder

### I. Electrical Neurostimulation of the Urinary Bladder

Following experimental studies, electrical neurostimulation of the urinary bladder was introduced into clinical practice by BURGHELE and ICHIM in 1967. Neurostimulation with a stimulus whose parameters are optimal produces long, powerful contraction of the detrusor, with intravesical pressures that exceed those of normal micturition, without injury to the nerves or fatigue of the neuromuscular complex.

Experimental research on electrical stimulation of the vesical motor nerves was conducted by GLENN et al. (1964), HALD, FREED and KANTROWITZ (1966), STAUBITZ et al. (1966), then by HOLMQUIST, STAUBITZ and GREATBACH (1967), HOLMQUIST and OLIN (1968) and HOLMQUIST, STAUBITZ and GREATBACH (1968).

### a) The Parameters of the Electric Stimulus

The optimal electrical stimulus for neurostimulation is of 4—10 mA intensity, 4—7 msec duration and 15 Hz frequency. Lower or higher values of the electrical stimulus either harm the stimulated nerves or cannot provoke voiding of the bladder. Similar values were found experimentally by STAUBITZ et al., in 1966 (frequency 20—25 Hz, duration 3—4 msec, voltage 2—3 V).

### b) Stimulation of the Pelvic Nerves in Man by Electromagnetic Induction

For stimulation of the pelvic nerves in man, BURGHELE, ICHIM and DEMETRESCU (1959) resorted to electromagnetic induction. This principle was subsequently applied by BRADLEY, WITMERS and CHOU (1963), KANTROWITZ and SCHAMAUN (1963), SUSETT et al. (1966), WISCHNEWSKY et al. (1967), HALD et al. (1967).

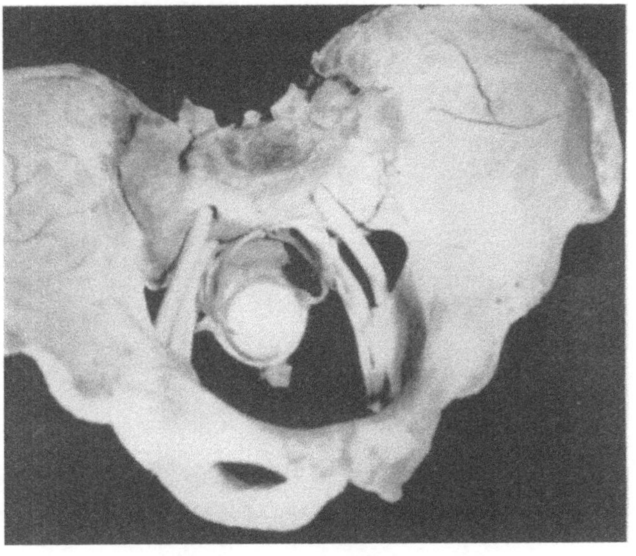

Fig. 27. Site of receptor and its relationship with the anterior aspect of the sacrum

Electromagnetic induction is obtained by means of a receiver introduced surgically on the anterior aspect of the sacrum and fitted with dual platinum electrodes placed on the pelvic nerves on both sides (BURGHELE, ICHIM and DEMETRESCU) (Fig. 27).

The receiver is acted upon by an external inductor whose antenna produces an electromagnetic field with great penetrability in the organism. Most authors implant the receiver below the skin of the abdomen.

The pelvic nerves are exposed by median, subumbilical laparotomy. After freeing the pelvic cavity, the site of the second and third anterior sacral foramens is determined by palpation.

The posterior parietal peritoneum is sectioned 5—6 cm along the anterior sacral foramens, the sigmoid being drawn to the right in order to expose the left side.

The second and third anterior sacral roots are carefully exposed. The pelvic nerves appear 1.5 to 2 cm after emergence of these roots from the foramens, and course in a postero-anterior direction. They are exposed up to their penetration within the pelvic plexus. A sample electrode is placed on each pelvic nerve and electrical stimulation is tested. The effect of stimulation is appraised by contraction of the detrusor and increase in intravesical pressure, the bladder being connected by means of a catheter connected with a water manometer. Normally, monolateral stimulation produces intravesical pressures of 35 to 40 cm of water.

After the control test, a dual platinum electrode is fixed on each pelvic nerve and covered with a thin polyethylene sheet to prevent irradiation of the electrical current to the neighbouring nervous and muscular formations.

The receiver, which is connected to the two electrodes by means of polyethylene-covered leads, is fixed retroperitoneally onto the anterior aspect of the sacrum. The parietal peritoneum is sutured, the receiver, leads and electrodes being placed retroperitoneally.

Function of the receiver is again tested by electrical stimulation. The signal is transmitted through the skin to the receiver by an antenna. Bilateral electrical stimulation raises intravesical pressure to 70—80 cm of water.

In order to lower the resistance of the bladder neck by contraction of the smooth sphincter, the hypogastric nerve is sectioned and the neck denervated surgically, or by alcohol or phenol infiltrations. The peritoneal cavity is closed and the bladder immediately emptied by electrical stimulation.

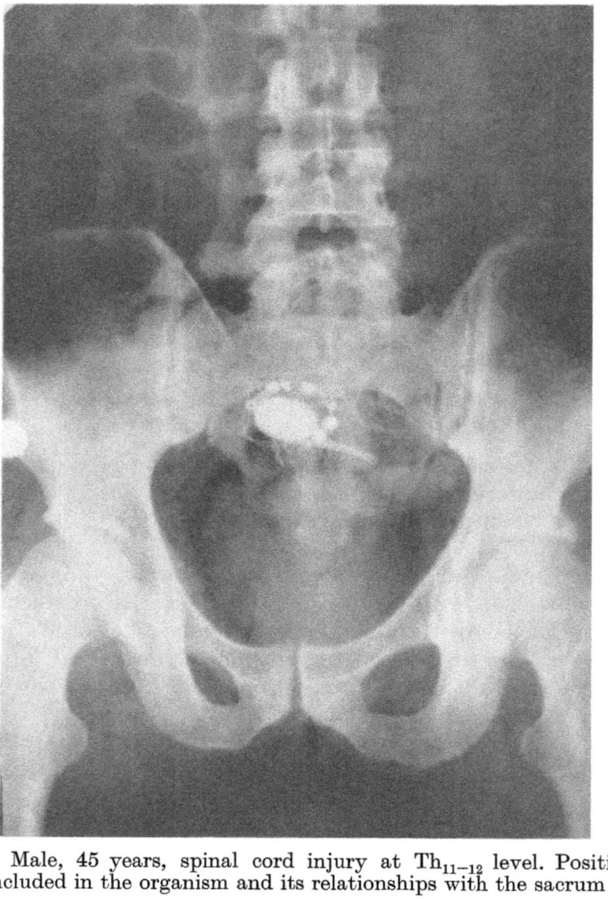

a

Fig. 28a and b. Male, 45 years, spinal cord injury at $Th_{11-12}$ level. Position of receptor included in the organism and its relationships with the sacrum 'able 2. *Neurostimulation of the urinary bladder by electromagnetic induction with an implanted receiver*

| Name | Age (years) | Level of lesion | Age of lesion | Cystometry | Uroculture | Results early | Results late | Side effects |
|---|---|---|---|---|---|---|---|---|
| T. V. | 45 | $Th_{11}$, $Th_{12}$ paraplegia | 22 days | areflex bladder | + | complete voiding of bladder | recovery of reflex activity | — |
| I. M. | 30 | $Th_8$ paraplegia | 26 days | areflex bladder | + | complete voiding of bladder | recovery of reflex activity | — |
| U. C. | 31 | $Th_9$ paraplegia | 31 days | areflex bladder | + | complete voiding of bladder | recovery of reflex activity | — |
| M. P. | 20 | $L_2$ paraplegia | 9 months | areflex bladder | + | No response to stimulation | Absent vesical reflectivity | |

## c) Clinical Cases

*Case 1.* The patient T.V. (case card No. 1728), aged 45, suffered a spinal cord injury on March 15, 1967, with fracture-luxation at $Th_{11}$—$Th_{12}$ level, with section of the spinal cord, observed at the decompression laminectomy performed.

After the accident, urine retention necessitated an urethral indwelling catheter. Cystometry revealed an areflex bladder. Bacillus proteus developed in the uroculture.

A bladder neurostimulator was implanted under general anaesthesia, 22 days after the accident (April 7, 1967), with section of the hypogastric nerve and denervation of the bladder neck by surgery and by infiltration with alcohol.

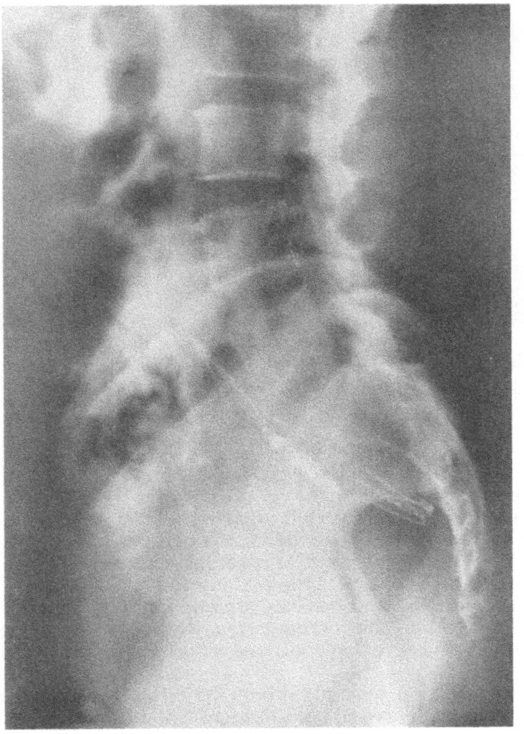

Fig. 28b

The front and side radiologic views of the pelvis showed the position of the receiver and leads to the dual platinum electrodes, attached to the pelvic nerves (Fig. 28a, b). The receiver was fixed to the promontory. In subsequent applications the receiver was placed more distally, on the anteror aspect of the sacrum. The change in the position of the receiver was dictated by the difficulty of obtaining a perfect parallelism between the antenna of the inductor and the receiver.

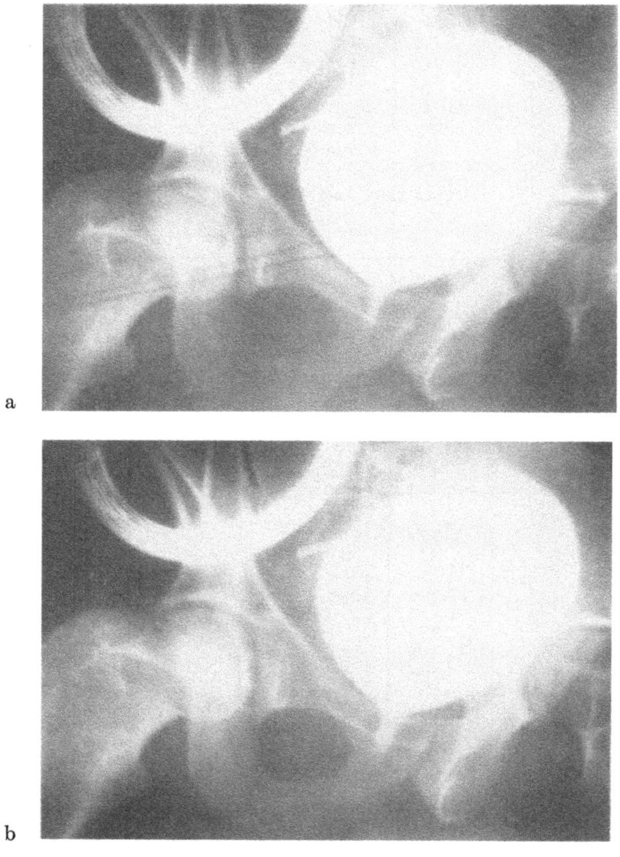

Fig. 29a and b. Male, 45 years, spinal cord injury. Voiding cystourethrogram following electrical stimulation of the pelvic nerves. Note opening of the bladder neck

Immediately after the operation the catheter was removed and the bladder emptied every 4—6 hours by electrical stimulation.

At each stimulation about 300 ml turbid urine was evacuated. Within 15 days the urine became clear and sterile. Two or three successive stimulations had to be applied to void the bladder of residual urine, because of urethral resistance produced by contraction of the perineal and sphincter striate musculature. Evacuation of the bladder was improved by novocaine infiltration of the pudendal nerves before stimulation (Fig. 29a, b).

Cystometry, performed after 5 days stimulation, showed gradual recovery of the bladder reflectivity. After 10 days, reflex vesical contractions occurred with spontaneous micturition, especially at night.

Thirty days later micturition took place only by reflex contractions, at intervals of an hour and a half — two hours. There was no residual urine. Electrical stimulation was given up. Urographic control eight months later was normal: no change in the position of the electrodes and receiver; good reflex voiding of the bladder; sterile uroculture; no residue.

*Case 2.* The patient I.M., aged 30 (case card 50,480), suffered a spinal cord injury with impaction of the 8th thoracal vertebra and consecutive section of the spinal cord, observed at decompression laminectomy, performed 24 hours after the accident. Urine retention developed immediately after the accident. Cystometry showed an areflex bladder. Urography performed 24 hours after the accident, interval during which a permanent catheter was introduced, showed moderate, bilateral uretero-pelvic dilatation. The bladder wall was thickened, the contrast medium stopping in the ureters at 2 cm distance from the bladder wall (Fig. 30).

Urinary infection was present: B. paracoli and Escherichia coli being isolated from the urine. The patient was febrile and eschars developed in the sacral and trochanteral regions.

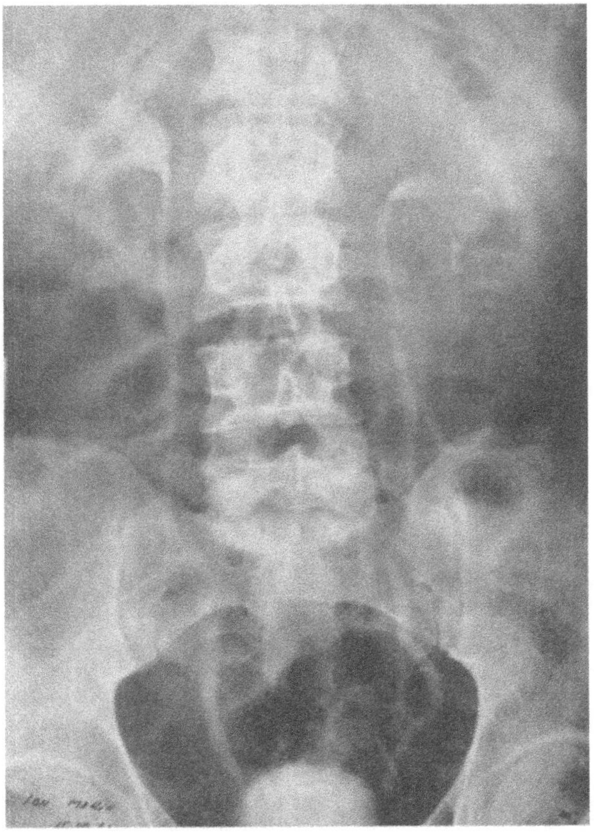

Fig. 30. Male, 30 years. Excretory urogram: bilateral ureteral reflux. Stenosis of the terminal ureter

On September 23, 1967 (26 days after the accident) a receiver was implanted for neurostimulation of the bladder by median subumbilical laparotomy. Marked thickening of the bladder wall was noted intraoperatively. Denervation of the bladder neck and section of the hypogastric nerve were performed. The catheter was removed immediately after the operation and electrical stimulation was started at 4—5 hours intervals. Slight erection occurred each time. The urine jet was at first strong, then gradually diminished and ceased after voiding 250—300 ml.

The roentgenogram (Fig. 31 a, b) shows the metallic part of the vesical neurostimulator on the anterior aspect of the sacrum. The two electrodes are wound round the pelvic nerves on both sides. The side view reveals the position of the neurostimulator with respect to the anterior aspect of the sacrum. Fig. 32 gives the details of the neurostimulator and inductor antenna in functional position. Complete voiding of the bladder was obtained by two or three interrupted stimulations.

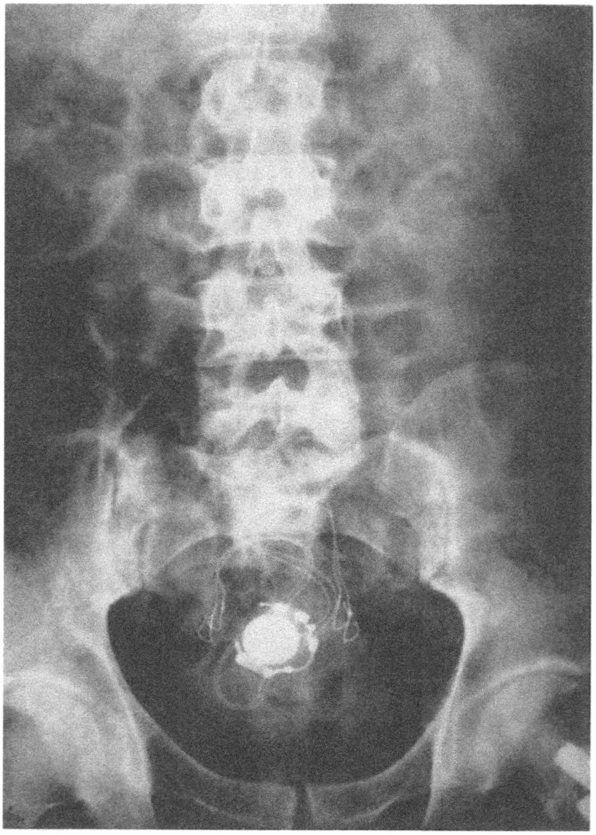

Fig. 31a and b. Male, 30 years, spinal cord injury. Radiography: front view and anterior oblique projection. Note metallic part of the receptor with electrodes applied upon the pelvic nerves

Twelve days after starting the electrical stimulations, reflex contractions of the bladder developed with elimination of a variable amount of urine. These contractions became increasingly more efficient and the whole bladder content was voided every one and a half — two hours.

Urography, performed 3 months after ceasing electric stimulation, showed maintenance of bilateral uretero-pelvic dilatation. The bladder appeared to be asymmetrical with a funnel-shaped, open neck and stenosed terminal ureters (Fig. 33).

These images demonstrate that hypertrophy of the detrusor occurred after application of the drainage, the catheter forming an obstacle in the way of the urinary uretero-vesical flow. Uretero-pelvic dilatation was produced both by the low ureteral stenosis and by section of the spinal cord. This dilatation was more evident a year later. The urograms in Fig. 34 show the evolution of the distension process due to the stasis created at the level of the terminal ureters by hypertrophy and sclerosis of the detrusor, generated by the 26 days bladder catheterism before the application of neurostimulation (Fig. 34).

Urography likewise revealed an interrupted lead close to the receiver. This interruption by micromovements was also noted by SUSSET and BOCTOR (1967).

*Case 3.* The patient U.C., aged 31 (case card No. 50,830) suffered spinal cord injury with fracture of the vertebral lamella of Th9 and section of the spinal cord, checked at decompression laminectomy. Flaccid paraplegia with an areflex bladder. An indwelling catheter was introduced immediately after the accident. The urine became infected with B. proteus and

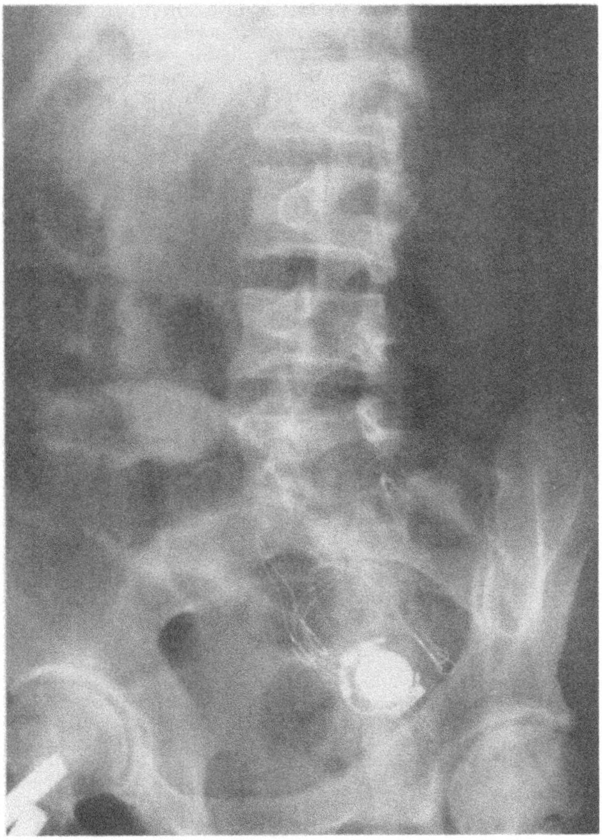

Fig. 31 b

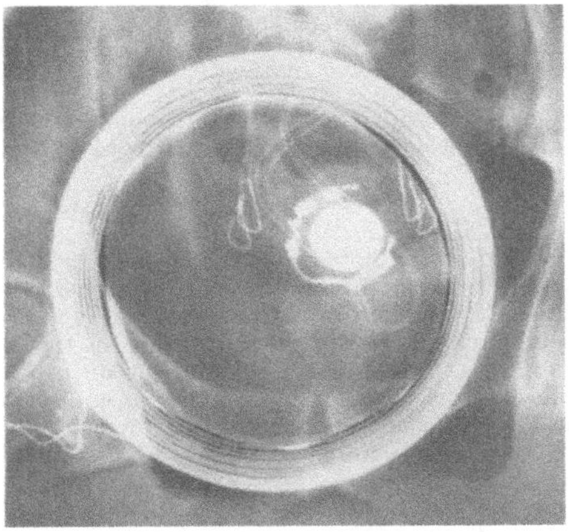

Fig. 32. Male, 30 years, spinal cord injury. Radiography of the pelvis. Details of the neurostimulator and inductor antenna

Escherichia coli. On January 31, 1968, bladder neurostimulation was started, introducing the receiver and leads according to the previously described technique, with section of the hypogastric nerve and surgical denervation of the ladder neck. Stimulation was done by means of two or three signals at 2—5 min interval.

The urine jet was very powerful and the urine became clear and limpid after 10 days.

Electrically-induced micturition was followed up by a video-recorder after filling the bladder with a contrast medium (Fig. 35).

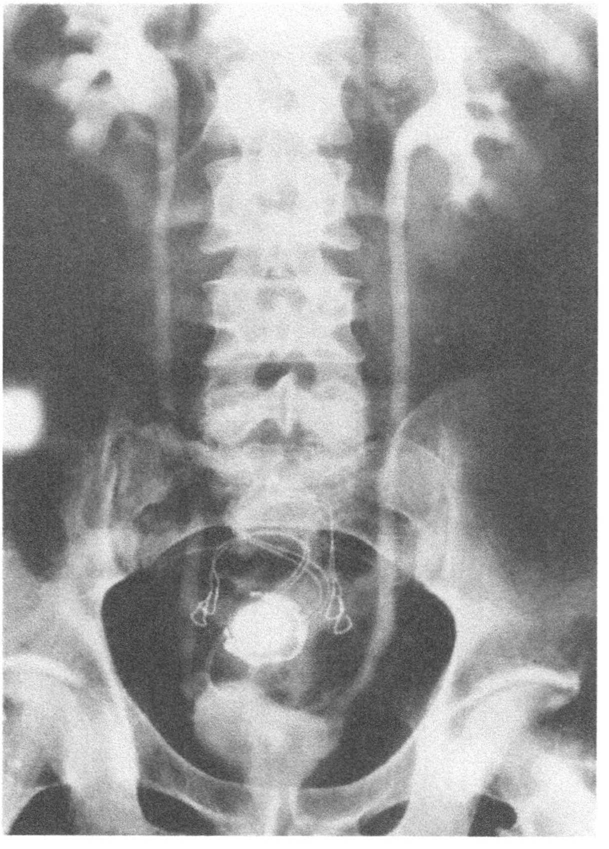

Fig. 33. Male, 30 years, spinal cord injury. Excretory urogram 3 months after ceasing electrical stimulation. Accentuation of the uretero-pelvic dilatation

At the onset of stimulation, it was noted that the base of the bladder was drawn upwards giving the bladder a spherical shape; the bladder neck gradually opened, the urine flowing into the posterior urethra and micturition was triggered normally. After about 30 seconds, when 300—350 ml were eliminated, the opaque substance in the posterior urethra became gradually narrower until it disappeared following contraction of the striate sphincter musculature and perineal musculature (last image). A new stimulation, at 2—5 min interval, produced contraction of the detrusor and opening of the bladder neck. After evacuation of the contrast medium, the neurostimulator could be discerned on the anterior aspect of the sacrum

In electrically-induced micturition the base of the bladder does not descend at the beginning of micturition, due to traction of the prostate by the detrusor muscular fibers. When intravesical pressure rises sufficiently it overcomes the resistance of the smooth and striate muscle.

Contraction of the perineal striate muscle is triggered at the beginning of electrical stimulation; however, urethral resistance is overcome for some time by pressure of the urine. The jet is interrupted by amplification of the contraction of the pelvic floor musculature and not by a decrease in the contraction force of the detrusor.

Automatism developed after 25 days electrical stimulation, which was then stopped, the bladder being evacuated by reflex contraction under control of the spinal sacral micturition center.

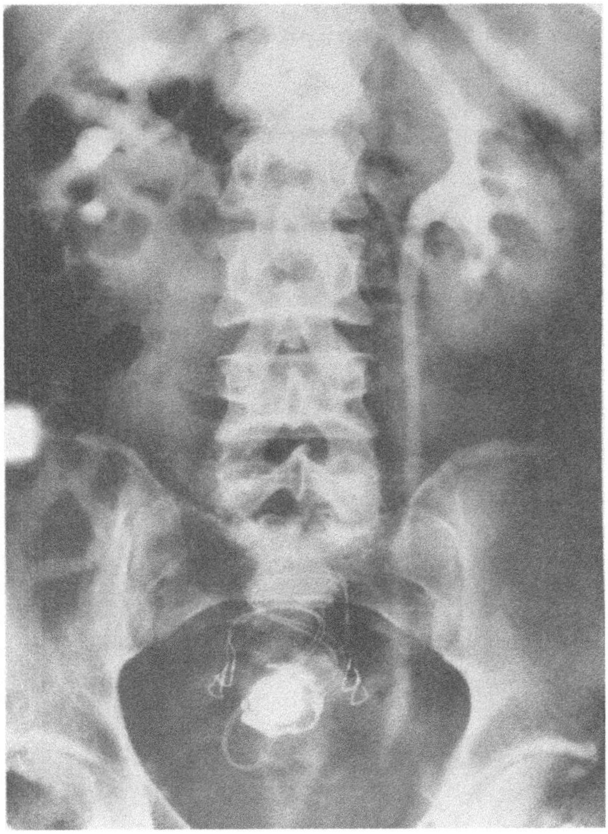

Fig. 34. Male, 30 years, spinal cord injury. Excretory urogram one year after ceasing electrical stimulation

At the control examination, 7 months after implantation of the neurostimulator, reflex automatic voiding of the bladder was efficient, the urine sterile and without any residue.

*Case 4.* The patient M.P., aged 20 years (case card No. 48,587) suffered from spinal cord trauma on March 30, 1967, with fracture of two lumbar vertebrae. Laminectomy also revealed involvement of the sacral micturition center. Flaccid paraplegia and urinary retention appeared immediately after the accident and an indwelling catheter was introduced. Escherichia coli developed in the uroculture. Nine months after the accident, the pelvic nerves were exposed for neurostimulation.

Intraoperative mono- and bilateral electric stimulation of the pelvic nerves gave no response; the detrusor did not contract and no changes occurred in intravesical pressure. Electrical stimulation, inefficient due to degeneration of the parasympathetic preganglionic nervous fibers, had to be given up. Consequently, electrical neurostimulation is contraindicated in lower motor neurone lesions, in the late phase of the accident.

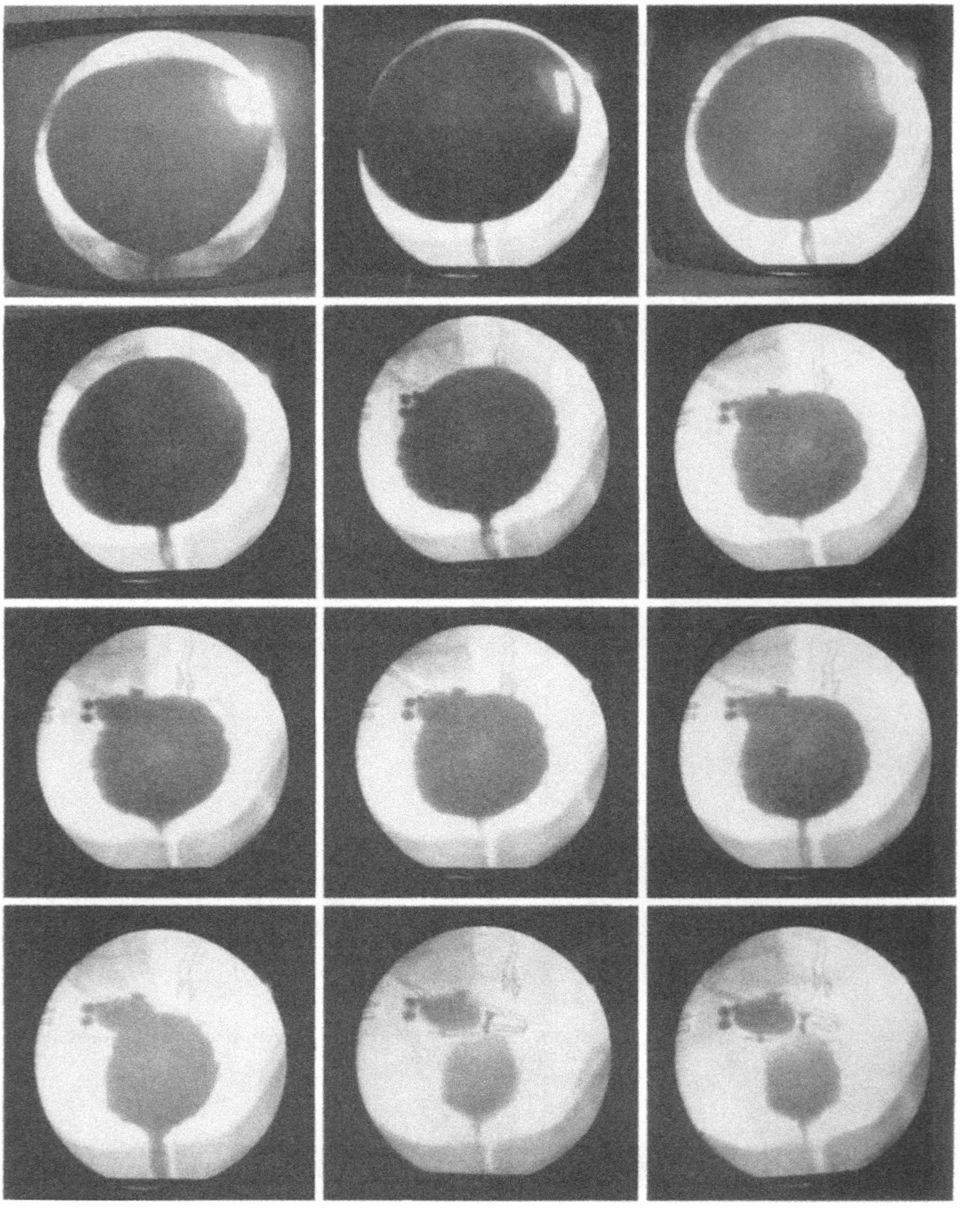

Fig. 35. Male, 31 years, spinal cord injury at $Th_9$ level, serial voiding cystourethrogram induced by electrical stimulation of the pelvic nerves and followed up in the videorecorder. Two successive stimulations. Note opening of the bladder neck and its closure by contraction of the striate sphincter. The neurostimulator can be seen behind the bladder

On analysing the clinical cases in which neurostimulation was applied (Table 2), it will be seen that the urinary disturbances developed in 3 patients after section of the spinal cord, above the micturition reflex center. In the fourth case the spinal injury destroyed the sacral micturition reflex center. The patients with lesion of the upper motor neurone were able to take up again bladder reflex activity after electrical stimulation.

### d) Deinhibition of the Sacral Micturition Reflex Center by Electrical Stimulation

In cases of spinal injury above the sacral reflex micturition center, electrical stimulation led to the recovery of vesical reflectivity within a short interval. This is of particular importance for the future of the urinary tract in spinal patients. Electric neurostimulation applied as early as possible after the spinal injury, when the sacral micturition center remains intact, deinhibits this center. The recovery of bladder reflectivity unquestionably takes place more rapidly following electrical stimulation. It is known that spinal shock, accompanied by vesical areflectivity may last 6—8 weeks or more.

Habib (1967) likewise noted that direct electrical stimulation of the detrusor in a patient with incomplete section of the spinal cord at the level of the 6th cervical vertebra provoked a return of spinal reflectivity.

Sternberg, Burnette and Bunts (1967) also observed that direct electrical stimulation of the bladder muscle influences the state of reflectivity of the detrusor, the reflex contraction of the bladder appearing after a period of 8 to 14 days in 3 patients with lesions above the sacral micturition center. The spinal lesions were located in two cases at the level of the 6th cervical vertebra and in one case at Th 10 level. In cervical lesions the interval from the accident up to electrical stimulation was of 11 and 8 months, and in the thoracic lesion, of 6 weeks, which implies that the spinal shock phase had passed but recovery of the bladder reflectivity was not efficient. Recovery of the bladder reflectivity after endovesical electrical stimulation was also noted by Ascoli and Federici (1964), who considered it indicated in the first week after the spinal injury or during the period when reflex contraction of the bladder is inefficient and the residue over 100 to 150 ml.

The fourth patient in Table 2 did not respond to intraoperative electrical stimulation of the pelvic nerves, due to degeneration of the sacral parasympathetic preganglionic neurone. Consequently, the major indication of direct stimulation of the detrusor is to be found in destructive lesions of the spinal sacral micturition center and in section of the motor or sensory pathways of the sacral micturition reflex arc.

Moreover, Staubitz et al. (1966) demonstrated experimentally that the excitability of the detrusor to stimulation of the pelvic nerves decreases in intensity and disappears after 7 days in animals with section of the cord at cauda equina level. Histologic examination revealed atrophy of the spinal ganglion without evident atrophy of the pelvic nerves.

## II. Electrical Myostimulation of the Urinary Bladder

Direct electrical myostimulation of the urinary bladder is done with electrodes fixed in the bladder wall.

The shape, number, size, site of implantation and material from which the electrodes are made vary from one author to another. Disk, wire or metal network electrodes have been used, and the number of the electrodes ranges from 2 to 10. The disk electrodes measure 0.5 to 1.5 cm in diameter and the length of the leads depends upon the size of the bladder. The best site for implantation of the electrodes is the trigger area, where a great number of vesical nervous fibers are to be found close to the uretero-vesical junctions. Experiments have been carried out with platinum, steel, gold, tantalum, iridium and graphite electrodes, but the best appear to be the platinum ones. The use of a large number of electrodes for direct stimulation of the bladder muscle produces stronger contractions of the bladder with a lower voltage of the electric current. The same effect can be obtained with a smaller number of electrodes if they are implanted in the area of greater concentration of nervous vesical fibers.

### a) The Parameters of the Electric Stimulus

Table 1 shows the parameters of the electrical stimuli used by different authors in experimental studies and in clinical applications for direct stimulation of the detrusor or for neurostimulation.

The values used for the electrical stimulus parameters vary very much; the voltage from 2.5 to 25 V, intensity from 20 to 60 mA, duration from 1 to 100 msec and frequency of the electrical stimulus from 20 to 60 Hz. This variability is due to the experimental conditions, the thickness and morphologic state of the bladder wall, the shape and site of implantation of the electrodes, the amount of fluid in the bladder and size of the bladder.

Eisenberg, Murno, Glenn and Hageman (1965) who carried out research work on the voltage in different kinds of stimulations, considered that for electrical stimulation of the urinary bladder via the sacral nerves 2.5 volts are necessary, via the pelvic nerves 5—10 volts and for direct stimulation of the detrusor 10—20 volts.

Schamaun and Kantrowitz (1963) relate that in spinal dogs evacuation of the urinary bladder by direct stimulation of the detrusor necessitates a voltage of 20—30 V.

Jonge, Kornelis and Berg (1966) demonstrated that the intravesical pressures obtained by direct stimulation of the detrusor in spinal animals, in chronic experiments, are greater the longer is the interval after transection of the cord. Although vesical pressure is superior to normal micturition pressures, urethral resistance cannot be overcome and requires a supplementary increase in pressure, obtained only by augmenting the voltage. This, on the other hand may lead to irradiation of the electrical current, that implicitly brings about an increased force of contraction of the perineal musculature.

Ellis, Parker and Hills (1964) drew attention to the fact that high values of the electrical stimulus parameters produce fibrosis at the level of the electrodes increasing the threshold of electric stimulation of the bladder muscle, which in turn leads to the use of more powerful stimuli, aggravating tissular destruction. Most authors report upon the negative effect of the electrical current when more than 10 volts are applied.

The optimal frequency and duration of the electrical stimulus in myostimulation established experimentally by Jonce, Kornelis and Berg (1966) are very close to the optimal values found by Burghele et al. for neurostimulation. However, they apply the electrodes in the area of maximum concentration of the vesical nerves.

According to Graber and Rutishauser (1965) the maximum value of the voltage should be of 4 V, since higher values produce pain and urethral resistance. An electrical current of more than 30 mA produces burns at the site of implantation of the electrodes. The great variety of the tension, duration and frequency of the stimulus to which the detrusor muscle responds following direct stimulation does not make it possible to establish mean values.

### b) Resistance of the Bladder to Electrical Stimulation

Kantrowitz and Schamaun (1963) established the resistance or impedance of the urinary bladder to be of 90 to 390 ohms, with an average value of 183 ohms, and Bradley, Wittmers and Chou (1963) found that impedance ranged between 40 and 100 ohms in terms of the number of electrodes used; the values of Potempa and Dittmar (1965) varied between 35 and 100 ohms, and of Alexander and Rowan (1965) between 70 and 370 ohms. An average value of 172 ohms was found between the electrodes, in the vicinity of the uretero-vesical junction by Hald et al. (1966). Resistance falls to 95 ohms when another two electrodes are placed, one on the anterior aspect and the other on the posterior aspect of the bladder.

Wear et al. (1967) give much higher values than the forementioned authors. Thus, between electrodes placed anterior and inferior to the ureteral orifices he found that resistance varies from 2000 to 5000 ohms, and between the electrodes placed on the vesical dome, from 7000 to 18,000 ohms. Still higher values were found (20,000 to 30,000 ohms) when the electrodes did not come in perfect contact with the bladder. The higher is the resistance the greater must the tension of the electrical current be to obtain efficient contractions of the bladder.

## III. Electrical Stimulation of the Anterior Sacral Roots

Electrical stimulation of the anterior sacral roots was practiced by Meirowsky et al. (1950) in order to determine the content of these roots in motor fibers innervating the bladder. They found that the third anterior sacral root contains several parasympathetic fibers and that their stimulation produces high intravesical pressures.

Habib (1963, 1965, 1967), following the unsatisfactory results obtained by direct stimulation of the detrusor, resorted to stimulation of the sacral roots for evacuation of the bladder. He found that electric stimulation of the second anterior sacral root produced tonic and clonic contractions of the lower limbs in man without increasing intravesical pressure or modifying urethral resistance.

Stimulation of the third anterior sacral root produces powerful erection, and unilateral electrical stimulation of the fourth anterior sacral root, on its emergence from the foramen, produces optimal evacuation of the bladder.

Electrical stimulation of the anterior sacral roots was applied by Habib to two patients with lesions of the superior motor neurone. However, in his publications he does not mention the interval between the accident and electrical stimulation, the quality of the detrusor contraction, the state of voiding of the bladder, the amount of vesical residue and resistance to evacuation due to contraction of the perineal musculature.

At variance with the data in literature is evacuation of the bladder obtained by unilateral stimulation of the fourth anterior sacral root which does not contain the largest number of motor fibers innervating the bladder.

Experimental investigations on electrical stimulation of the anterior sacral roots were likewise carried out by Hald, Agrawal and Kantrowitz (1966), who reported on the powerful effect of stimulation upon the striate musculature innervated by the sacral plexus and incomplete evacuation of the bladder, the vesical residue being of more than 30 ml. They also found that the pressures obtained by electrical stimulation of the anterior sacral roots falls from 81 cm of water to 20 cm of water after 32 days. A higher intravesical pressure can only be obtained by increasing the voltage, but emptying of the bladder is incomplete and a residue of 120 ml remains.

## IV. Transrectal Electrical Stimulation of the Urinary Bladder

Dees (1965, 1967) and Grice and Makow (1965) experimented on the possibility of evacuating the urinary bladder by transrectal electrical stimulation with a bipolar electrode placed on the anterior wall of the rectum, in the zone of higher concentration of the nervous fibers of the pelvic plexus.

In mice, cats and dogs transrectal stimulation produces evacuation of the bladder but only at high tensions. The stimulation provokes pain and contraction of the perineal and abdominal muscles and of the hind legs.

Dees applied transrectal stimulation in the clinic to 4 patients, one normal and the other three with spinal cord lesions, but did not obtain evacuation of the bladder. In the normal individual, a stimulus of 2 mA produces contraction of the levator ani and bulbocavernosus muscles. Increase of the current to 3,5 mA propuces rectal pain and powerful contraction of the perineal musculature. Rectal pain becomes unbearable at 3.5 mA.

In the patients with spinal cord lesions the transrectal electrical stimulation applied did not produce voiding of the bladder in spite of the high intensity of the stimulus. In two patients the spinal cord was sectioned at C6 and respectively Th6 level and in the third patient intervertebral disk hernia produced compression of the spinal cord at the level of the fifth cervical vertebra.

Transrectal electric stimulation of the urinary bladder is not applicable in the clinic.

## V. Neuro- or Myo-Electrical Stimulation of the Urinary Bladder?

The experimental and clinical studies carried out up to the present in electrical stimulation of the detrusor or of the pelvic nerves permit a comparison of the two methods.

In clinical applications, American authors prefered myostimulation (30 applications). As may be seen from Table 3 the results cannot be considered to plead for the unreserved application of myostimulation. There are still many drawbacks to be eliminated before complete evacuation of the bladder can be obtained by myostimulation without the untoward side effects described.

Although the clinical statistics of neurostimulation only includes four cases, the results obtained in lesions of the upper motor neurone are homogenous, with complete emptying of the bladder and without side-effects. Contraction of the perineal musculature, that occurs with both kinds of stimulation, did not prevent complete emptying of the bladder on stimulation of the pelvic nerves.

In all the cases of lesion of the upper motor neurone, stimulation of the pelvic nerves favoured deinhibition of the sacral parasympathetic micturition center. Similarly, perfect tolerance of the receiver included within the organism was noted.

Susset and Boctor (1967) consider that stimulation of the nerves results in lesion of the nerves, pain, erection and incomplete evacuation of the bladder, because of concomitant contraction of the striate sphincter and striate perineal musculature.

Graber and Rutishauser (1965) demonstrated experimentally the more rapid and superior response of the bladder to stimulation of the pelvic nerves in comparison to stimulation of the detrusor, as well as the difference in tension necessary for the two stimuli. In stimulation of the pelvic nerves, an intravesical pressure of 100 mm Hg was obtained with a stimulus of 4 V, whereas in myostimulation a tension of 16 V was necessary to obtain a pressure of 70 mm Hg.

According to Hald, Agrawall and Kantrowitz (1966) neurostimulation rather than myostimulation produces contraction of the external sphincter and perineal musculature, although they believe that irradiation of the current occurs directly from the detrusor to the urethra and not by nervous pathways.

As demonstrated, irrespective of the way in which the electric current is produced, irradiation occurs more readily when the tension of the current is higher. From this point of view, neurostimulation has the advantage of producing artificial micturition with an electrical stimulus of 2.5 V.

Staubitz et al. (1966) noted the advantage of neurostimulation, whose effect on intravesical pressure is more evident when some time has elapsed after the accident, due to hypertrophy of the detrusor that contracts reflexly or by electrical induction. Applying an electrical stimulus 20 weeks after the accident they obtained an intravesical pressure of 85 mm Hg, whereas in the acute experiment a pressure of 27.5 mm Hg, was obtained following stimulation of the pelvic nerves. In neurostimulation, the response of the detrusor diminishes when deterioration due to overdistension and sclerosis occurs.

A contradictory opinion exists on the opportunity of either one or other form of neurostimulation in terms of the level of the spinal cord lesion. Susset and Boctor (1967) consider that neurostimulation is not indicated in lesions of the lower motor neurone because of involvement of the micturition reflex arc. This was demonstrated in the clinic by Burghele and Ichim. According to Bradley et al. (1963) myostimulation is particularly indicated in lesion of the lower motor neurone, of traumatic origin, and may also be applied in spina bifida, tabes, diabetes and congenital or acquired flaccid bladder.

Graber and Rutishauser (1965) likewise recommend myostimulation in lesions of the lower motor neurone, considering that paralysis of the striate perineal musculature prevents it from opposing any resistance to evacuation of the bladder to the same extent as in lesions of the upper motor neurone. Moreover, in these cases, transection of the pudendal nerves for lowering urethral resistance is more readily accepted, erection being compromised by the spinal cord lesion.

Although Susset and Boctor (1967) believe that myostimulation is not applicable in the spinal shock phase, Bradley et al. (1963) consider that electrical stimulation of the bladder must be applied as early as possible after injury to the spinal cord. Application of electrical stimulation immediately after paralysis of the bladder prevents overdistension, inactivity of the detrusor or infection of the bladder, hence substitution of the smooth vesical muscle by cicatricial tissue, hypertrophy of the detrusor due to excessive autonomic activity or involvement of the blood or lymph circulation leading to nutritional disturbances of the smooth muscle.

## VI. The Indications of Electrical Stimulation of the Urinary Bladder

Following the accumulate experience in clinical application of electrical stimulation of the urinary bladder via the pelvic nerves and directly on the bladder muscle, the indications of this stimulation can be outlined.

### 1. Spinal Cord Injury

a) Lesions of the upper motor neurone: stimulation of the pelvic nerves immediately after the injury.

b) Lesions of the lower motor neuron: stimulation of the detrusor as early as possible after spinal transection.

## 2. Neurologic Diseases of the Spinal Cord

a) Tabes: stimulation of the pelvic nerves or detrusor applied in the reversible phase of the bladder lesions produced by overdistension or infection.

b) Transverse myelitis: neuro- or myostimulation according to the level of the lesion as in spinal injury.

c) Demyelinating diseases of the central nervous system, multiple sclerosis, amyotrophic lateral sclerosis with areflex neurogenic bladder; neuro- or myostimulation in terms of the involvement of the spinal micturition reflex center.

d) Meningomyelocele with areflex neurogenic bladder; neuro- or myostimulation.

e) Compression of the spinal cord by disk hernia or of other origin: neuro- or myostimulation according to the site, degree and age of the compression.

Table 3. *Clinical application of electrical stimulation*

| Author | Year | Level of lesion | Interval after the accident |
|---|---|---|---|
| SCOTT, QUESADA, CARDUS, LASKOWSKI | 1965 | 1. $Th_3$—$Th_4$ | 12 months |
| DEES | 1965 | 2. $Th_6$<br>3. $C_6$ | $4^1/_2$ months<br>24 hours |
| MARKLAND, CHOU, BRADLEY, WESTGATE, WOLFSON | 1966 | 4. $Th_{10}$ | 40 days |
| WISCHNEWSKY, LIWSCHITZ, CHODOROV | 1967 | 5. $Th_{12}$—$L_1$ | 6 months |
| SUSSET, BOCTOR | 1967 | 6. $Th_4$ | 44 months |
| HABIB | 1967 | 7. $C_6$<br>8. $C_6$<br>9. $Th_7$ | not reported<br>not reported<br>not reported |
| HALD, MEIER, KHALILI, AGRAWAL, BENTON, KANTROWITZ | 1967 | 10. $Th_{12}$ incomplete | 26 months |
| CHOU, BRADLEY, MARKLAND | 1967 | 11. $L_1$, $Th_{12}$<br>12. $Th_{11}$<br>13. cervical<br>14. cervical<br>15. conus<br>16. $C_6$<br>17. $Th_{10}$—$Th_{11}$<br>18. $C_6$ | not reported<br>not reported<br>not reported<br>not reported<br>not reported<br>not reported<br>not reported<br>not reported |
| BURGHELE, ICHIM | 1967 | 19. $Th_{11}$—$Th_{12}$ spinal shock<br>20. $Th_8$ spinal shock<br>21. $Th_9$ spinal shock<br>22. $L_2$ | 22 days<br>26 days<br>31 days<br>9 months |
| STERNBERG, BURNETTE, BUNTS | 1967 | 23. $C_6$<br>24. $Th_{10}$ spinal shock<br>25. $C_6$<br>26. $C_6$ | 11 months<br>6 weeks<br>9 months<br>8 months |

## VII. The Results of Electrical Stimulation of the Urinary Bladder

Electrical stimulation of the urinary bladder was applied in 39 patients, of whom 26 with spinal cord injuries and 13 with diseases of the nervous system accompanied by micturition disturbances (Tables 3 and 4).

Stimulation of the detrusor was performed in 30 cases, of the pelvic nerves in 4 cases, of the sacral nerves in 2 cases, and transrectal stimulation in 3 cases.

Stimulation of the detrusor was followed by complete evacuation of the bladder in 4 cases, incomplete evacuation in 9 cases (a residue of 175 ml being found in a single patient) and failure in 17 cases.

Stimulation of the pelvic nerves was applied in 4 cases, with complete evacuation of the bladder in 3 and failure in 1 case. The effect of stimulation of the

*of the urinary bladder in spinal cord injuries*

| Site of stimulation | Evacuation of the bladder | Side effects |
|---|---|---|
| detrusor | absent | Contraction of perineal muscles |
| transrectal | absent | absent |
| transrectal | absent | erection |
| detrusor | absent | contraction of striate m. of the lower limbs |
| detrusor | complete | absent |
| detrusor | incomplete | absent |
| detrusor | incomplete | clonic contractions of lower limbs |
| sacral III | not reported | absent |
| sacral IV | not reported | not reported |
| detrusor | incomplete residue 175 $cm^2$ | not reported |
| detrusor | absent | absent |
| detrusor | absent | absent |
| detrusor | absent | needle-like sensation in the lower limbs absent |
| detrusor | absent | absent |
| detrusor | absent | absent |
| detrusor | absent | absent |
| detrusor | absent | absent |
| detrusor | absent | absent |
| pelvic nerves | complete (2—3 successive stimulations) | contraction of external sphincter |
| pelvic nerves | complete (2—3 successive stimulations) | contraction of external sphincter |
| pelvic nerves | complete (2—3 successive stimulations) | contraction of external sphincter |
| pelvic nerves | absent | absent |
| detrusor | absent | not reported |
| detrusor | incomplete | not reported |
| detrusor | absent | contraction of perineal muscles |
| detrusor | absent | not reported |

Table 4. *Clinical application of electrical stimulation of the urinary bladder in diseases of the nervous system*

| Author | Year | No. | Diagnosis and level of lesion | Site of stimulation | Evacuation of the bladder | Side effects |
|---|---|---|---|---|---|---|
| BOYCE, LATHEM, HUND | 1964 | 1 | not reported | detrusor | absent | pain + muscular contractions |
| | | 2 | not reported | detrusor | incomplete evacuation | absent |
| | | 3 | degeneration of the spinal conus | detrusor | complete | absent |
| PEDERSEN, JAKOBSEN, GRYNDERUP | 1965 | 4 | multiple sclerosis | detrusor | incomplete | pain with a tenesmus caracter |
| DEES | 1965 | 5 | disk hernia $C_5$ | trans-rectal | absent | rectal pain |
| HABIB | 1967 | 6 | meningo-myelocele | detrusor | incomplete Residue 150—200 ml | strong pains. Discomfort |
| HALD, MEIER, KHALILI, AGRAWAL, BENTON, KANTROWITZ | 1967 | 7 | spina bifida meningomyelo-cele | detrusor | complete | needle-like sensation in the lower abdomen |
| | | 8 | transverse myelitis $Th_9$ | detrusor | incomplete | absent |
| | | 9 | spinal metastasis $Th_{12}$ schiso-stomiasis | detrusor | incomplete | contraction of striate sphinc-terial muscula-ture. Pain |
| CHOU, BRADLEY, MARKLAND | 1967 | 10 | metastatic tumor $Th_5$ | detrusor | absent | absent |
| | | 11 | cerebral tumor | detrusor | complete evacuation | absent |
| | | 12 | meningo-myelocele $T_{10}$ | detrusor | complete evacuation | absent |
| | | 13 | meningo-myelocele | detrusor | absent | pain |

sacral nerves has not been reported. Transrectal stimulation did not induce voiding of the bladder.

Complete evacuation of the bladder on myostimulation was obtained in a case of spinal cord injury (WISCHNEWSKY et al., 1967) and 3 cases of diseases of the nervous system: 2 meningomyoceles (HALD et al., 1967; CHOU et al., 1967) and a cerebral tumor (CHOU et al., 1967). The parameters of the electrical stimulus used in the case of spinal cord injury were of 10 V, 1 msec and 20 Hz. In one of the cases of meningocele the electrical signal was of 40 mA, but produced a sensation of "pins and needles" in the lower abdomen.

Evacuation of the bladder was incomplete following stimulation of the detrusor in 4 cases of spinal injury and 5 cases of neurologic conditions. The voltage or intensity of the electrical stimulus was variable, but as a rule the values were

Table 5. *Results of clinical electrical stimulation in cases of spinal cord injury and neurologic diseases*

| Stimulation of | Voiding of the bladder | | No. voiding | Not stated |
|---|---|---|---|---|
| | complete | incomplete | | |
| Detrusor | 4 | 9 | 17 | — |
| Pelvic nerves | 3 | — | 1 | — |
| Sacral nerves | — | — | — | 2 |
| Transrectal | — | — | 4 | — |

high. For instance, Habib (1967) used 25—40 V for stimulation of the sacral nerves, and Dees (1965) 40 mA for transrectal stimulation.

The failures met with in clinical applications occurred in 16 cases of spinal cord injury and 4 cases of neurologic disease, following direct stimulation of the detrusor (17 cases), stimulation of the pelvic nerves (1 case) and transrectal stimulation (3 cases). Whenever the parameters of the electrical signal are given, the values are high. Hence, it may be deduced that failure or incomplete evacuation was brought about by concomitant contraction of the striate sphincter and perineal musculature following irradiation of the electrical stimulus.

Failure may also be attributed to the interval elapsing after the accident or the onset of the neurological disease, up to application of electrical stimulation. The longer this interval is, the greater is the alteration of the bladder caused by infection and sclerosis. Only two patients were subjected to myostimulation in the phase of spinal shock (Markland et al., 1966; Sternberg et al., 1967). In all the other cases a period of 6 to 44 months elapsed after the accident or onset of the neurologic disease sufficient for the period of spinal shock to have come to an end. Normally, in such cases the bladder must take up its reflex activity, efficient to a greater or lesser extent in terms of the destruction of the bladder wall brought about by infection and sclerosis.

Drainage was applied in all the cases before myostimulation and the detrusor was modified by infection, overdistension or prolonged inactivity. It is known that overdistension or prolonged drainage modifies the excitability of the detrusor, the smooth vesical muscle being replaced by collagen tissue, as demonstrated by Bradley, Chou, Markland and Swaiman (1965) who injected sclerosing solutions into the bladder wall. The contraction force of the detrusor was appraised by recording intravesical pressures, and histologic or biochemical studies for the determination of collagen proteins. Although increase of the fibrous tissue to the detriment of the muscular tissue is difficult to detect histologically, it is certain that fibrozing of the bladder wall significantly lowers the response to direct stimulation of the detrusor.

Diminution of the excitability of the detrusor demands an increase in the tension of the electrical current which, however, amplifies irradiation and hence contraction of the perineal striate musculature, rendering electrical stimulation inoperative.

A vicious circle is thus created, that can only be prevented by applying myostimulation before the onset of structural alterations of the detrusor, therefore as early as possible after the spinal trauma.

Although Susset and Boctor (1967) do not consider that myostimulation is indicated in the spinal shock phase when the bladder may recover its reflectivity, in lesions of the upper motor neurone the reflex activity of the detrusor and its future function depend upon the duration of drainage. To avoid this drainage, electric stimulation becomes a necessity even in the spinal shock phase. In diseases of the nervous system, with micturition disorders and an infected, distended bladder with chronic retention, the chances of success in myostimulation are conditioned by the possibility of the detrusor to contract.

Stimulation of the pelvic nerves in 3 cases of lesion of the upper motor neurone, 22, 26 and respectively 31 days after the accident, was followed by complete voiding of the bladder after 2—3 successive stimulations and recovery of the reflex activity of the bladder by deinhibition of the micturition reflex center, 10—15 days after starting neurostimulation.

Deinhibition of the reflex micturition center by electrical stimulation was first observed by Habib (1967) and Hald et al. (1967). This is an important argument in favour of applying electrical stimulation of the urinary bladder as early as possible after the accident.

Electrical stimulation of the pelvic nerves in lesions of the lower motor neurone becomes inefficient after degeneration of nerves. Degeneration of the preganglionic nervous fibers, consequent to destruction of the sacral parasympathetic micturition reflex center lowers conduction of the electric impulses also at the level of the uretero-vesical junctions, as reported by Jonce, Kornelis and Berg (1966), who demonstrated experimentally by myostimulation that an intensity of up to 90 mA is necessary in order to obtain complete evacuation of the bladder content in such situations.

The level of the lesion cannot be incriminated as a cause of failure in direct electrical stimulation of the detrusor. Failures were recorded in lesions of both the upper and the lower motor neurone. Electrical stimulation was applied in 8 cases of cervical spinal lesions, 7 thoracic lesions and 3 lumbar lesions, i.e. 15 cases of lesion of the upper motor neurone and 3 cases of lesions of the lower motor neurone.

The effect of stimulation of the sacral nerves on evacuation of the bladder is not described in detail by Habib. It appears paradoxical that he should have obtained contractions of the bladder by stimulating with a fairly low voltage the fourth anterior sacral root, which contains only a small number of fibers coursing towards the detrusor.

Transrectal stimulation was not followed by voiding of the bladder and the method is contraindicated in the clinic because of the pain and contraction of the perineal striate musculature generated by the high voltage and intensity of the stimulus.

The clinical results of electrical stimulation of the neurogenic urinary bladder emphasize the complex problems to which this method gives rise, and to which no satisfactory solution has yet been found, in spite of the long and minute experimental studies carried out.

## References

### *A. The Architectonics of the Musculature of the Urinary Bladder, Terminal Ureters, Trigone and Urethra*

Bro-Rasmussen, F., Halborg Sørensen, A., Bredahl, E., Kelstrup, A.: The structure and function of the bladder. Urol. int. (Basel) **19**, 280—285 (1965).

Burghele, Th., Ichim, V., Demetrescu, M.: L'électroexcitation de la vessie médullaire. Étude expérimentale. J. Urol. méd. chir. **64**, 317 (1958).

— — — Contribution à la physiologie de la miction. Étude expérimentale. J. Urol. méd. chir. **65**, 43 (1959).

Cooper, E. R. A.: Human histology. London: H. K. Lewis & Co. 1948.

DEBLED, G.: La fonction normale et pathologique de la musculature ureterotrigonale. Acta urol. belg. **36**, 366 (1968).

DENNY-BROWN, D.: Nervous disturbances of vesical sphincter. New Engl. J. med. **15**, 647 (1936).

DIESE, J.: Harnorgane. In: Bardelebens Handbuch der Anatomie des Menschen. Jena: Gustav Fischer 1902.

EINHORNING, G.: Simultaneous recording of intravesical and intraurethral pressure. A study on urethral closure in normal and stress incontinent women. Acta chir. scand., Suppl. 276 (1961).

GIL VERNET: Physiologie der Miktion. Z. Urol. **53**, 180—202, 223—251 (1960).

GRIFFITHS, J.: Observations on the urinary bladder and urethra. J. Anat. and Physiol. **25**, 535 (1891).

GRUBER, C. M.: Function of uretero-vesical valve and experimental production of hydroureters without obstruction. J. Urol. (Baltimore) **23**, 161 (1930).

HANCOCK, H.: On normal micturition. Lancet **1852 I**, 211—215.

HUNTER, W. D. DE, JR.: New concept of urinary bladder musculature. J. Urol. (Baltimore) **71**, 695 (1954).

— Musculature of the prostate gland. Brit. J. Urol. **40**, 278 (1968).

HUTCH, J. A.: Nonobstructive dilatation of upper urinary tract. J. Urol. (Baltimore) **71**, 412 (1954).

— Panel on ureteral reflux in children. J. Urol. (Baltimore) **85**, 119 (1961).

— A new theory of the anatomy of the internal urinary sphincter and the physiology of micturition. Invest. Urol. **3**, 36 (1965).

— A new theory of the anatomy of the internal urinary sphincter and the physiology of micturition. II. The base plate. J. Urol. (Baltimore) **96**, 182 (1966).

— RAMBO, O. N., JR.: A new theory of the anatomy of the internal urinary sphincter and the physiology of micturition. III. Anatomy of the urethra. J. Urol. (Baltimore) **97**, 696 (1967).

— — IV. The urinary sphincter mecanism. J. Urol. (Baltimore) **97**, 705 (1967).

KALISCHER, O.: Die Urogenitalmusculatur des Dammes, mit besonderer Berücksichtigung des Harnblasenverschlusses. XIII. Berlin: Karger 1900.

KJELLBERG, S. R., ERICSSON, N. O., RUDHE, U.: The lower urinary tract in childhood. Chicago: The Yearbook Publ., Inc. 1957.

KOHLRAUSCH, O.: Zur Anatomie und Physiologie der Beckenorgane. Leipzig 1854.

LAPIDES, J.: Structure and function of the internal vesical sphincter. J. Urol. (Baltimore) **80**, 341 (1958).

— Further observations on the kinetics of the urethrovesical sphincter. J. Urol. (Baltimore) **84**, 86 (1960).

— HODGSON, N. B., BOYD, R. E., SHOOK, E. L., LICHTWARDT, J. R.: Further observations on pharmacologic reactions of the bladder. J. Urol. (Baltimore) **79**, 707 (1958).

— SWEET, R. B., LEWIS, L. W.: Role of striated muscle in urination. J. Urol. (Baltimore) **77**, 247 (1957).

LEARMONTH, J. R.: A contribution to the neurophysiology of the urinary bladder in man. Brain **54**, 147 (1931).

LE GROS CLARK, E.: Some remarks on the anatomy and physiology of the urinary bladder and the sphincter of the rectum. J. Anat. and Physiol. **17**, 445 (1883).

MACLEOD, D.: Posterior wall of prostate gland. Brit. J. Urol. **14**, 153 (1942).

McCREA, E. D'ARCY: The musculature of the bladder. Proc. roy. Soc. Med. **19**, 35 (1926).

MELLICK, W. F., BRODEUR, A. E., KARELLOS, D. N.: A suggested classification of ureteral reflux and suggested treatment based on cineradiografic findings and simultaneous pressure recording by means of the strain gauge. J. Urol. (Baltimore) **88**, 35 (1962).

— — — NARYKA, J. J.: Abnormal hydrodynamics of the bladder and ureters as a cause of ureteral reflux. J. Urol. (Baltimore) **88**, 38 (1962).

— NARYKA, J. J.: Pressure studies of the normal and abnormal ureter in children by means of the strain gauge. J. Urol. (Baltimore) **83**, 267 (1960).

PRATHER, G. C.: Vesico-ureteral reflux. Report of case cured by operation. J. Urol. (Baltimore) **52**, 437 (1954).

SCHER, S.: Some observations on the anatomy of the bladder neck and posterior urethra with reference to the prostatic obstruction. Brit. J. Urol. **22**, 116 (1950).

TANAGHO, E. A., HUTCH, J. A.: Primary reflux. J. Urol. (Baltimore) **93**, 158 (1965).

— — MEYERS, F. H., RAMBO, O. N., JR.: Primary vesicoureteral reflux: experimental studies of its etiology. J. Urol. (Baltimore) **93**, 165 (1965).

— MEYERS, F. H., SMITH, D. R.: The trigone: anatomical and physiological considerations. 1. In relation to the ureterovesical junction. J. Urol. (Baltimore) **100**, 623 (1968).

Tanagho, E. A., Miller, E. R., Meyers, F. H., Corbett, R. K.: Observations on the dynamics of the bladder neck. Brit. J. Urol. **38**, 72 (1966).
— Pugh, R. C. B.: The anatomy and function of the ureterovesical junction. Brit. J. Urol. **35**, 151 (1963).
— Smith, D. R.: The anatomy and function of the bladder neck. Brit. J. Urol. **38**, 54 (1966).
— — Mechanism of urinary continence. 1. Embryologic, anatomic and pathologic considerations. J. Urol. (Baltimore) **100**, 640 (1968).
— — Meyers, F. H.: The trigone: Anatomical and physiological considerations. 2. In relation to the bladder neck. J. Urol. (Baltimore) **100**, 633 (1968).
Uhlenhuth, E., Hunter, W. T., Loechel, W. E.: Problems in the anatomy of the pelvis. Philadelphia: J. B. Lippincott Co. 1953.
Versari, R.: Richerche sulla tonaca muscolare della vesica urinaria specialmente sul musculo spihnctero interno. Ric. fatte lab. anat. norm. Univ. Roma **6**, 59 (1897—1898).
Wesson, M. B.: Anatomical, embryological and physiological studies of the trigone and neck of the bladder. J. Urol. (Baltimore) **9**, 279 (1920).
Woodburne, R. T.: Structure and function of the urinary bladder. J. Urol. (Baltimore) **84**, 79 (1960).
— Anatomy of the bladder. The neurogenic bladder. Baltimore: Williams & Wilkins Co. 1967.
— Anatomy of the bladder and bladder outlet. J. Urol. (Baltimore) **100**, 474 (1968).

### *B. Innervation of the Urinary Bladder and Sphincters*

Adler, A.: Über organisch-(kortikale) und funktionell-nervöse Blasenstörungen. Dtsch. Z. Nervenheilk. **65**, 72 (1920).
Anand, B. K., Dua, S.: Electrical stimulation of the limbic system of brain (visceral brain) in the waking animals. Indian J. med. Res. **44**, 107 (1956).
Barrington, F. J. F.: The relation of the hind-brain to micturition. Brain **44**, 23 (1921).
— The localization of the paths subserving micturition in the spinal cord of the cat. Brain **56**, 126 (1933).
Beattie, J., Kerr, A. S.: The effects of the encephalic stimulation on urinary bladder tonus. Brain **59**, 302 (1936).
Bechterew, W., Mislawsky, N.: Die Hirncenter für die Bewegung der Harnblase. Neurol. Zbl. **7**, 505 (1888).
Bors, E.: Segmental peripheral innervation of the urinary bladder. J. nerv. ment. Dis. **116**, 572 (1952).
Chambers, W. W., Jr.: Electrical stimulation of the interior of the cerebellum in the cat. Amer. J. Anat. **80**, 55 (1947).
Czyhlarz, E. V., Marburg, O.: Über cerebrale Blasenstörungen. Jb. Psychiat. Neurol. **20**, 134 (1901).
Elliot, T. R.: The innervation of the bladder and urethra. J. Physiol. (Lond.) **35**, 367 (1907).
Friedmann, M.: Zur Kenntnis der zerebralen Blasenstörungen und namentlich des Rindenzentrums für die Innervation der Harnblase. Münch. med. Wschr. **50**, 1591 (1903).
Gjone, R., Setekleiv, J.: Excitatory and inhibitory bladder responses to stimulation of the cerebral cortex in cat. Acta physiol. scand. **59**, 337 (1963).
Hamberger, B., Norberg, K. A.: Adrenergic synaptic terminals and nerve cells in bladder ganglia of the cat. Int. J. Neuropharm. **4**, 441 (1965).
Henneman, E.: Trans. Amer. neurol. Ass. **150** (1948). Cit. in ref. Kaada, B. R. (1951).
Hess, W. R., Brügger, M.: Der Miktions- und der Defäkationsakt als Erfolg zentraler Reizung. Helv. physiol. Acta **1**, 511 (1943).
Kaada, B. R.: Somato-motor, autonomic and electrocorticographic responses to electrical stimulation of "rhinencephalic" and other structures in primates, cat and dog. Study of responses from limbic, subcallosal, orbito-insular, piriform and temporal cortex, hippocampus, fornix and amygdala. Acta physiol. scand. **24**, Suppl. 83, 1—285 (1951).
— Andersen, P., Jansen, J., Jr.: Stimulation of amygdaloid nuclear complex in a unanesthetized cats. Neurology **4**, 48 (1954).
Kabat, H., Magoun, W., Ranson, S. W.: Reaction of the bladder to stimulation of points in the forebrain and mid-brain. J. comp. Neurol. **63**, 211 (1936).
Kabat, H. B., Anson, B. J., Magoun, H. W., Ranson, S. W.: Stimulation of the hypothalamus with special reference to the effect on gastrointestinal motility. Amer. J. Physiol. **12**, 214 (1935).
Katsuki, S., Okajina, T., Matsumoto, T.: Experimental studies on the autonomic function of the preoptic area. 1. Influences of electrical stimulation of the preoptic area upon the blood pressure and the mouvement of pelvic organs (urinary bladder, rectum and uterus). Kumamoto med. J. **8**, 180 (1955).

KLEIST, K.: Die Hirnverletzungen in ihrer Bedeutung für die Lokalisation der Hirnfunktionen. Neurol. Zbl. **12**, 414 (1918).

KOIKEGAMI, H., DODO, T., MOCHIDA, Y., TAKAHASHI, H.: Stimulation experiments on the amygdaloid nuclear complex and related structures. Effects upon the renal volume, urinary secretion, movements of the urinary bladder, blood pressure and respiratory movements. Folia psychiat. neurol. jap. **11**, 157 (1957).

KOYAMA, Y., MAKUYA, A., KURU, M.: Vesico-motor areas in the cat midbrain. Jap. J. Physiol. **12**, 63 (1962).

KREMER, W. F.: Autonomic and somatic reactions induced by stimulation of the cingular gyrus in dogs. J. Neurophysiol. **10**, 371 (1947).

KUNTZ, A.: The autonomic nervous system. Philadelphia: Lea & Febiger 1953.

— SACCOMANNO, G.: The sympathetic innervation of the detrusor muscle. J. Urol. (Baltimore) **51**, 535 (1944).

KURU, M.: Über die bulbären Endungen des anterolateral ascendierenden Bündels, unter besonderer Berücksichtigung eines neuen spino-bulbären Systems des Tractus spino-juxtasolitaris. Jap. J. med. Sci. I. Anat. **8**, 135 (1940a).

— Kritik des Chordotomieeffektes vom anatomischen Standpunkt aus. Dtsch. Z. Chir. **235**, 325 (1940b).

— The spino-bulbar tracts and the pelvic sensory vagus. Further contributions to the theory of the sensory dual innervation of the viscera. J. comp. Neurol. **104**, 207 (1956).

— HUKAYA, G.: Contributions to the knowledge of bulbar autonomic centers. I. Vesicorectal responses to electrical stimulation of the medulla oblongata. Jap. J. Physiol. **4**, 175 (1954).

— KAMIKAWA, K.: Unit discharges recordet from the medullary vesico-motor centers in response to filling and isometric contraction of the urinary bladder. Jap. J. Physiol. **10**, 142 (1960).

— KOYAMA, Y., OZAKI, H.: Part of the brain stem controlling the tone of external urethral sphincter. Proc. Jap. Acad. **39**, 530 (1963).

— OZAKI, H.: Evidence presented for the existence of the micturition center in the medulla. Proc. Jap. Acad. **35**, 186 (1959).

— YAMAMOTO, H.: Fiber connections of the pontine detrusor nucleus (Barrington). J. comp. Neurol. **123**, 161 (1964).

LANGWORTHY, O. R., KOLB, L. C.: Demonstration of encephalic control of micturition by electric stimulation. Bull. Johns Hopk. Hosp. **56**, 37 (1935).

— — LEWIS, L. G.: Physiology of micturition. Baltimore: Williams & Wilkins 1940.

— MURPHY, E. L.: Nerve endings in the urinary bladder. J. comp. Neurol. **71**, 487 (1939).

LEARMONTH, J. R.: A contribution to the neurophysiology of the urinary bladder in man. Brain **54**, 147 (1931).

MACLEAN, P. D., DELGADO, J. M. R.: Electrical and chemical stimulation of fronto-temporal portion of the limbic system in the waking animal. Electroencephalog. Clin. Neurophysiol. **5**, 91 (1953).

MATSUMOTO, H.: On the autonomic control of superior colliculus and limbic area to the bladder and rectum. Wakayama Igaku **8**, 65 (1957).

MOCHIDA, Y.: Stimulation of the amygdaloid nuclear complex, orbital surface of the frontal lobe and pes hippocampi, with special reference to its effects upon the movements of urinary bladder. Niigata Iggakkai Zasshi **71**, 767 (1957).

MUKAI, K.: Experimental studies on the bladder contraction point in gyrus cinguli and projection fibers from this point. Osaka Dagaku Igaku Zasshi **11**, 1645 (1959).

NESBIT, R. M., LAPIDES, J.: Tonus of the bladder during spinal shock. Arch. Surg. **56**, 139 (1948).

NICULESCU, I. T., ENACHESCU, A., COSOVEANU-VOINESCU, S.: Contribuţiuni la studiul terminaţiilor nervoase din vezica urinară şi ureter. Bul. st. S.S.M. **8**, 775 (1956).

NISHIYAMA, K.: Experimental studies on the bladder responses following electrical stimulation of the hypothalamus and its descending pathways. Osaka Daigaku Igaku Zasshi **11**, 4801 (1959).

PETERSEN, I., FRANKSSON, C.: Electromyographic study of the striated muscle of the male urethra. Brit. J. Mol. **27**, 148 (1955).

PFEIFER, B.: Über corticale Blasenstörungen und deren Lokalisation bei Hirnverletzten. Neurol. Zbl. **46**, 173 (1919).

PRESSMAN, YM. SHITOV, F. M.: On the relation between the cerebellum and the centers of the autonomous nervous system. Bull. exp. Biol. Med. **9**, 43 (1940).

RANSON, S. W., KABAT, H., MAGOUN, H. W.: Autonomic responses to electrical stimulation of hypothalamus, preoptic region and septum. Arch. Neurol. Psychiat. (Chic.) **33**, 467 (1935).

Riddoch, J.: Conduction of sensory impulses from the bladder by the inferior hypogastricus and the central afferents connections of the nerves. J. Physiol. (Lond.) **24**, 134 (1921).
Shearly, C. N., Peele, T. L.: Studies on amygdaloid nucleus of vat. J. Neurophysiol. **20**, 125 (1957).
Taber, E.: The cytoarchitecture of the brain stem of the cat. 1. Brain stem nuclei of cat. J. comp. Neurol. **116**, 27 (1961).
Takebayashi, H., Kobai, Y., Ushida, A., Matsumoto, H., Yoshioka, T., Arimoto, K. Shimizu, K., Matsuda, A., Kawashima, A., Jinya, Y., Fujita, I., Maeshima, S.: Superior colliculus, playing roles in the optokinetic and neuro-vegetative mechanism. Wakayama med. Rep. **4**, 1 (1937).
Tang, P. C.: Levels of brain stem and diencephalon controlling micturition reflex. J. Neurophysiol. **18**, 583 (1955).
— Ruch, T. C.: Localisation of brain stem and diencephalic areas controlling the micturition reflex. J. comp. Neurol. **196**, 213 (1956).
Tokunaga, S., Kuru, M.: Vesico-constrictor center and vesico-relaxer center in the medulla. Jap. J. Physiol. **9**, 365 (1959).
Uvnäs, B.: Effect of frequency of hypothalamic stimulation upon bladder responses. Proc. Soc. exp. Biol. (N.Y.) **64**, 181 (1947).
Wang, S. R., Ranson, S. W.: Autonomic responses to electrical stimulation of the lower brain stem. J. comp. Neurol. **71**, 437 (1939).
Yamaguchi, K.: Supplementary study on the sensory nerve supply of the human urinary bladder. Arch. Histol. Japan **19**, 6677 (1960).
Yokoyama, S., Ban, T., Korotsu, T.: Urinary bladder responses to the biolelectrical stimulation of the hypothalamus, preoptic areas in rabbits. Med. J. Osaka Univ. **11**, 191 (1960).
— Inoue, K., Ban, T.: Urinary bladder responses to the electrical stimulation of the cerebellum in rabbits. Med. J. Osaka Univ. **13**, 271 (1963).

### *C. Physiology of the Urinary Bladder and Sphincters*

Arbuckle, L. D., Paquin, A. J., Jr.: Experimental bladder neck obstruction. Invest. Urol. **1**, 173 (1963).
Bettex, M.: Le reflux vésico-uréteral chez l'enfant. Urol. int. (Basel) **22**, 97 (1967).
Bradley, W., Clarren, S., Shapiro, R., Wolfson, J.: Air cystometry. J. Urol. (Baltimore) **100**, 451 (1968).
Denny-Brown, D., Robertson, E. G.: On the physiology of micturition. Brain **56**, 149 (1933).
Emmet, J. L.: Urology. Philadelphia and London: W. B. Saunders Co. 1954.
Fister, G. M., Nichols, R. L., Zabriskie, C. V., Stucki, J. F.: Dynamic urethrography. A cineradiographic method. J. Urol. (Baltimore) **84**, 733 (1960).
Garrelts, B. von: Analysis of micturition. A new method of recording the voiding of the bladder. Acta chir. scand. **112**, 326 (1956).
— Intravesical pressure and urinary flow during micturition in normal subject. Acta chir. scand. **114**, 49 (1957).
Gleason, D. M., Lattimer, J. K.: A miniature radio transmitter which is inserted into the bladder and which records voiding pressure. J. Urol. (Baltimore) **87**, 507 (1962).
— — Bauxbaum, C.: Bladder pressure telemetri. J. Urol. (Baltimore) **94**, 254 (1965).
Goetzen, F. J., Boeminghaus, H.: Die nerval gestörte Harnblase. Z. Urol. **47**, 129 (1954).
Holm, H. H.: Micro-manometer for measurement of intravesical pressure. J. Urol. (Baltimore) **86**, 280 (1961).
Lapides, J.: Structure and function of the internal vesical sphincter. J. Urol. (Baltimore) **80**, 341 (1958).
— Sweet, R. B., Lewis, L.W.: Fonction of striated muscles in control of urination. II. Effect of complete sceletal muscle paralysis. Surg. Forum **6**, 613 (1955).
Laux, G., Marchal, G.: Le parasympathique pelviperinéal. Montpellier méd. **46**, 114 (1954).
Learmonth, J. R.: A contribution to the neurophysiology of the urinary bladder in man. Brain **34**, 147 (1931).
Pierce, J. M., Braun, E., Sniderman, A J., Lewis, H. Y.: The concept of resistance to flow applied to the lower urinary tract. Surg. Gynec. Obstet. **116**, 217 (1963).
Rankin, J. T.: Concepts of urethral resistance. Brit. J. Urol. **39**, 594 (1967).
Retief, P. J. M.: Physiology of micturition and ejaculation. S. Afr. med. J. **24**, 509 (1950).
Sandøe, E., Bryndorf, J., Gertzt, C.: Cystometry. Dan. med. Bull. **6**, 194 (1959).
— Smith, D. R.: The anatomy and function of the bladder neck. Brit. J. Urol. **38**, 54 (1966).

TANAGHO, E. A., MEYERS, F. H., SMITH, D. R.: The trigone: anatomical and physiological considerations. 1. In relation to the uretero-vesical junction. J. Urol. (Baltimore) **100**, 623 (1968).

WOODBURNE, R. T.: Structure and function of the urinary bladder. J. Urol. (Baltimore) 84, 79 (1960).

## *D. Electrophysiology of the Urinary Bladder and Sphincters*

ABUREL, E., CHAUCHARD, H., CHAUCHARD, B.: Recherches physiologiques sur l'innervation motrice de la vessie. C.R. Soc. Biol. (Paris) **23**, 1036 (1931).

BUDGE, J.: Über den Einfluß des Nervensystems auf die Bewegung der Blase. Z. rat. Med. **21**, 1 (1864).

BURGHELE, TH., ICHIM, V., DEMETRESCU, M.: L'éléctroexcitation de la vessie médullaire. Étude expérimentale. J. Urol. Néphrol. **64**, 317 (1958).

— — — Experimental study of empting of cord bladder. Transcutaneous stimulation of pelvic nerves by electromagnetic induction apparatus. Therapeutic deduction. Digest of the 1962 15th Annual Conference on engineering in Medicine and Biology, Nov. 5—7, 1962.

ECKHARD, C.: Untersuchungen über die Erektion des Penis beim Hunde. Beitr. Anat. Physiol. **3**, 123 (1863).

EVANS, I. R.: The physiologic basis of the neurgenic bladder. J. Amer. med. Ass. **117**, 1927 (1941).

GASTAUD, H.: Correlations entre le system nerveux végétatif et lesysteme de la vie de relation dans le rhinencephale. J. Physiol. (Paris) **44**, 431 (1952).

GIANUZZI, J.: Note sur les nerfs moteurs de la vessie. C.R. Acad. Sci., Janvier 1963.

GRABER, P., RUTISHAUSER, G.: Vorversuche im Hinblick auf eine klinisch anwendbare elektrische Blasenentleerung. Urol. int. (Basel) **19**, 410 (1965).

— — WOLLF, G.: Experimentelle Untersuchungen über den Öffnungs- und Schließmechanismus der elektrisch stimulierten Blase. Urol. int. **21**, 182 (1966).

GRIFFITHS, J.: Observations on the urinary bladder and urethra. J. Anat. and Physiol. **25**, 535 (1891).

HEGRE, E. S., INGERSOLL, E. H.: An analysis of regional variations in response of detrusor muscle to electrical stimulation of the hypogastric nerves. J. Urol. (Baltimore) **61**, 1037 (1949).

HENNEMAN, E.: Trans. Amer. neurol. Ass. 150 (1948). Zit. in Acta physiol. scand. **24**, Suppl. 83, 1—285 (1951).

INGERSOLL, E. H.: Urinary bladder response to unilateral stimulation of hypogastric nerve. J. Urol. (Baltimore) **72**, 178 (1954).

— Effect on urinary bladder of unilateral stimulation. Amer. J. Physiol. **189**, 166 (1957).

— JONES, L. L., HEGRE, E. S.: Response to unilateral stimulation of hypogastric nerves. J. Urol. (Baltimore) **12**, 178 (1955).

KABAT, H., MAGUN, H. W., RANSON, S. W.: Somato-motor, autonomic and electrocorticographic responses to electrical stimulation of rhinencephalic and other structures in primates, cat, and dogs. Acta physiol. scand. **24**, 3 (1951).

KREMER, W. F.: Autonomic and somatic reactions induced by stimulation of the cingular gyrus in dogs. J. Neurophysiol. **10**, 371 (1947).

LANGWORTHY, O. R., KOLB, L. C., LEWIS, L. G.: Physiology of micturition. Experimental and clinical studies with suggestion as to diagnosis and treatment. Baltimore: Williams & Wilkins 1940.

MACDONALD, A. D., MACCREA, L. E.: Observations on the control of the bladder. The effect of nervous stimulations and of the drugs Quart. J. exp. Physiol. **20**, 379 (1930).

MUELLNER, S. R.: The physiology of micturition. J. Urol. (Baltimore) **65**, 805 (1951).

STEWART, O. W.: The neurogenic bladder. Combined tidal irrigator and cystometer. Lancet **1942**, 672.

## *E. Electrical Stimulation of the Neurogenic Bladder*

ALEXANDER, S., ROWAN, D.: Experimental evacuation of the bladder by means of implanted electrodes. Brit. J. Surg. **52**, 10, 808 (1965).

ASCOLI, R., FEDERICI, B.: La stimulazione elettrica della vescica urinaria nell practica clinica. Urologia (Italia) **31**, 654 (1964).

BOYARSKY, S.: The neurogenic bladder. Baltimore. The Williams & Wilkins Co. 1967.

BOYCE, W. H., LATHEM, J. E., HUND, L. D.: Research related to the development of an electrical stimulator for the paralyzed human bladder: A review. Trans. Amer. Ass. gen.-urin. Surg. **55**, 81 (1963).

Boyce, W. H., Lathem, J. E., Hund, L. D.: Research related to the development of an artificial electrical stimulation for the paralyzed human bladder. J. Urol. (Baltimore) **91**, 41 (1964).

Bradley, W. E., Chou, S. N., French, L. A.: Further experience with the radiotransmitter receiver unit for the neurogenic bladder. J. Neurosurg. **20**, 953 (1963b).

— — Markland, C., Swaiman, K.: Biochemical assay technique for estimation of bladder fibrosis. Invest. Urol. **3**, 59 (1965).

— Wingrove, R., Chou, S. N.: Use of an implantable R.F. powered receiver for evacuation of the neurogenic bladder. Proc. on Eng. of the 15th annual Conf. in Med. and Biol., Nov. 5—6, 59 (1962a).

— Wittmers, L. E., Chou, S. N.: An experimental study of the traetment of the bladder. J. Urol. (Baltimore) **90**, 575 (1963a).

— — — French, L. A.: Use of a radio transmitter receiver unit for the treatment of neurogenic bladder. Preliminary report. J. Neurosurg. **19**, 782 (1962b).

Burghele, Th., Ichim, V.: Tulburările vezicale în traumatismele medulare. Bucureşti: Edit. Academiei Republicii Socialiste Romania 1963.

— — Demetrescu, M.: L'électroexcitation de la vessie médullaire. Étude expérimentale. J. Urol. Néphrol. **64**, 317 (1958a).

— — — Contribution à la physiologie de la miction. Etude expérimentale. Acta urol. belg. **26**, 289 (1958).

— — — Etude expérimentale sur l'évacuation de la vessie médullaire. Méthode d'excitation transcutanée des nerfs pelviens par un dispositif utilisant l'induction électromagnetique. Déduction thérapeutiques. Urol. int. (Basel) **8**, 32 (1959a).

— — — Experimental studies on the physiology of micturition and the emptying of the urinary bladder in patients with lesions of the spinal cord. Artificial micturition through distant electromagnetic induction. Rum. med. Rev. **3**, 48 (1959b).

Carpenter, F. G.: Excitation of rat urinary bladder by coaxial electrodes and by chemical agents. Amer. J. Physiol. **204**, 724 (1963).

Chou, S. N., Bradley, W. E., Markland, L.: Pain with radio frequency stimulation of the neurogenic bladder. Baltimore: Williams & Wilkins Co. 1967.

Dees, J. E.: Contraction of the urinary bladder produced by electric stimulation. Preliminary report. Invest. Urol. **2**, 539 (1965).

— Contraction of the urinary bladder produced by electrical stimulation. Baltimore: Williams & Wilkins Co. 1967.

Eisenberg, L., Munro, A., Glenn, W. W., Hageman, J. H.: Radio frequency stimulation: a research and clinical tool. Science **147**, 578 (1965).

Ellis, F., Parker, J., Hills, M.: Experimental electrical stimulation of the bladder. Brit. J. Surg. **51**, 857 (1964).

— — Lale, P. G.: The treatment of experimental cord bladder by electrical stimulation. Brit. J. Urol. **37**, 129 (1965).

Glenn, W. W. L., Hageman, J. H., Munro, A., Eisenberg, L., Flanigan, S., Harvard, M.: Electrical stimulation of excitable tissues by radio frequency transmission. Ann. Surg. **160**, 338 (1964).

Graber, P., Rutishauser, G.: Vorversuche im Hinblick auf eine klinisch anwendbare elektrische Blasenentleerung. Urol. int. (Basel) **19**, 401 (1965).

— — Vorversuche im Hinblick auf eine klinisch anwendbare elektrische Blasenentleerung. Z. Urol. **58**, 73 (1965).

Graber, R., Rutishauser, G., Wollf, G.: Experimentelle Untersuchungen über den Öffnungs- und Schließmechanismus der elektrisch stimulierten Blase. Urol. int. (Basel) **21**, 182 (1966).

Grice, H. C., Makow, D. H.: Bladder evacuation by electrical stimulation of the rectum. J. Urol. (Baltimore). **94**, 5 (1965).

Habib, H. H.: Neural trigger points for evacuation ofneurogenic bladder by electrostimulation. Surg. Forum **14**, 489—491 (1963).

— Experience and recent contributions in sacral nerve stimulation for voiding in both human and animal. Baltimore: Williams & Wilkins Co. 1967a.

— Experience and recent contribution in sacral nerve stimulation for voiding in both human and animal. Brit. J. Urol. **33**, 1, 73 (1967b).

Hald, T., Agrawal, G., Kantrowitz, A.: Studies in stimulation of the bladder and its motor nerves. Surgery **60**, 4, 848 (1966).

— Freed, P. S., Agrawal, G., Kantrowitz, A.: Urethral resistance during electrical stimulation. Invest. Urol. **3**, 247 (1966).

— — Kantrowitz, A.: Urinary bladder: Mode of excitation during stimulation. Invest. Urol. **4**, 3, 439 (1966).

HALD, T., MEIER, W., KHALILI, A., AGRAWAL, G., BENTON, J., KANTROWITZ, A.: Clinical experience with a radio-linked bladder stimulator. J. Urol. (Baltimore) **97**, 1, 73 (1967).
— MYGIND, T.: Radiological study of electrically induced micturition. Invest. Urol. **4**, 2, 152 (1966).
— — Effect of curare on canine micturition. J. Urol. (Baltimore) **97**, 101 (1967).
— ROSSEL, I.: Electrostimulation of the urinary bladder in normal cats. Acta chir. scand. **128**, 414 (1964).
— — Electrostimulation of the urinary bladder in the paraplegic cats. Acta chir. scand. **130**, 247 (1965).
HOLMQUIST, B., OLIN, T.: Electromicturition in male dogs at pelvic nerve stimulation. An urethro-cystographic study. Scand. J. Urol. Nephrol. **2**, 115 (1968a).
— — Electromicturition in female dogs at pelvic nerve stimulation. An urethro cystographic study. Scand. J. Urol. Nephrol. **2**, 129 (1968b).
— STAUBITZ, W. J.: The role of the pudendal nerve in connection with electronic emptying of the neurogenic cord bladder in dogs. J. Urol. (Baltimore) **98**, 198 (1967).
— — GREATBACH, W.: The use of dual electrodes for electro-micturition by pelvic nerve stimulation in dogs. Invest. Urol. **5**, 1, 1 (1967).
— — — The significance voltage and wave duration of the stimuli in electromicturition, induced by electric nerve stimulation in dogs. Scand. J. Urol. Nephrol. **2**, 137 (1968).
JONGE, M. C., KORNELIS, J. A., VAND DEN BERG: Electrically induced evacuation of the neurogenic bladder. Acute and longterm experiments (2 years) with paraplegic dogs. Acta neurol. scand., Suppl. **20**, 42, 155 (1966).
KANTROWITZ, A., SCHAMAUN, M.: Paraplegic dogs: Urinary bladder evacuation with direct electric stimulation. Science **139**, 115 (1963).
— — Bladder evacuation in paraplegic dogs by direct electric stimulation. J. Amer. med. Ass. **187**, 8, 595 (1964).
KATONA, F.: Electric stimulation in the diagnosis and therapy of bladder paralysis. Orv. Hetil. **99**, 277 (1958).
LEARMONTH, J. R.: A contribution to the neurophysiology of the urinary bladder in man. Brain **34**, 147 (1931).
MARKLAND, C., CHOU, S., BRADLEY, W., WESTGATE, H., WOLFSON: Some problems in the use of intermittent vesical electronic stimulation. Invest. Urol. **4**, 2, 168 (1966).
— CHOU, S. N., SWAIMAN, K., WESTGATE, A., BRADLEY, W. E.: Evaluation of neurologic urinary dysfunction. Surg. Forum **16**, 504 (1965).
MALLOY, T., KOMINS, J., ROHNER, T., SCHOENBERG, H.: The effect of retropubic revision of the bladder neck upon electrical stimulation of the neurogenic bladder. J. Urol. (Baltimore) **98**, 347 (1967).
MEIROWSKY, A. M., SCHEIBERT, C. D., HINCKEY, T. R.: Studies on the sacral reflex arc in paraplegia, response of the bladder to surgical elimination of sacral nerve impulses by rhisotomy. J. Neurosurg. **7**, 33 (1950).
MONTGOMERY, W. G., BOYCE, W. H.: Problems related to the physiology of micturition in attempting artificial electrical stimulation of the urinary bladder. Baltimore: Williams & Wilkins Co. 1967.
PEDERSEN, E., JAKOBSEN, B. E., GRYNDERUP: In: The neurogenic bladder. Copenhagen: Munksgaard 1966.
POTEMPA, J., DITTMAR, A.: Aktive Entleerung der neurogen gestörten Blase mittels eines elektrischen Schrittmachers. Verhandlungsbericht der deutschen Gesellschaft für Urologie. Berlin-Heidelberg-New York: Springer 1965.
ROHNER, H. W., SCHOENBERG, H. W.: The effect of retropubic revision of the bladder neck upon voiding induced by electrical stimulation. J. Urol. (Baltimore) **96**, 919 (1966).
SCHAMAUN, M., KANTROWITZ, A.: Management of neurogenic urinary bladder in paraplegic dogs by direct electric stimulation of the detrusor. Surgery **54**, 4, 460 (1963).
SCHOENBERG, H. W., MURPHY, J. J., YOUNG, D. G.: Electrical stimulation of the bladder. J. Urol. (Baltimore) **89**, 820 (1963).
— YOUNG, D. G., JR., MURPHY, J. J.: Electrical stimulation of urinary bladder. Surg. Forum **13**, 509 (1962).
SCOTT, F. B., QUESADA, E. M., CARDUS, D., LASKOWSKI, T.: Electronic bladder stimulation: dog and human experiments. Invest. Urol. **3**, 231 (1965).
STAUBITZ, W. J., CHENG, S. F., GILEEN, H. W., HOLMQUIST, B., ZURLO, P., GRATBACH, W.: Management of neurogenic bladder in paraplegic dogs by electrical stimulation of pelvic nerves. Invest. Urol. **4**, 20 (1966).
STERNBERG, C. C., BURNETTE, H. W., BUNTS, R. C.: Electrical stimulation of human neurogenic bladder: Experience with 4 patients. J. Urol. (Baltimore) **97**, 1, 79 (1967).
SUSSET, G. J., BOCTOR, Z. N.: Implantable electrical vesical stimulator. Clinical experience. J. Urol. (Baltimore) **98**, 6, 673 (1967b).

SUSSET, G. J., BOCTOR, Z. N.: Electrical stimulation of the bladder: An experimental study. Invest. Urol. **5**, 20 (1967a).

— — RABINOVITCH, NAGLER, B., MACKINNON, K. J.: Implantable, electrical, vesical stimulation: Review of the literature and report of a successful case. Canad. med. Ass. J. **95**, 1128 (1966).

TORBEY, K., LEADBETER, W. F.: Innervation of the bladder and lower ureter: Studies on pelvic nerve section and stimulation in the dog. J. Urol. (Baltimore) **90**, 395 (1963).

WEAR, J. B., KREUTZMANN, R., BARQUIN, F., BERNHARDT, N.: Observations on electrical stimulation of the canine bladder. J. Urol. (Baltimore) **97**, 469 (1967).

WISCHNEWSKY, A. A., LIWSCHITZ, A. W., CHODOROW, B.: Radiofrequente Stimulation der Harnblase im Experiment und in der Klinik. Zbl. Chir. **92**, 48, 2917 (1967).

— — CHODOROV, B. I.: Electrical stimulation of the bladder. Exp. Hir. Anest. **5**, 5 (1966).

YOUNG, H. H., WESSON, M. B.: The anatomy and surgery of the trigone. Arch. Surg. **3**, 1 (1921).

Editorial: Electrical stimulation of the bladder: a new prospect after spinal injury. Lancet **1965 I**, 851.

# Author Index

The numbers shown in square brackets are the numbers of the references in the bibliography. Page numbers in *italics* refer to the bibliography.

# Subject Index

REPRINT FROM

HANDBUCH DER UROLOGIE
ENCYCLOPEDIA OF UROLOGY
ENCYCLOPÉDIE D'UROLOGIE

EDITED BY

C. E. ALKEN · V. W. DIX · W. E. GOODWIN · E. WILDBOLZ

BAND XIII/2

SPRINGER-VERLAG/BERLIN · HEIDELBERG · NEW YORK 1970
(PRINTED IN GERMANY) NOT IN CIRCULATION

---

# RENOVASCULAR SURGERY

BY

J. J. KAUFMAN AND A. N. LUPU

WITH 22 FIGURES

REPRINT FROM

**HANDBUCH DER UROLOGIE**
**ENCYCLOPEDIA OF UROLOGY**
**ENCYCLOPÉDIE D'UROLOGIE**

EDITED BY

**C. E. ALKEN · V. W. DIX · W. E. GOODWIN · E. WILDBOLZ**

BAND XIII/2

SPRINGER-VERLAG/BERLIN · HEIDELBERG · NEW YORK 1970
(PRINTED IN GERMANY) NOT IN CIRCULATION

# RENAL TRANSPLANTATION

BY

**D. C. MARTIN**

WITH 60 FIGURES

REPRINT FROM

**HANDBUCH DER UROLOGIE**
**ENCYCLOPEDIA OF UROLOGY**
**ENCYCLOPÉDIE D'UROLOGIE**

EDITED BY

**C. E. ALKEN · V. W. DIX · W. E. GOODWIN · E. WILDBOLZ**

BAND XIII/2

SPRINGER-VERLAG/BERLIN · HEIDELBERG · NEW YORK 1970
(PRINTED IN GERMANY) NOT IN CIRCULATION

# OPEN SURGERY OF THE PROSTATE

BY

**R. F. GITTES**

WITH 15 FIGURES

REPRINT FROM

HANDBUCH DER UROLOGIE
ENCYCLOPEDIA OF UROLOGY
ENCYCLOPÉDIE D'UROLOGIE

EDITED BY

C. E. ALKEN · V. W. DIX · W. E. GOODWIN · E. WILDBOLZ

BAND XIII/2

SPRINGER-VERLAG/BERLIN · HEIDELBERG · NEW YORK 1970
(PRINTED IN GERMANY) NOT IN CIRCULATION

# THE NEUROGENIC BLADDER IN SPINAL CORD INJURY

BY

TH. BURGHELE AND V. ICHIM

WITH 35 FIGURES

SPRINGER-VERLAG
BERLIN · HEIDELBERG · NEW YORK

## Handbuch der allgemeinen Pathologie

Herausgeber: H.-W. Altmann, F. Büchner, H. Cottier, E. Grundmann, G. Holle, E. Letterer, W. Masshoff, H. Meessen, F. Roulet, G. Seifert, G. Siebert, A. Studer

# VII. Band Reaktionen

# 3. Teil Immunreaktionen

## Immune Reactions

Mit 129 Abbildungen
Etwa 540 Seiten
Erscheint Dezember 1970
Neun Beiträge, davon fünf in englischer Sprache
Gebunden DM 265,—
US $ 76.20
**Subskriptionspreis:**
**Gebunden DM 212,—**
**US $ 61.00**

Bearbeitet von H. Bürki, K. Bürki, H. Cottier, E. Diener, H. Gerster, M. W. Hess, P. Koldovský, J. Laissue, N. A. Mitchison, J. Oort, J. J. T. Owen, B. Roos, A. Schauer, J. L. Turk
Redigiert von Professor Dr. **A. Studer,** Basel, und Professor Dr. **H. Cottier,** Bern

Das Werk ist ein Fortschrittsbericht, in dem Wissenschaftler aus dem deutschen und englischen Sprachbereich die neuesten Ergebnisse auf ihrem Arbeitsgebiet schildern und diskutieren. Es werden Themen behandelt, die in den Bänden „Entzündung und Immunität" (1956) und „Überempfindlichkeit und Immunität" (1967) bereits besprochen sind. Jetzt werden besonders die Forschungsgebiete berücksichtigt, die wertvolle Erweiterungen erfahren haben. Bei der Darstellung der neuen Erkenntnisse in zusammenfassender Form wurde Wert auf persönliche Meinungsäußerung gelegt, auch dort, wo unkonventionelle Auffassungen vertreten werden.

**Inhaltsübersicht**

Makrophagen: Herkunft, Entwicklung und Funktion. — Ontogenesis of Immunobiological Systems. — Lymphatischer Apparat, insbesondere Thymus, in der Pathogenese der Defektimmunopathien. — Die cellulären Grundlagen der immunbiologischen Reizbeantwortung: Cellular and Molecular Recognition Mechanism Prior to the Immune Response. — Produktion humoraler Antikörper: The Primary Immune Response and Immunilogical Tolerance. — Mit Bildung humoraler Antikörper einhergehende Immunreaktionen: Die anamnestische Reizbeantwortung. — The Production of Sensitized Cells in Cell-Mediated Immunity. — Die Mastzelle bei akuten Überempfindlichkeitsreaktionen. — The Significance of Immunology in Oncology.

■ **Bitte Prospekt anfordern!**

Universitätsdruckerei H. Stürtz AG, Würzburg

GPSR Compliance
The European Union's (EU) General Product Safety Regulation (GPSR) is a set of rules that requires consumer products to be safe and our obligations to ensure this.

If you have any concerns about our products, you can contact us on

ProductSafety@springernature.com

In case Publisher is established outside the EU, the EU authorized representative is:

Springer Nature Customer Service Center GmbH
Europaplatz 3
69115 Heidelberg, Germany

www.ingramcontent.com/pod-product-compliance
Ingram Content Group UK Ltd.
Pitfield, Milton Keynes, MK11 3LW, UK
UKHW052339030826
474029UK00003B/146

* 9 7 8 3 6 4 2 6 5 0 6 2 8 *